ACP | MKSAP® 17

Medical Knowledge Self-Assessment Program®

Dermatology

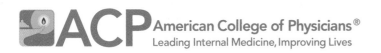

ACP **American College of Physicians®**
Leading Internal Medicine, Improving Lives

Welcome to the Dermatology Section of MKSAP 17!

In these pages, you will find updated information on approaches to various dermatologic diseases and therapeutic principles in dermatology. Included are more than 200 color images of dermatologic diseases. We review rashes and other eruptions, skin and nail infections, neoplasms, pruritus and urticaria, autoimmune bullous diseases, and other clinical challenges. All of these topics are uniquely focused on the needs of generalists and subspecialists *outside* of dermatology.

The publication of the 17th edition of Medical Knowledge Self-Assessment Program (MKSAP) represents nearly a half-century of serving as the gold-standard resource for internal medicine education. It also marks its evolution into an innovative learning system to better meet the changing educational needs and learning styles of all internists.

The core content of MKSAP has been developed as in previous editions—newly generated, essential information in 11 topic areas of internal medicine created by dozens of leading generalists and subspecialists and guided by certification and recertification requirements, emerging knowledge in the field, and user feedback. MKSAP 17 also contains 1200 all-new, psychometrically validated, and peer-reviewed multiple-choice questions (MCQs) for self-assessment and study, including 72 in Dermatology. MKSAP 17 continues to include *High Value Care* (HVC) recommendations, based on the concept of balancing clinical benefit with costs and harms, with links to MCQs that illustrate these principles. In addition, HVC Key Points are highlighted in the text. Also highlighted, with blue text, are *Hospitalist*-focused content and MCQs that directly address the learning needs of internists who work in the hospital setting.

MKSAP 17 Digital provides access to additional tools allowing you to customize your learning experience, including regular text updates with practice-changing, new information and 200 new self-assessment questions; a board-style pretest to help direct your learning; and enhanced custom-quiz options. And, with MKSAP Complete, learners can access 1200 electronic flashcards for quick review of important concepts or review the updated and enhanced version of Virtual Dx, an image-based self-assessment tool.

As before, MKSAP 17 is optimized for use on your mobile devices, with iOS- and Android-based apps allowing you to sync your work between your apps and online account and submit for CME credits and MOC points online.

Please visit us at the MKSAP Resource Site (mksap.acponline.org) to find out how we can help you study, earn CME credit and MOC points, and stay up to date.

Whether you prefer to use the traditional print version or take advantage of the features available through the digital version, we hope you enjoy MKSAP 17 and that it meets and exceeds your personal learning needs.

On behalf of the many internists who have offered their time and expertise to create the content for MKSAP 17 and the editorial staff who work to bring this material to you in the best possible way, we are honored that you have chosen to use MKSAP 17 and appreciate any feedback about the program you may have. Please feel free to send us any comments to mksap_editors@acponline.org.

Sincerely,

Philip A. Masters, MD, FACP
Editor-in-Chief
Senior Physician Educator
Director, Content Development
Medical Education Division
American College of Physicians

Dermatology

Committee

Misha Rosenbach, MD, Section Editor[2]
Assistant Professor of Dermatology and Internal Medicine
Perelman School of Medicine at the University of
   Pennsylvania
Philadelphia, Pennsylvania

Jack Ende, MD, MACP, Associate Editor[1]
The Schaeffer Professor of Medicine
Perelman School of Medicine at the University of
   Pennsylvania
Philadelphia, Pennsylvania

Joslyn S. Kirby, MD[1]
Associate Professor of Dermatology
Penn State Milton S. Hershey Medical Center
Department of Dermatology
Hershey, Pennsylvania

James Treat, MD[2]
Assistant Professor of Pediatrics and Dermatology
Perelman School of Medicine at the University of
   Pennsylvania
Fellowship Director, Pediatric Dermatology
Children's Hospital of Philadelphia
Philadelphia, Pennsylvania

Karolyn Wanat, MD[1]
Assistant Professor of Dermatology and Pathology
University of Iowa Health Center
Department of Dermatology
Iowa City, Iowa

Andrew Werchniak, MD[1]
Assistant Professor of Dermatology
Harvard Medical School
Department of Dermatology
Brigham and Women's Hospital
Boston, Massachusetts

Editor-in-Chief

Philip A. Masters, MD, FACP[1]
Director, Clinical Content Development
American College of Physicians
Philadelphia, Pennsylvania

Director, Clinical Program Development

Cynthia D. Smith, MD, FACP[2]
American College of Physicians
Philadelphia, Pennsylvania

Dermatology Reviewers

Kevin K. Brown, MD[2]
Elizabeth Cerceo, MD, FACP[2]
Richard A. Fatica, MD[1]
Faith T. Fitzgerald, MD, MACP[1]
Jerry L. Spivak, MD, FACP[2]

Dermatology ACP Editorial Staff

Randy Hendrickson[1], Production Administrator/Editor
Margaret Wells[1], Director, Self-Assessment and Educational
   Programs
Becky Krumm[1], Managing Editor

ACP Principal Staff

Patrick C. Alguire, MD, FACP[2]
Senior Vice President, Medical Education

Sean McKinney[1]
Vice President, Medical Education

Margaret Wells[1]
Director, Self-Assessment and Educational Programs

Becky Krumm[1]
Managing Editor

Valerie A. Dangovetsky[1]
Administrator

Ellen McDonald, PhD[1]
Senior Staff Editor

Katie Idell[1]
Digital Content Associate/Editor

Megan Zborowski[1]
Senior Staff Editor

Randy Hendrickson[1]
Production Administrator/Editor

Linnea Donnarumma[1]
Staff Editor

Susan Galeone[1]
Staff Editor

Jackie Twomey[1]
Staff Editor

Kimberly Kerns[1]
Administrative Coordinator

---

1. Has no relationships with any entity producing, marketing, reselling, or distributing health care goods or services consumed by, or used on, patients.

2. Has disclosed relationship(s) with any entity producing, marketing, reselling, or distributing health care goods or services consumed by, or used on, patients.

Disclosure of Relationships with any entity producing, marketing, reselling, or distributing health care goods or services consumed by, or used on, patients:

Patrick C. Alguire, MD, FACP
Board Member
Teva Pharmaceuticals
Consultantship
National Board of Medical Examiners
Royalties
UpToDate
Stock Options/Holdings
Amgen Inc, Bristol-Myers Squibb, GlaxoSmithKline, Covidien, Stryker Corporation, Zimmer Orthopedics, Teva Pharmaceuticals, Express Scripts, Medtronic

Kevin K. Brown, MD
Consultantship
Actelion, Altitude Pharma, Amgen, Biogen/Stromedix, Boehringer Ingelheim, Celgene, Centocor, Fibrogen, Genenetech, GeNO, Genoa Pharma, Gilead, Medimmune, Mesoblast, Novartis, Pfizer, Promedior, Vascular Biosciences, Veracyte, Sanofi/Genzyme

Elizabeth Cerceo, MD, FACP
Honoraria
Scientific Therapeutic Information, Inc.

Misha Rosenbach, MD
Research Grants/Contracts
Centocor, Johnson & Johnson

Cynthia D. Smith, MD, FACP
Stock Options/Holdings
Merck and Co.; spousal employment at Merck

Jerry L. Spivak, MD, FACP
Consultantship
Novartis

James Treat, MD
Royalties
UpToDate

Acknowledgments

The American College of Physicians (ACP) gratefully acknowledges the special contributions to the development and production of the 17th edition of the Medical Knowledge Self-Assessment Program® (MKSAP® 17) made by the following people:

Graphic Design: Michael Ripca (Graphics Technical Administrator) and WFGD Studio (Graphic Designers).

Production/Systems: Dan Hoffmann (Director, Web Services & Systems Development), Neil Kohl (Senior Architect), Chris Patterson (Senior Architect), and Scott Hurd (Manager, Web Projects & CMS Services).

MKSAP 17 Digital: Under the direction of Steven Spadt, Vice President, Digital Products & Services, the digital version of MKSAP 17 was developed within the ACP's Digital Product Development Department, led by Brian Sweigard (Director). Other members of the team included Dan Barron (Senior Web Application Developer/Architect), Chris Forrest (Senior Software Developer/Design Lead), Kara Kronenwetter (Senior Web Developer), Brad Lord (Senior Web Application Developer), John McKnight (Senior Web Developer), and Nate Pershall (Senior Web Developer).

The College also wishes to acknowledge that many other persons, too numerous to mention, have contributed to the production of this program. Without their dedicated efforts, this program would not have been possible.

MKSAP Resource Site (mksap.acponline.org)

The MKSAP Resource Site (mksap.acponline.org) is a continually updated site that provides links to MKSAP 17 online answer sheets for print subscribers; the latest details on Continuing Medical Education (CME) and Maintenance of Certification (MOC) in the United States, Canada, and Australia; errata; and other new information.

ABIM Maintenance of Certification

Check the MKSAP Resource Site (mksap.acponline.org) for the latest information on how MKSAP tests can be used to apply to the American Board of Internal Medicine for Maintenance of Certification (MOC) points.

Royal College Maintenance of Certification

In Canada, MKSAP 17 is an Accredited Self-Assessment Program (Section 3) as defined by the Maintenance of Certification (MOC) Program of The Royal College of Physicians and Surgeons of Canada and approved by the Canadian Society of Internal Medicine on December 9, 2014. Approval extends from July 31, 2015 until July 31, 2018 for the Part A sections. Approval extends from December 31, 2015 to December 31, 2018 for the Part B sections.

Fellows of the Royal College may earn three credits per hour for participating in MKSAP 17 under Section 3. MKSAP 17 also meets multiple CanMEDS Roles, including that of Medical Expert, Communicator, Collaborator, Manager, Health Advocate, Scholar, and Professional. For information on how to apply MKSAP 17 Continuing Medical Education (CME) credits to the Royal College MOC Program, visit the MKSAP Resource Site at mksap.acponline.org.

The Royal Australasian College of Physicians CPD Program

In Australia, MKSAP 17 is a Category 3 program that may be used by Fellows of The Royal Australasian College of Physicians (RACP) to meet mandatory Continuing Professional Development (CPD) points. Two CPD credits are awarded for each of the 200 *AMA PRA Category 1 Credits*™ available in MKSAP 17. More information about using MKSAP 17 for this purpose is available at the MKSAP Resource Site at mksap.acponline.org and at www.racp.edu.au. CPD credits earned through MKSAP 17 should be reported at the MyCPD site at www.racp.edu.au/mycpd.

Continuing Medical Education

The American College of Physicians (ACP) is accredited by the Accreditation Council for Continuing Medical Education (ACCME) to provide continuing medical education for physicians.

The ACP designates this enduring material, MKSAP 17, for a maximum of 200 *AMA PRA Category 1 Credits*™. Physicians should claim only the credit commensurate with the extent of their participation in the activity.

Up to 12 *AMA PRA Category 1 Credits*™ are available from July 31, 2015, to July 31, 2018, for the MKSAP 17 Dermatology section.

Learning Objectives

The learning objectives of MKSAP 17 are to:
- Close gaps between actual care in your practice and preferred standards of care, based on best evidence
- Diagnose disease states that are less common and sometimes overlooked or confusing
- Improve management of comorbid conditions that can complicate patient care

- Determine when to refer patients for surgery or care by subspecialists
- Pass the ABIM Certification Examination
- Pass the ABIM Maintenance of Certification Examination

Target Audience
- General internists and primary care physicians
- Subspecialists who need to remain up-to-date in internal medicine and in areas outside of their own subspecialty area
- Residents preparing for the certification examination in internal medicine
- Physicians preparing for maintenance of certification in internal medicine (recertification)

Earn "Instantaneous" CME Credits Online

Print subscribers can enter their answers online to earn instantaneous Continuing Medical Education (CME) credits. You can submit your answers using online answer sheets that are provided at mksap.acponline.org, where a record of your MKSAP 17 credits will be available. To earn CME credits, you need to answer all of the questions in a test and earn a score of at least 50% correct (number of correct answers divided by the total number of questions). Take any of the following approaches:

1. Use the printed answer sheet at the back of this book to record your answers. Go to mksap.acponline.org, access the appropriate online answer sheet, transcribe your answers, and submit your test for instantaneous CME credits. There is no additional fee for this service.

2. Go to mksap.acponline.org, access the appropriate online answer sheet, directly enter your answers, and submit your test for instantaneous CME credits. There is no additional fee for this service.

3. Pay a $15 processing fee per answer sheet and submit the printed answer sheet at the back of this book by mail or fax, as instructed on the answer sheet. Make sure you calculate your score and fax the answer sheet to 215-351-2799 or mail the answer sheet to Member and Customer Service, American College of Physicians, 190 N. Independence Mall West, Philadelphia, PA 19106-1572, using the courtesy envelope provided in your MKSAP 17 slipcase. You will need your 10-digit order number and 8-digit ACP ID number, which are printed on your packing slip. Please allow 4 to 6 weeks for your score report to be emailed back to you. Be sure to include your email address for a response.

If you do not have a 10-digit order number and 8-digit ACP ID number or if you need help creating a user name and password to access the MKSAP 17 online answer sheets, go to mksap.acponline.org or email custserv@acponline.org.

Permission/Consent for Use of Figures Shown in MKSAP 17 Dermatology Multiple-Choice Questions

Figures shown in Self-Assessment Test Items 1 and 48 appear courtesy of Dr. Christopher J. Miller.

Figure shown in Self-Assessment Test Item 5 appears courtesy of Dr. John Hillstein.

Figure shown in Self-Assessment Test Item 34 appears courtesy of Dr. William D. James.

Figure shown in Self-Assessment Test Item 50 appears courtesy of CDC Public Health Image Library.

Figure shown in Self-Assessment Test Item 56 appears courtesy of Dr. Adam Rubin.

Figures shown in Self-Assessment Test Items 23, 46, and 61 are reprinted with permission from Physicians Information and Education Resource (ACP PIER). Philadelphia, PA: American College of Physicians.

Disclosure Policy

It is the policy of the American College of Physicians (ACP) to ensure balance, independence, objectivity, and scientific rigor in all of its educational activities. To this end, and consistent with the policies of the ACP and the Accreditation Council for Continuing Medical Education (ACCME), contributors to all ACP continuing medical education activities are required to disclose all relevant financial relationships with any entity producing, marketing, re-selling, or distributing health care goods or services consumed by, or used on, patients. Contributors are required to use generic names in the discussion of therapeutic options and are required to identify any unapproved, off-label, or investigative use of commercial products or devices. Where a trade name is used, all available trade names for the same product type are also included. If trade-name products manufactured by companies with whom contributors have relationships are discussed, contributors are asked to provide evidence-based citations in support of the discussion. The information is reviewed by the committee responsible for producing this text. If necessary, adjustments to topics or contributors' roles in content development are made to balance the discussion. Further, all readers of this text are asked to evaluate the content for evidence of commercial bias and send any relevant comments to mksap_editors@acponline.org so that future decisions about content and contributors can be made in light of this information.

Resolution of Conflicts

To resolve all conflicts of interest and influences of vested interests, the American College of Physicians (ACP) precluded members of the content-creation committee from deciding on any content issues that involved generic or trade-name products associated with proprietary entities with which these committee members had relationships. In addition, content was based on best evidence and updated clinical care guidelines, when such evidence and guidelines were available. Contributors' disclosure information can be found with the list of contributors' names and those of ACP principal staff listed in the beginning of this book.

Hospital-Based Medicine

For the convenience of subscribers who provide care in hospital settings, content that is specific to the hospital setting has been highlighted in blue. Hospital icons (H) highlight where the hospital-based content begins, continues over more than one page, and ends.

High Value Care Key Points

Key Points in the text that relate to High Value Care concepts (that is, concepts that discuss balancing clinical benefit with costs and harms) are designated by the HVC icon (**HVC**).

Educational Disclaimer

The editors and publisher of MKSAP 17 recognize that the development of new material offers many opportunities for error. Despite our best efforts, some errors may persist in print. Drug dosage schedules are, we believe, accurate and in accordance with current standards. Readers are advised, however, to ensure that the recommended dosages in MKSAP 17 concur with the information provided in the product information material. This is especially important in cases of new, infrequently used, or highly toxic drugs. Application of the information in MKSAP 17 remains the professional responsibility of the practitioner.

The primary purpose of MKSAP 17 is educational. Information presented, as well as publications, technologies, products, and/or services discussed, is intended to inform subscribers about the knowledge, techniques, and experiences of the contributors. A diversity of professional opinion exists, and the views of the contributors are their own and not those of the American College of Physicians (ACP). Inclusion of any material in the program does not constitute endorsement or recommendation by the ACP. The ACP does not warrant the safety, reliability, accuracy, completeness, or usefulness of and disclaims any and all liability for damages and claims that may result from the use of information, publications, technologies, products, and/or services discussed in this program.

Publisher's Information

Unauthorized Use of This Book Is Against the Law

MKSAP 17 ISBN: 978-1-938245-18-3
(Dermatology) ISBN: 978-1-938245-20-6

Printed in the United States of America.

For order information in the United States or Canada call 800-523-1546, extension 2600. All other countries call 215-351-2600, (M-F, 9 AM – 5 PM ET). Fax inquiries to 215-351-2799 or email to custserv@acponline.org.

Errata

Errata for MKSAP 17 will be available through the MKSAP Resource Site at mksap.acponline.org as new information becomes known to the editors.

Table of Contents

Dermatology High Value Care Recommendations

The American College of Physicians, in collaboration with multiple other organizations, is engaged in a worldwide initiative to promote the practice of High Value Care (HVC). The goals of the HVC initiative are to improve health care outcomes by providing care of proven benefit and reducing costs by avoiding unnecessary and even harmful interventions. The initiative comprises several programs that integrate the important concept of health care value (balancing clinical benefit with costs and harms) for a given intervention into a broad range of educational materials to address the needs of trainees, practicing physicians, and patients.

HVC content has been integrated into MKSAP 17 in several important ways. MKSAP 17 now includes HVC-identified key points in the text, HVC-focused multiple choice questions, and, for subscribers to MKSAP Digital, an HVC custom quiz. From the text and questions, we have generated the following list of HVC recommendations that meet the definition below of high value care and bring us closer to our goal of improving patient outcomes while conserving finite resources.

High Value Care Recommendation: A recommendation to choose diagnostic and management strategies for patients in specific clinical situations that balance clinical benefit with cost and harms with the goal of improving patient outcomes.

Below are the High Value Care Recommendations for the Dermatology section of MKSAP 17.

- Dermatologic treatments are highly variable in cost; generic topical medications should be considered for a cost-effective approach.
- Food allergies are an uncommon cause of flares in atopic dermatitis; routine food testing without a reliable history of flaring with a particular food should be avoided.
- Less frequent handwashing and application of a thick emollient such as petrolatum are the treatments of choice for irritant hand dermatitis caused by overwashing (see Item 67).
- Systemic therapy, such as phototherapy, traditional systemic agents, or biologics should be reserved for severe (>10% body surface area) psoriasis, psoriatic arthritis, or psoriasis unresponsive to topical therapy.
- Systemic glucocorticoids, systemic retinoids, and phototherapy should be reserved for severe or recalcitrant lichen planus.

- Seborrhea can be treated with over-the-counter selenium sulfide or zinc pyrithione shampoos that are lathered into the skin and allowed to work for a few minutes and then washed out; ketoconazole shampoo and topical cream are also very effective.
- First-line therapy for cellulitis without a draining wound or abscess is a course of antibiotics against both *Streptococcus* spp. and *Staphylococcus* spp. (cephalexin or dicloxacillin, clindamycin, or a macrolide); a 5-day course of antibiotics is as effective as a 10-day course.
- Treatment of most superficial dermatophyte infections includes topical antifungal agents; however, over-the-counter preparations are cost-effective options with good efficacy.
- Minor wounds and burns may be treated with thorough cleansing, application of topical sterile petrolatum, and the application of a nonadherent bandage; nonstick silicone dressings are a more expensive option.
- Dysplastic nevi are benign melanocytic lesions most commonly found on the trunk and extremities; removal should be reserved for those lesions that are changing, symptomatic, or stand out from the patient's other nevi (see Item 32).
- Seborrheic keratoses, solar lentigines, acrochordons, melanocytic nevi, cherry angiomata, dermatofibromas, lipomas, and epidermal inclusion cysts are benign lesions that usually do not require biopsy or treatment.
- Surgical excision is the mainstay of treatment for basal cell carcinoma; Mohs surgery should be reserved for head and neck lesions, large or recurrent tumors, or when cosmetic outcome is crucial; superficial lesions may be treated topically.
- Squamous cell carcinomas typically present as red scaly papules and nodules on sun-exposed skin and are treated with excision; Mohs surgery should be reserved for large tumors with high-risk characteristics in the head and neck region.
- Uncomplicated acute urticaria is a clinical diagnosis based on the presence of pruritic wheals; laboratory studies are almost always normal, and no further diagnostic evaluation is required in most patients before initiating therapy, if needed (see Item 55).
- Management of black hairy tongue consists of tongue brushing as part of aggressive oral hygiene (see Item 5).

Dermatology

Approach to the Patient with Dermatologic Disease

Introduction

Skin conditions account for a substantial number of physician visits, with patients presenting to internists for evaluation and management of primary dermatologic issues, the skin manifestations of internal disease, or cutaneous adverse reactions from therapeutic regimens. Thus, the ability to recognize common skin findings and the cutaneous clues associated with underlying disorders or their treatment is an important skill required of internists. This section will cover key aspects of dermatology for the internist, with an emphasis on diagnostic recognition, early evaluation, and initial management. This will also include a focus on "when to refer," with an emphasis on recognizing key cutaneous signs that suggest a patient may be more acutely ill or require a more thorough evaluation and consultation with an experienced dermatologist.

Physical Examination

The U.S. Preventive Services Task Force (USPSTF) states that there is insufficient evidence to recommend dedicated screening for skin cancer in the general population. However, there is a growing body of evidence suggesting that patients who are screened have earlier, more treatable skin cancers, and that counseling these patients about preventive measures and self-examination can reduce the number or severity of skin cancers and lead to earlier detection. A sensible approach in average-risk patients is to perform an "integrated skin examination," evaluating the skin during the course of the routine physical examination. While checking blood pressure and pulse, look at the arms; while examining the abdomen, look at the skin of the torso; and while listening to the lungs, look at the back. High-risk patients may warrant more comprehensive and regular evaluation (**Table 1**). A comprehensive skin examination, which takes on average only 1 to 2 minutes, should include evaluation of the scalp below the hair, the mucosa, and the genitals, including looking between skin folds, digits, and on the soles of the feet. Patients should be counseled about how to perform skin self-examinations (generally done once monthly, in a systematic fashion) and to use sun protection (**Table 2**).

The language of dermatology is often a point of confusion for many internists, but recognizing and describing primary lesions is critical to forming an accurate differential diagnosis and can help dermatologists triage referred patients based on the acuity of their lesions.

TABLE 1. Skin Cancer Risk Factors That Warrant Regular Skin Cancer Screening
History of multiple blistering sunburns
Red or light hair; light-colored eyes
Multiple atypical nevi
History of melanoma
History of nonmelanoma skin cancers
Family history of skin cancers or melanoma
Immunosuppression
History of phototherapy

TABLE 2. Sun Protection
Use broad-spectrum ultraviolet protective sunscreen
Use chemical or physical sun blocking agents (or combination)
Use SPF 30 or greater
Apply 30 minutes before sun exposure, reapply every 2 hours; more frequently if wet
Avoid the peak hours (11 AM to 2 PM)
Consider ultraviolet protective clothing

SPF = sun protection factor.

The "primary lesion" refers to the morphology of a skin eruption as it first starts and is an essential clue to a specific diagnosis. Lesions often evolve over time and may cause secondary changes to the skin, either due to the process itself or to external factors such as trauma and scratching; these findings are called "secondary lesions" (**Table 3**). When describing skin lesions, focus on the color, location, and distribution of the lesion, including the primary morphology. "Erythema" implies transient redness of the skin due to inflammation that blanches or lightens with pressure. It is often essential to distinguish erythema from nonblanching purpura, which implies damage to vessels and a substantially different differential diagnosis.

It is not uncommon for patients to have pictures of their lesions or for physicians to have access to mobile devices that allow photography and image transmission. Physicians should be cautious in taking pictures and sending them and must ensure that any patient photography is protected as patient information and sent only through secure telecommunication services or as encrypted e-mail. Photographs are part of the patient's medical record, and copies of all pictures should be maintained with the patient's chart. Whereas teledermatology

TABLE 3.	Lesion Morphology
Primary Lesions	**Description**
Macule	Small size, flat, change in skin color
	Circular, oval, or irregular
	Border may be distinct or gradually fade to normal skin
Patch	Larger than a macule, 1 cm or larger
	May have very faint fine scale or minimal surface change
Papule	Small bumps, from pinpoint to 1 cm
	Discrete raised lesions
	Lack fluid or pus
	May be flat, umbilicated, grouped, filiform, or scaly
Maculopapular	An eruption with overlapping morphologies
	Admixture of small, flat areas with pinpoint slightly raised bumps
Plaque	Larger raised lesion, 1 cm or larger
	Often flat topped
	"Like a plateau"
Nodule	Larger than a papule
	Usually indistinct borders
	Often arises deeper under the skin and pushes up
Wheal	Transient, edematous, erythematous plaques
	Often oval, arcuate, serpiginous, circular
	"Hives"
Vesicle	Small, fluid-filled papules, ranging from pinpoint to 1 cm
	Often translucent or slightly yellow
	Whitish vesicles are termed "pustules"
Bullae	Larger than vesicles, often 1 cm or larger
	May be thin walled and rupture easily ("flaccid") or tense with thicker top ("tense")
	"Blisters"
Secondary Lesions	**Description**
Scale	Excess keratin from stratum corneum
	May be a fine dusting, a moist greasy scale, or a thick silvery scale
Crust	Dried out serum, blood, or inflammatory cells, often mixed with epidermis and surface bacteria
	May be hemorrhagic (from blood), orange-yellow (from serum or *Staphylococcus* colonization), or thick and black (eschar from chronic wound)
	Ulcers may develop a fibrinous biofilm with polymicrobial colonization, which may represent a moist "crust"
Excoriation	Linear erosions, often crusted, may suggest external trauma and scratching that can lead to loss of the epidermis
Fissure	Linear crack exposing dermis
	Generally occurs where skin is moist and macerated, such as folds, or where skin is very thick and rigid, such as tips or edges of acral sites
Erosion	Loss of the epidermis alone leads to a small, often "punched-out," shallow, moist depression
	Heals without scarring
Ulcer	Complete loss of the epidermis into the dermis
	Can be varying depths, including to deeper tissues in the subcutis
	Heals with scarring
Scar	Skin damaged beyond the basement membrane of the epidermis will generally heal with scarring
	Certain anatomic sites and some black persons are more prone to thicker scarring

is a valuable tool and holds promise for expanding access in the future, studies are ongoing to determine the accuracy of teledermatology for triage and patient management, and at this time most insurers do not reimburse for teledermatology services.

As in all of medicine, a primary responsibility is to determine the level of acuity of a disorder and whether a patient requires immediate intervention or a higher level of care. This holds true for dermatology as well, and although most dermatologic diseases lack urgency, some disorders represent true emergencies (**Table 4**).

KEY POINTS

- Screening for skin cancer in patients who are at increased risk may allow for diagnosis at a more treatable stage.

- For average risk patients, an "integrated skin examination" involves evaluating the skin for abnormalities during the course of the routine physical examination.

Therapeutic Principles in Dermatology

The initial management of skin conditions is based on the type and severity of the cutaneous lesions. In stable patients, treatment with topical medications is an appropriate approach. Most topical therapies for dermatologic conditions will be "off label" as there is a paucity of evidence for many of these conditions, and most treatment regimens are not FDA approved.

When prescribing topical therapy, patients should be evaluated according to the morphology of the cutaneous eruption, their skin type, and for tolerance of different vehicles. As some dermatologic treatments are highly variable in cost, consideration of the resources available to the patient should also be a factor in shared treatment decision making. Generic topical medications are generally similar in efficacy and should be considered for a cost-effective approach, although formal comparative effective studies are lacking.

The optimal medication and vehicle depend on the type of condition (**Table 5**). For many skin conditions, the vehicle through which a medication is delivered is extremely important. A cream may severely irritate an acutely inflamed eczematous eruption, whereas an ointment will be soothing and well tolerated. A thick, scaly eruption in the scalp is best treated using a foam, allowing easy penetration through the hair onto the inflamed skin. Ointments are the most moisturizing, include the fewest ingredients, and are the least likely to burn when put on inflamed skin. Ointments often have higher potency when compared with the same medication and concentration in a cream or lotion. Patients may prefer creams, gels, and lotions for their feel. Solutions and foams may be easier to apply in hair-bearing areas, especially the scalp. It is important to ask patients what they prefer, as compliance is essential. Patients with different skin types or ethnic backgrounds may have a preference for specific vehicles.

Patients who do not respond to topical therapy should be carefully reevaluated. Skin biopsy is a rapidly available diagnostic test with very low associated morbidity and may provide important information about the pattern of inflammation to help guide treatment. Referral to a dermatologist is appropriate for any skin condition of unclear cause that fails to respond to initial therapy. Additionally, widespread eruptions that are inflammatory, painful, or associated with vesicles, bullae, or purpura, or those occurring in immunosuppressed patients, should also be referred to a dermatologist for rapid evaluation.

TABLE 4. Dermatologic Emergencies
Widespread erythema or erythroderma (drug eruption, bacterial toxin-mediated disease, severe psoriasis)
High fever and widespread rash (severe drug eruptions, rickettsial diseases)
Diffuse peeling or sloughing of skin (toxic epidermal necrolysis, infection)
Dark, dusky, purple areas of painful skin (impending skin loss from infection or severe drug eruption)
Mucosal inflammation, erosions, or ulceration (severe drug eruption, autoimmune blistering disease with high risk of morbid scarring)
Widespread blistering (autoimmune blistering disease, infection, severe drug eruption)
Purpura, particularly "retiform" or lacey, patterned purpura (vasculitis, vasculopathy, infection, autoimmune disease)
Broad areas of exquisitely painful skin out of proportion to clinical examination findings (necrotizing fasciitis)
Angulated purpura of the distal extremities (sepsis, autoimmune phenomena)
Palpable purpura (small vessel vasculitis from infection, medications, or autoimmune reactions)
Immunosuppressed, particularly patients with neutropenia, with skin lesions of unknown cause in the setting of fever, particularly red or purple nodules (skin signs of infection in immunosuppressed hosts)
Purple or necrotic skin lesions in immunosuppressed hosts (angioinvasive fungal infection)
Rapidly growing lesions in immunosuppressed hosts (infection, malignancy)
Worrisome pigmented lesions warrant urgent (not emergent) referral and evaluation (melanoma)

Vehicle	Description
Cream	Mixture of oil and water; often appears white and smooth
	Easily applied, rubs in, and is absorbed; high rates of compliance
	May be irritating to acutely inflamed, raw, eroded, open skin; may not penetrate thick scale
Ointment	More oil than water; thick and greasy
	Often leaves a thick and messy residue; hard to put on before clothing
	Most moisturizing emollient; hydrophobic, traps water on the skin
	Less irritating than creams; may be used on actively inflamed, raw skin
Solution	Very liquid, minimally viscous, feels mostly like water
	Easy to use when applying medications over large areas or hair-bearing areas
	If alcohol based, may be drying; certain preservatives lead to irritation but generally solutions are well tolerated
Lotion	Texture between a solution and a cream; somewhat thicker than a solution
	Very variable in terms of irritation and tolerance, depending on brand and medication
	Easy to apply over broad areas
Gel	Semisolid thick preparation; firmer than a solution
	May dry out the skin and frequently may sensitize the skin, often causes stinging, burning, or irritation when applied to inflamed skin
	High rates of compliance when used appropriately on noninflamed skin
Foam	Generally used specifically for hair-bearing areas; easier to apply to places like the scalp than other vehicles
Powder	Often used in skin folds, as it is easy to apply and may dry out moist areas of skin-on-skin friction and sweating

TABLE 5. Topical Medication Vehicles

Topical Glucocorticoids

Topical glucocorticoids are important anti-inflammatory medications that, because they can be applied directly to the affected area, can offer a powerful treatment with fewer side effects than systemic glucocorticoids. Topical glucocorticoids are grouped into classes from 7 (weak) to 1 (ultrapotent) based on their ability to cause vasoconstriction (**Table 6**).

The choice of a topical glucocorticoid should be made by evaluating the location and thickness of the rash, the age of the patient, and how long the therapy is likely to be needed. In general, thicker dermatoses such as psoriasis, lichen planus, or lichenified atopic dermatitis will require higher potency topical glucocorticoids and longer courses of therapy. Prescribing enough topical glucocorticoid for adequate therapy is vital. Thirty grams of a topical glucocorticoid is enough for one application to the entire body of an adult male. This amount can be extrapolated down to the appropriate amount for a more localized eruption. For widespread eruptions, 454-gram tubs of hydrocortisone and triamcinolone can be dispensed. Fifteen or 30 grams can be prescribed if there is concern for overuse (for example, on the face).

Side effects from topical glucocorticoids include thinned skin, striae distensae (stretch marks), and easy bruising, all mediated in part by decreased collagen production. These side effects are most likely to occur when more potent topical glucocorticoids are used under occlusion, in skin folds, or for extended periods of time. Hypothalamic-pituitary axis sup-pression has also been documented from even short courses of potent and ultrapotent topical glucocorticoids, especially if occluded or used in areas of thinned skin or over large body surface areas. Topical glucocorticoid use around the eyes can lead to glaucoma and cataracts, and therefore their use should be limited. Although topical glucocorticoids are often implicated in hypopigmentation, more commonly the color change is caused by postinflammatory pigment loss once the primary eruption resolves.

Tachyphylaxis occurs when an individual topical gluco-corticoid stops being effective because of prolonged use, and simply switching to a different topical glucocorticoid, even one with the same strength, may be effective.

It is important to understand the potential risks of using topical glucocorticoid and antifungal combinations. Clotrimazole-betamethasone combines an azole antifungal agent with a potent topical glucocorticoid. There are reports of failure in treating dermatophyte infections. If tinea is suspected, using a topical antifungal agent alone is preferred. Fungal infections also often occur in skin folds, such as under the breast or in the inguinal fold, which would be an inappropriate place to apply betamethasone for extended periods owing to the risk of atrophy. Clotrimazole-betamethasone is only approved for 2 weeks when applied in the perineum. There is also a preparation with nystatin and triamcinolone. Nystatin is an anticandidal agent that is ineffective against dermatophytes, and again triamcinolone may lead to stretch marks if overused in skin folds.

Group	Generic Name	Brand Name
I	Flurandrenolide tape	Cordran tape
	Clobetasol propionate (0.05%)	Cormax
		Temovate
		Temovate-E
		Olux foam
	Halobetasol propionate (0.05%)	Ultravate
	Augmented betamethasone dipropionate (0.05%)	Diprolene
	Diflorasone diacetate (0.05%)	Psorcon
II	Betamethasone dipropionate (0.05%)	Diprosone
	Halcinonide (0.1%)	Halog
	Fluocinonide (0.05%)	Lidex
		Lidex-E
	Desoximetasone (0.25%)	Topicort
III	Triamcinolone acetonide (0.5%)	Aristocort A
	Betameth valerate (0.1%)	Betatrex
	Fluticasone propionate (0.005%)	Cutivate
	Amcinonide (0.1%)	Cyclocort
	Mometasone furoate (0.1%)	Elocon
IV	Triamcinolone acetonide (0.1%)	Aristocort
		Kenalog
	Flurandrenolide (0.05%)	Cordran
	Amcinonide (0.1%)	Cyclocort
	Prednicarbate (0.1%)	Dermatop-E
	Mometasone furoate (0.1%)	Elocon
	Betamethasone valerate (0.12%)	Luxig foam
	Fluocinolone acetonide (0.025%)	Synalar
	Hydrocortisone valerate (0.2%)	Westcort
V	Triamcinolone acetonide (0.1%)	Aristocort
		Kenalog
	Betamethasone valerate (0.1%)	Betatrex
	Clocortolone pivalate (0.1%)	Cloderm
	Flurandrenolide	
	(0.05%)	Cordran SP
	(0.05%)	Cordran
	(0.025%)	Cordran
	Fluticasone propionate (0.05%)	Cutivate
	Prednicarbate (0.1%)	Dermatop-E
	Desonide (0.05%)	DesOwen
	Hydrocortisone butyrate (0.1%)	Locoid
	Fluocinolone acetonide (0.025%)	Synalar
		Synemol
	Desonide (0.05%)	Tridesilon
	Hydrocortisone valerate (0.2%)	Westcort

(Continued on the next page)

TABLE 6. Classes and Strengths of Topical Glucocorticoids *(Continued)*

Group	Generic Name	Brand Name
VI	Prednicarbate (0.05%)	Aclovate
	Triamcinolone acetonide (0.025%)	Kenalog
	Fluocinolone acetonide (0.01%)	Synalar
		Capex
		Dermasmooth
		FS
	Flurandrenolide (0.025%)	Cordran SP
	Desonide (0.05%)	DesOwen
VII	Hydrocortisone	
	(2.5%)	Hytone
	(1.0%)	Lacticare HC
	Hydrocortisone + pramoxine	
	(1.0%)	
	(2.5%)	
	5 g Hydrocortisone powder in 454 g acid mantle cream	Pramosone

KEY POINTS

HVC

- Dermatologic treatments are highly variable in cost; generic topical medications should be considered for a cost-effective approach.

- The choice of a topical glucocorticoid should be made by evaluating the location and thickness of the rash, the age of the patient, and how long the therapy is likely to be needed.

- Side effects from topical glucocorticoids include thinned skin, striae distensae (stretch marks), and easy bruising, and are likely to occur when they are used for extended periods of time, especially in skin folds or areas of occlusion.

Common Rashes

Eczematous Dermatoses

Eczematous dermatitis is a type of inflammation characterized by inflamed, dry, red, itchy skin. The terms eczema and dermatitis are often used interchangeably. There are multiple types of eczematous dermatoses (**Table 7**).

In all types of eczematous dermatoses, patients should be told to take short showers or baths in warm (but not hot) water, use a mild soap, and apply moisturizer liberally within 3 minutes of getting out of the bathtub. The skin loses the hydration gained from bathing within 3 minutes, and if moisturizer is delayed longer than this, the skin becomes drier than it was before bathing. There are newer moisturizers containing ceramides that may provide extra benefit in healing the skin barrier. Washcloths, buff puffs, loofahs, and other abrasive cleaning implements should be avoided in patients with eczematous dermatitis because they can inappropriately exfoliate the skin. They may also act as fomites and harbor sources for infection, especially with repeated use.

Atopic Dermatitis

Atopic dermatitis (AD) is characterized by xerotic, pink, scaly skin and is most commonly seen on the periocular areas, posterior neck, antecubital and popliteal fossae, wrists, and ankles (**Figure 1**). The rash often waxes and wanes. Many patients with

TABLE 7. Types of Eczematous Dermatoses

Atopic dermatitis	A specific type of eczematous dermatitis that is genetically driven and often affects areas such as the antecubital and popliteal fossae; typically presents in childhood
Allergic contact dermatitis	A type IV hypersensitivity reaction to an allergen that comes into contact with the skin
Irritant contact dermatitis	Inflammation caused by a direct caustic or irritant effect of a chemical
Xerotic eczema	Extremely dry skin that results in inflammation and pruritus
Nummular dermatitis	An acute and extremely pruritic dermatitis characterized by coin-shaped plaques
Stasis dermatitis	An acute inflammation of the skin caused by chronic venous stasis

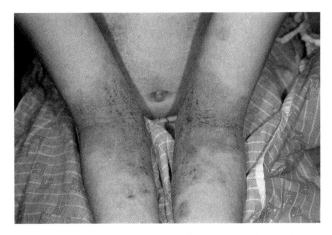

FIGURE 1. Subacute eczema of the flexural folds showing erythema with crusts typical of atopic dermatitis.

AD have a defective skin barrier because of a mutation in filaggrin, which is a protein that helps the epidermis provide a barrier against allergens and irritants. Therefore, patients with a filaggrin mutation often have dry, scaly skin and are at higher risk for contact dermatitis. Patients with AD also have downregulated innate immunity, and therefore their skin is locally immunosuppressed and more susceptible to infection. Because of the impaired barrier, the circulating Langerhans cells in the skin are more easily in contact with environmental antigens, and patients are more likely to become sensitized to environmental allergens such as dust mites, ragweed pollen, and animals. They are also more likely to become sensitized to chemicals put onto their skin leading to contact dermatitis. Staphylococcal colonization of AD is very common. When the skin is scratched, there are breaks in the epidermis that can become infected, as evidenced by honey-colored crusting, oozing erosions, and pustules. Food allergies are an uncommon cause of flares in AD, and blood and skin IgE tests for these allergens have high false-positive rates. Therefore, random food testing without a reliable history of flaring with a particular food can lead to inappropriate food avoidance and patient frustration.

Contact Dermatitis

Although contact dermatitis is common and causes significant morbidity, it is also curable by avoiding the causative chemical. There are two types of contact dermatitis, allergic and irritant. Allergic contact dermatitis is a type IV delayed hypersensitivity reaction to a specific chemical. With repeated exposure to the chemical, a pruritic eczematous dermatitis develops on the exposed area (**Figure 2**). In exuberant cases, the localized inflammation can lead to a secondary "id" reaction, a generalized acute cutaneous reaction in which pinpoint flesh-colored to red papules develop diffusely on the body. Id reactions may be centered on the initial allergic site but may also induce uniform monomorphous small papules especially on the extensor arms, legs, or neck. Irritant contact dermatitis is caused by a direct toxic effect on the epidermis from exposure to a chemical such

as a cleaning agent, other caustic substances, or repeated wetting and drying and is not mediated by the immune system. For example, overwashing with harsh soap will often lead to dry, irritated skin, which is not immune mediated.

Causes of Allergic Contact Dermatitis

Urushiol is an allergen in the *Toxicodendron* (formerly classified as *Rhus*) genus of plants. Examples of these plants include poison ivy, poison oak, and poison sumac. Typically this rash presents with geometric lines or splatters of red papules and vesicles, especially on exposed areas. If the urushiol resin oxidizes to the skin, it will turn black and is often mistaken for a spider bite ("black dot poison ivy").

Nickel metal allergy is also very common, especially with the increasingly frequent practice of piercing. Nickel is typically found in jewelry, belts, or snaps, including the inside button on jeans, which rubs against the lower abdomen.

Neomycin and bacitracin are commonly used over-the-counter topical antibiotics that with repeated use, especially on abraded or lacerated skin, can lead to contact sensitization. Patients and physicians often mistake this for a wound infection, but if the area is itchy and there is a geometric, sharply bordered pattern, a contact allergy should be suspected. Transdermal medications such as clonidine or buprenorphine have also been associated with allergic contact dermatitis.

Fragrances such as eugenol, geraniol, and cinnamic aldehyde are common causes of contact dermatitis when used in perfumes and colognes as well as in soaps and moisturizers. Contact dermatitis to aerosolized fragrances will present in an airborne pattern (involving the face, especially the eyelids; neck; and arms). Patients who are allergic to fragrances in soaps and moisturizers will have a more diffuse eruption on the trunk and extremities.

Rubber and chemicals used in the processing of rubber can be found in labels or emblems on clothing, nonslip grips, gloves, or other workplace exposures and may also cause contact allergies.

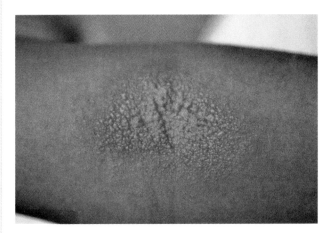

FIGURE 2. Pinpoint vesicles on a red base on the antecubital fossa are characteristic of acute contact dermatitis.

Plant materials such as tea tree oil and balsam of Peru, as well as other organic ingredients, have become more popular as people are choosing to use more organic products. These can be potent allergens and go unnoticed by patients who are often using them as topical agents to treat a primary skin eruption, resulting in secondary sensitization.

There are many other allergens, including preservatives in medicines and soaps. When an obvious causative agent cannot be identified, epicutaneous patch testing can be very helpful. This test involves putting small commercially available concentrations of the potential causative chemicals on the back. The allergens are removed after 48 hours, and the areas are evaluated for a rash at 48 hours and again at 72 or 96 hours. The decision about which allergens to apply is based on the distribution of the contact dermatitis. Often the causative agent is not easy to identify prior to testing. For example, a patient may develop a rash because of irritation or rubbing from a new pair of shoes and then apply topical medications or moisturizers and develop a secondary contact dermatitis on the original rash. Therefore, most patients are tested using a standard panel of the most commonly described allergens. Epicutaneous patch testing is not the same as scratch or prick testing, which is used to identify immediate type I IgE-mediated wheal and flare responses.

Hand Dermatitis

Hand dermatitis is characterized by inflamed, scaling, and sometimes fissured skin on the palmar or dorsal hand (**Figure 3**). The most common causes are overwashing, allergic or irritant contact dermatitis, AD, dyshidrotic eczema (pompholyx), and tinea. Repeated or extended washing with soap causes hand dermatitis by friction, removal of the protective skin barrier, and irritation from the surfactant properties of the soap. People who are required to repeatedly wash their hands (such as medical professionals) or those who wash repeatedly because of obsessive-compulsive or autism spectrum disorders often have extremely pronounced hand dermatitis. This

type of irritant dermatitis will be especially marked on the dorsal hands where the stratum corneum is thinner than that of the palms. Many chemicals found in common products can cause allergic contact dermatitis. Hairdressers, rubber workers, health care workers, or others exposed to many different chemicals have a higher risk of becoming sensitized. Allergic contact dermatitis manifests with extreme itching and redness. Dyshidrotic eczema (pompholyx) is an extremely itchy eruption of small vesicles on the sides of the fingers and palms that can occur from frequent wetting and drying, sweating, allergies, or as a reaction to tinea pedis. AD typically affects the hands, but other areas may often be affected as well; therefore, the entire body should be examined. Patients who wear rings often have soap and water trapped underneath the ring after washing. This leads to an irritant dermatitis. Removing the ring prior to washing or making sure that no soap or water residue is left under the ring after washing are effective preventive measures.

Therapy for hand dermatitis starts with identifying a cause. For irritant hand dermatitis, avoiding the irritant by washing less, moisturizing more, and wearing cotton gloves inside of rubber gloves when around chemicals or during activities such as dishwashing can prevent development of a rash. If rubber gloves are worn alone, the hands often sweat and the water is trapped against the skin, leading to further flares of dyshidrosis. Topical petrolatum jelly is an inexpensive and effective way of repairing the damaged skin barrier. A topical glucocorticoid may be necessary for a short period while the triggers are identified or if the skin is very inflamed. Allergic contact dermatitis, AD, and dyshydrotic eczema can all be treated the same way but nearly always require a short course of topical glucocorticoids for symptom relief. Tinea manuum, a fungal infection that characteristically involves the hands, is often recalcitrant to topical therapy because the infection involves an anatomic site with very thick stratum corneum; often topical keratolytic agents are added to help antifungal agents penetrate the skin, and some patients require oral medications.

Xerotic Eczema

Xerotic eczema, also called asteatotic eczema or "winter itch," is characterized by very dry skin that upon close examination may be slightly fissured. Typical areas include the anterior shins, trunk, back, and arms (**Figure 4**). The eruption is extremely pruritic. Aggressive moisturization, along with changing to soaps that contain less surfactant, may be all that is needed to treat the eczema.

Nummular Dermatitis

Nummular dermatitis is characterized by round (not annular or ring-like) scaling plaques that are intensely itchy (**Figure 5**). The skin is so inflamed that pinpoint vesiculation from serum accumulating in the inflamed skin often occurs and can simulate infection. Tinea corporis can be differentiated from

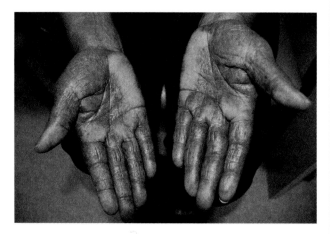

FIGURE 3. Dyshidrotic hand eczema, characterized by acute episodes of an intensely pruritic eruption on the palms.

FIGURE 4. Extensive fine scaling with minimal erythema on the back in a patient with severe xerotic eczema.

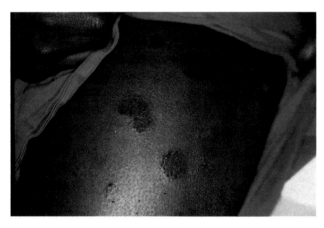

FIGURE 5. Nummular dermatitis is characterized by extremely pruritic round or oval patches of eczematous dermatitis, consisting of papules, scaling, crusting, and often serous oozing. Most lesions appear on the trunk or legs and are 2 to 10 cm in diameter.

nummular dermatitis because the rash of tinea corporis is often annular with at least a partially cleared center and scaling at the periphery. Psoriasis is often located on the elbows, knees, scalp, or intergluteal cleft but has larger, thicker white scale. Allergic contact dermatitis can also present with small, round, intensely itchy plaques. The patient therefore should be asked if the location of the rash aligns with any outside

contactant (for example, metal from a belt or chair) or if anything is being applied (for example, neomycin, bacitracin, herbal moisturizers, or tea tree oil) that may help to differentiate the rash of nummular dermatitis from that of allergic contact dermatitis. Nummular dermatitis is often recalcitrant to therapy and may require potent topical glucocorticoid treatment.

Stasis Dermatitis

Stasis dermatitis manifests with red, inflamed skin on the lower legs in patients with venous stasis or other causes of lower extremity edema. Decreased venous drainage results in venous hypertension and increased vascular permeability and edema. Because the shins are often one of the driest parts of the body and are easily excoriated, dermatitis in this area related to venous stasis is common. The red area on the anterior shins in patients with stasis dermatitis is often bilateral and warm to the touch but typically is not tender (**Figure 6**). Although stasis dermatitis can simulate infection, cellulitis usually is not present. Patients will often have a normal leukocyte count and be afebrile. Conversely, cellulitis is almost always unilateral and is usually accompanied by fever and leukocytosis. Therapy includes optimizing total body fluids, using compression stockings, elevating the legs, and applying frequent emollients. Topical glucocorticoids sometimes help if severe pruritus or inflammation is present.

KEY POINTS

- Food allergies are an uncommon cause of flares in atopic   **HVC**
  dermatitis; routine food testing without a reliable history of flaring with a particular food should be avoided.
- Allergic contact dermatitis is a type IV delayed hypersensitivity reaction to a specific chemical, and epicutaneous patch testing can help to identify the causative allergen.   *(Continued)*

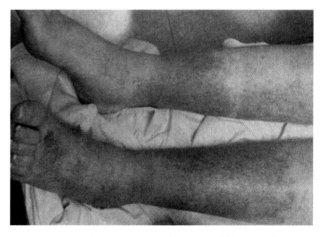

FIGURE 6. Stasis dermatitis causing erythematous, pebbly, oozing plaques on the bilateral lower legs of a patient hospitalized for cellulitis.

KEY POINTS (continued)

KEY POINTS (continued)

- Hand dermatitis is characterized by inflamed, scaling, and sometimes fissured skin on the palmar or dorsal hand and is most commonly caused by overwashing, allergic or irritant contact dermatitis, atopic dermatitis, dyshidrotic eczema (pompholyx), and tinea.

- Stasis dermatitis is sometimes confused with cellulitis; however, patients with stasis dermatitis do not have tender skin, will have a normal leukocyte count, and will be afebrile.

Papulosquamous Dermatoses

Papulosquamous dermatoses are characterized by scaling papules and plaques due to inflammation of the epidermis.

Psoriasis

Psoriasis is a chronic inflammatory dermatosis that manifests with scaling, variably pruritic plaques that may be recalcitrant to topical therapy (**Figure 7** and **Figure 8**). A total of 1% to 2% of the population is affected, and there is a genetic predisposition given that 50% of offspring will have psoriasis if both parents

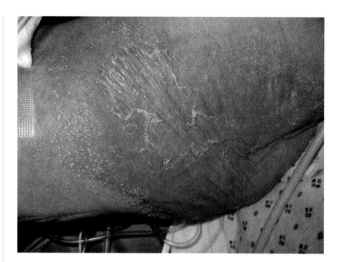

FIGURE 8. Scaling patch with pustules at the edge typical of a pustular flare of psoriasis.

are affected. The incidence of psoriasis peaks at around age 20 years and again at age 60 years. There are many different patterns of psoriasis (**Table 8**). Patients with psoriasis have increased inflammatory Th1, Th17, and Th22 cells. This likely explains why psoriasis may be considered to be a multisystem inflammatory response rather than being limited to the skin. A total of 6% to 11% of patients with psoriasis also have psoriatic arthritis. Psoriatic arthritis can be severe and debilitating (see MKSAP 17 Rheumatology). Patients with psoriasis, especially those who have widespread disease, have an increased risk of myocardial infarction and other major cardiovascular events. Emerging data suggest that psoriasis may be associated with the metabolic syndrome, and some have shown links between psoriasis and diabetes mellitus, hypertension, and hyperlipidemia. Therefore, patients with psoriasis should be monitored more closely for cardiovascular disease and other associated risk factors. Psoriasis seems to be more common in obese patients and those who smoke. Weight loss may lead to improvement. Smoking tobacco may worsen psoriasis, and

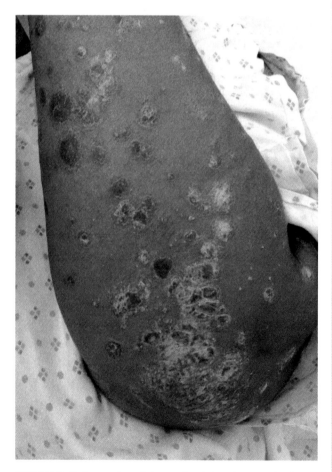

FIGURE 7. Scaling papules and plaques of psoriasis coalescent on the elbow and extensor forearm.

TABLE 8.	Types of Psoriasis
Psoriasis vulgaris	Red, thick, scaling plaques concentrated on the elbows, knees, ankles, shins, and trunk
Inverse psoriasis	Red, thin plaques with variable amount of scale in the axillae, under the breasts or pannus, intergluteal cleft, and perineum
Sebopsoriasis	Red, thin plaques in the scalp, eyebrows, nasolabial folds, central chest, and pubic area
Guttate psoriasis	0.5- to 2-cm red plaques that erupt suddenly on the trunk often after a group A streptococcal infection
Nail psoriasis	Indentations and "oil spots" often involving multiple nails

patients should also be counseled against smoking especially because of the elevated risk of cardiovascular disease. Patients with psoriasis often perceive that their disease has greater impact on their lives than more severe medical conditions such as hypertension and diabetes, and many feel that their skin condition is undertreated.

The choice for therapy for psoriasis is based primarily on location and severity. Topical therapy is the preferred choice for localized disease and usually consists of intermittent pulses of medium- to high-potency topical glucocorticoids either alternating with or in conjunction with topical vitamin D analogues or keratolytic agents. A typical regimen might be a medium-potency glucocorticoid applied once or twice a day on the weekdays and a topical vitamin D analogue applied on the weekends for flares. Topical glucocorticoids applied continuously pose a higher risk of atrophy and striae, so having "steroid holidays" a few days each week may allow the medications to be used more safely over time. The vitamin D analogues have some benefit in psoriasis but do not cause the same side effects as glucocorticoids. Ointments and creams are preferred on the body, whereas solutions and foams are more appropriate for the scalp. Calcineurin inhibitors are used topically "off label" for inverse psoriasis (psoriasis in the perineum, axillae, or under the breasts).

Patients with psoriasis covering more than 10% body surface area or those with psoriatic arthritis, recalcitrant palmoplantar psoriasis, pustular psoriasis, or psoriasis in challenging anatomic areas (groin, scalp) may be considered for systemic therapy. Systemic agents include phototherapy, traditional systemic agents (retinoids, methotrexate, cyclosporine), or biologic agents, most often tumor necrosis factor (TNF)-α inhibitors and interleukin-12 or interleukin-23 inhibitors. Phototherapy does not cause immunosuppression but requires multiple visits per week; phototherapy does not impact psoriatic arthritis. There may be a long-term risk of skin cancer associated with light therapy, although this is primarily a risk with psoralen-ultraviolet A (PUVA) phototherapy, so light therapy may be safer in patients with darker skin types who have lower initial risk. Systemic therapy with retinoids, methotrexate, or cyclosporine has been used for many years in appropriate patients. TNF-α inhibitors and interleukin-23 inhibitors are also FDA-approved alternatives for psoriasis. Therapy with any of the systemic agents should be guided by a clinician experienced in their use, including appropriate evaluation for contraindications and careful monitoring. The impact of these treatments on the psoriasis-associated comorbidities is as yet unknown.

> **KEY POINTS**
>
> - Psoriasis can be a multisystem inflammatory response limited not just to the skin, and patients who have widespread disease have an increased risk of myocardial infarction and other major cardiovascular events.

(Continued)

> **KEY POINTS** *(continued)*
>
> - Topical therapy is the preferred treatment for localized psoriasis and consists of intermittent pulses of medium- to high-potency topical glucocorticoids either alternating with or in conjunction with topical vitamin D analogues or keratolytic agents.
>
> - Systemic therapy, such as phototherapy, traditional systemic agents, or biologics should be reserved for severe (>10% body surface area) psoriasis, psoriatic arthritis, or psoriasis unresponsive to topical therapy.

HVC

Lichen Planus

Lichen planus (LP) is an acute eruption of purple, pruritic, polygonal papules that most commonly develops on the flexural surfaces, especially the wrists and ankles (**Figure 9**). LP can also occur in the mucous membranes (mouth, vaginal vault, and penis) with white plaques that, if uncontrolled, may ulcerate. The eruption can also develop in the nails, leading to thickening and distortion of the nail plate. LP is most commonly idiopathic but may be induced by medications or possibly infection. LP has been reported in up to 20% of patients with hepatitis C infection in some studies, but other reports have failed to show an association. Medications implicated in causing LP or lichenoid drug reactions are gold salts, captopril, hydrochlorothiazide, and hydroxychloroquine.

LP tends to remit after 1 to 2 years with or without therapy but may last longer, especially if erosive. Therapy with potent topical glucocorticoids is often effective in lessening the lesions and decreasing pruritus but may not be curative. Erosive LP that is active for many years may degenerate into squamous cell carcinoma as a result of chronic inflammation; therefore therapy to control erosive LP is very important. Systemic glucocorticoids, systemic retinoids, and phototherapy can be considered for treatment of severe or recalcitrant LP.

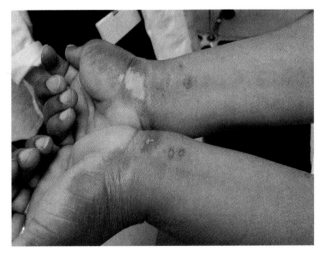

FIGURE 9. Lichen planus presenting as hyperpigmented purple, pruritic polygonal papules and plaques on the ventral wrists.

- Lichen planus is an acute eruption of purple, pruritic, polygonal papules that most commonly presents on the flexural surfaces; topical glucocorticoids are often effective at decreasing the size of the lesions and the associated itch but may not be curative.

HVC • Systemic glucocorticoids, systemic retinoids, and phototherapy should be reserved for severe or recalcitrant lichen planus.

Pityriasis Rosea

Pityriasis rosea (PR) is a reactive eruption of unknown cause, although some experts have suggested an association with a previous viral eruption. It is more commonly seen in the spring and fall and has a predilection for young adults. Clinically, PR often presents with one scaling patch that is a few centimeters wide (herald patch) and is typically mistaken for an area of tinea corporis or contact dermatitis. Many 0.5- to 2.0-cm red scaling patches then erupt along the skin cleavage lines in a "Christmas tree" distribution on the back a few days later and last 1 to 3 months (**Figure 10**). The eruption is often mildly pruritic. The clinical appearance of scaling papules and plaques is similar to that of secondary syphilis, although PR typically spares the face, palms, and soles, whereas the rash of secondary syphilis often affects the palms and soles. Testing should be performed if there is any clinical concern for syphilis. Therapy for PR is challenging, although there are off-label reports of the use of sunlight (allowing the patient to tan with natural light without burning), phototherapy, and systemic macrolide antibiotics. Topical glucocorticoids and antihistamines may help with the pruritus.

Seborrheic Dermatitis

Seborrheic dermatitis is an inflammatory scaling, itchy dermatosis that most commonly affects the scalp but can also affect the eyebrows, nasolabial folds, chin, central chest, and perineum (**Figure 11**). Seborrhea is thought to be an overreaction of the body to commensal *Malassezia* yeasts that live on the skin. Seborrhea is characterized by waxy, scaling, red patches. The rash often starts in puberty and waxes and wanes over months and years. The rash on the face is very common, especially in the elderly, in immunosuppressed patients (particularly in patients with HIV infection), and in patients with neurologic disorders such as Parkinson disease. Patients will often think they just have consistently dry skin on the face; however, the distribution of a scaling rash on the eyebrows and nasolabial folds extending onto the cheeks and chin is typical of seborrhea and often does not respond to moisturization only.

Seborrhea can be treated with over-the-counter selenium sulfide or zinc pyrithione shampoos that are lathered into the skin and allowed to work for a few minutes and then washed out. Ketoconazole shampoo and topical ketoconazole cream are also very effective. When the skin is more inflamed, a short course of low-potency topical glucocorticoids can be used, but patients should be warned against continued use around the eyes to avoid side effects.

Drug Reactions

There are many different manifestations of medication reactions in the skin. Morbilliform or type IV hypersensitivity reactions are the most common and manifest as pink-to-red macules and papules (often called maculopapular) that are often very pruritic (**Figure 12**). The typical onset is within 7 to 14 days of starting the medication, but if exposure is recurrent, it may be faster. The therapy is to stop the medication and treat

FIGURE 10. Pink macules with a collar of scale consistent with pityriasis rosea.

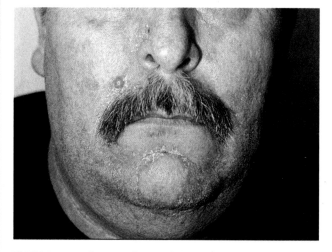

FIGURE 11. Erythematous plaques with dry scale occurring in the beard area and nasolabial folds characteristic of seborrheic dermatitis.

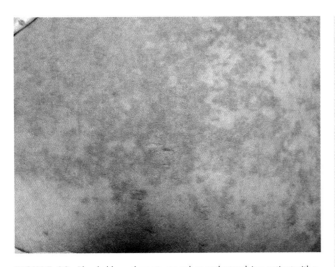

FIGURE 12. Blanchable erythematous patches on the trunk in a patient with a morbilliform drug eruption.

symptomatically with antihistamines and medium-potency topical glucocorticoids for a brief time while the reaction resolves. Patients should be warned to alert their clinician if they develop fevers, skin pain, blisters, pustules, or mucous membrane involvement.

Drug reaction with eosinophilia and systemic symptoms (DRESS) syndrome (or drug hypersensitivity syndrome [DHS]) is a severe drug-induced hypersensitivity syndrome characterized by a papular eruption, facial edema, lymphadenopathy, internal organ involvement, and hematologic abnormalities such as eosinophilia, lymphocytosis, or thrombocytopenia. The most common implicated drugs are allopurinol, sulfonamides, anticonvulsant agents, and minocycline. DRESS is managed by discontinuing the causative medication immediately and providing symptomatic supportive care. Systemic glucocorticoids should be given because of the high risk of end organ damage. For a more detailed discussion of DRESS or DHS, see Dermatologic Urgencies and Emergencies. ⊞

Acute generalized exanthematous pustulosis (AGEP) is an acute eruption of pinpoint pustules that often starts on the head and neck and extend down. The pustules are so minute that sometimes only the resultant peeling is noted (**Figure 13**). AGEP is caused by various medications (most commonly antibiotics, especially penicillins, cephalosporins, and macrolides) or viruses. The list of causative drugs is long and ever-growing and includes such hard-to-identify triggers as contrast dye and dialysates. Therefore, if AGEP is suspected, the clinician should obtain a thorough history of all possible exposures. Generally AGEP begins within 48 to 72 hours of beginning a new drug, which may help identify the culprit. Patients will usually have a fever, and laboratory results will show leukocytosis and occasionally excess bands. The disease self-resolves; however, it may result in extensive peeling, which may be alleviated by the use of emollients.

Fixed drug eruptions (FDE) are purple patches that occur in the same location (fixed) each time a patient is exposed to

the same medication. Severe eruptions may have central bullae. Lips, genitals, and hands are commonly involved, but only one spot may develop with the first exposure. If reexposed, however, the original spot will recur along with new areas. Common drug culprits include over-the-counter medications such as pseudoephedrine, NSAIDs, sulfonamides, and other antibiotics, but there is a very long list of medications that are frequently responsible.

Pigmented purpuric dermatoses are characterized by lesions that look like petechiae but are arranged into small patches or plaques (**Figure 14**). The lesions are sometimes itchy but may be asymptomatic. There is no associated platelet abnormality. The lesions are often compared to "cayenne pepper" and tend to resolve with some rust-colored pigmentation. Pigmented purpura may be caused by exposure to viruses or medications such as NSAIDs. The eruption is asymptomatic. There is no specific work-up indicated and no satisfactorily consistent therapy.

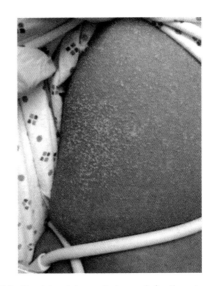

FIGURE 13. Pinpoint pustules on a background of erythema in a patient with acute generalized exanthematous pustulosis.

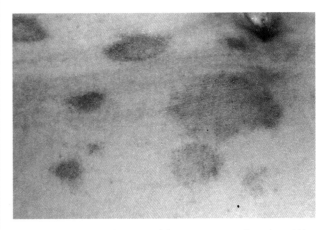

FIGURE 14. Pigmented purpura with fine "cayenne pepper" petechiae within pigmented patches of skin, usually appearing on the extremities.

KEY POINTS

- Seborrhea can be treated with over-the-counter selenium sulfide or zinc pyrithione shampoos that are lathered into the skin and allowed to work for a few minutes and then washed out; ketoconazole shampoo and topical cream are also very effective.

- Drug hypersensitivity syndrome (or drug reaction with eosinophilia and systemic symptoms) is a severe life-threatening, idiosyncratic medication reaction.

- The most common medications causing drug hypersensitivity syndrome are sulfonamides, allopurinol, anti-convulsant agents, and minocycline.

- Therapy for drug hypersensitivity syndrome consists of stopping the causative medication immediately; due to the high risk of end organ damage, systemic glucocorticoids are typically needed.

Miliaria

Miliaria is colloquially called "heat rash" or "prickly heat" and is characterized by clogging of the eccrine sweat glands. The clogging may be partially due to overgrowth of *Staphylococcus epidermidis*. The location along the sweat gland that is clogged will determine what type of miliaria is seen. When the gland is clogged superficially, there are minute pustules that are ruptured easily and can be wiped off (miliaria crystallina) (**Figure 15**). Miliaria rubra causes deeper red papules and some pustules when the clog is deeper, and more inflammation is present. Miliaria is often seen in the setting of fever and occlusion. A typical clinical situation is a patient who is immobilized, either from pain or following surgery, and sweat glands are occluded as a result. Therapy is guided toward cooling the affected area, allowing air circulation. If the eruption is severe, topical antibiotics such as clindamycin solution or low-potency topical glucocorticoids may be used.

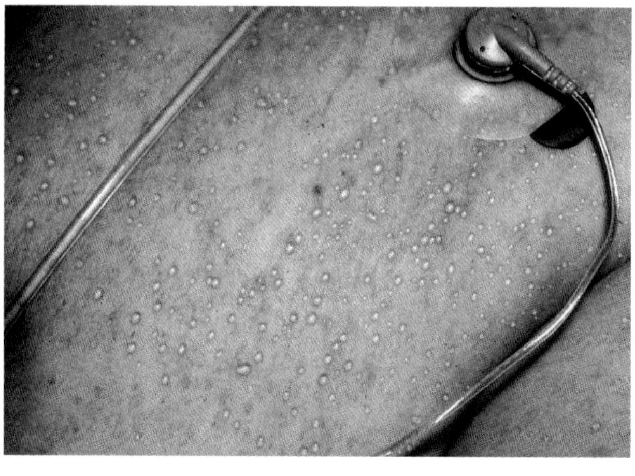

Acantholytic Dermatosis (Grover Disease)

Acantholytic dermatosis (Grover disease) is a benign pruritic eruption of papules or papulovesicles on the central chest, flanks, and back (**Figure 16**). It is often seen in middle-aged to elderly patients and may be induced by sweating or extreme dryness of the skin. The eruption often flares seasonally. Acantholytic dermatosis is typically self-limited, but therapy with topical glucocorticoids or moisturizers may be effective.

Acneiform Eruptions

Acne

Acne is a chronic inflammatory skin condition characterized by open and closed comedones (blackheads and whiteheads, respectively) and inflammatory lesions, including papules, pustules, and nodules (**Figure 17**). Androgens stimulate increased sebum production; thus, when acne develops in patients outside the typical age range or when the acne is difficult to manage, it is important to look for signs of hyperactivity of the hypothalamic-pituitary-adrenal or the hypothalamic-pituitary-gonadal axis. Examples include Cushing syndrome, congenital adrenal hyperplasia, and polycystic ovary syndrome. Depending on the suspected underlying disorder, measurement of free testosterone, dehydroepiandrosterone sulfate (DHEAS), luteinizing hormone (LH), and follicle-stimulating hormone (FSH) levels may be appropriate.

The microcomedone is the precursor to acne lesions and is caused by the proliferation and accumulation of keratinocytes that block the outflow of sebum. If sebum accumulation continues, an open or closed comedone will form. The anaerobic bacterium *Propionibacterium acnes* proliferates in the comedone

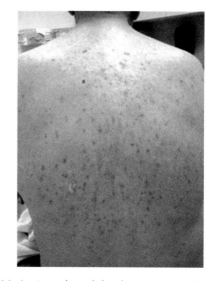

FIGURE 16. A patient with acantholytic dermatosis (Grover disease) showing recurrent outbreaks of itchy red bumps with peripheral scale on the back.

FIGURE 15. Miliaria crystallina with clear, fragile vesicles but no inflammation.

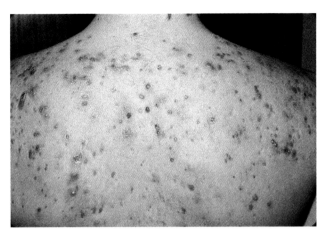

FIGURE 17. Extensive acne involvement of upper and mid-back with papules, pustules, nodules, granulation tissue, postinflammatory erythema, hyperpigmentation, and scarring.

and can incite inflammation if there is leakage of the contents into the dermis. This manifests as papules, pustules, and in severe cases, deep cysts, nodules, and interconnecting sinus tracts. Scarring can occur and be disfiguring. Rarely, severe acne may be associated with systemic inflammation (acne fulminans) or sterile inflammation of the bones or joints (**Table 9**).

Treatment begins by considering the types and distribution of lesions, as well as the pregnancy status of the female patient (**Figure 18** and **Table 10**, on page 17). Interventions are selected with the goal of modifying the main causal factors, such as follicular occlusion, sebum production, *P. acnes* proliferation, and inflammation. It is important to educate patients about the expectations of therapy; treatments often take 6 to 8 weeks to demonstrate an effect, need to be used regularly during this time, and are not capable of complete clearance in all patients. In addition, patients can be counseled that neither dietary restriction nor excessive face washing has been shown to be beneficial.

Treatment of acne is important, not only to avoid complications but also because acne has been shown to significantly reduce quality of life measures for those affected. Patients with moderate acne report more mental health and social problems than those with asthma, epilepsy, or diabetes mellitus. Complications from acne are postinflammatory hyperpigmentation and scarring including hypertrophic scars and keloids. Treatment of acne scarring can be performed by dermatologists or plastic surgeons; however, mitigating scar development by early and appropriate treatment is preferred.

First-line treatment for most patients is topical retinoid and topical antimicrobial therapy. Benzoyl peroxide is available over the counter and is an excellent complement to

TABLE 9. Differential Diagnosis of Acne and Acneiform Skin Disorders	
Disease	**Characteristics**
Acne (acne vulgaris)	Very common in adolescents, but also occurs in preadolescents and adults. Women may have premenstrual flare-ups. Physical examination: coexisting open and closed comedones, papules, pustules, and nodular lesions located primarily on face, neck, and upper trunk.
Rosacea	Not true acne; primary lesion is not a comedone but an inflammatory papule; rhinophyma (bulbous, red nose) is a variant. Physical examination: central facial erythema, telangiectasias, papules, and pustules.
Medication-induced acneiform eruption	Onset weeks to months after start of the medication. Comedones are absent; inflammatory papules and pustules commonly appear on the upper trunk and arms when the cause is systemic.
	Possible triggers are glucocorticoids, anabolic steroids, bromides, iodides, isoniazid, phenytoin, azathioprine, cyclosporine, disulfiram, phenobarbital, quinidine, vitamins B_1, B_2, B_6, B_{12}, and D_2, testosterone, progesterone, lithium, epidermal growth factor inhibitors.
Bacterial folliculitis	Common in athletes. Physical examination: follicular papules, pustules, occasional furuncles on any hair-bearing area, especially scalp, buttocks, and thighs. Positive culture for pathogenic bacteria. Most common cause is *Staphylococcus aureus*.
Gram-negative folliculitis	Caused by overgrowth of bacteria during prolonged systemic antibiotic treatment for acne and presents as exacerbation of preexisting acne. Physical examination: many inflamed pustules, most often on the face. Positive culture for gram-negative bacteria, often *Escherichia coli*.
Periorificial dermatitis, idiopathic	More common in women. Physical examination: small (<2 mm) papules and pustules around mouth or eyelids. Similar to acne but without comedones.
Periorificial dermatitis, iatrogenic	Frequent causes are prolonged topical glucocorticoid therapy for atopic dermatitis and inappropriate use of these agents to treat acne. Similar in appearance to idiopathic type.
Cutaneous proliferations	Adenoma sebaceum: numerous pink or skin-colored papules clustered around the nose and chin, associated with tuberous sclerosis. Patients without tuberous sclerosis may have one or up to several fibrous papules on the nose and central face.
	Follicular tumors (fibrofolliculomas and trichodiscomas): numerous skin-colored papules on the face and ears, associated with Birt-Hogg-Dubé syndrome (kidney cancer risk).

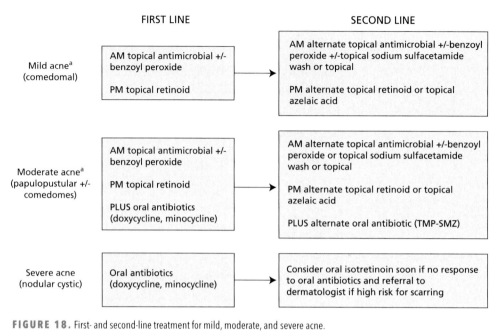

	FIRST LINE	SECOND LINE
Mild acne[a] (comedomal)	AM topical antimicrobial +/- benzoyl peroxide PM topical retinoid	AM alternate topical antimicrobial +/-benzoyl peroxide +/-topical sodium sulfacetamide wash or topical PM alternate topical retinoid or topical azelaic acid
Moderate acne[a] (papulopustular +/- comedomes)	AM topical antimicrobial +/- benzoyl peroxide PM topical retinoid PLUS oral antibiotics (doxycycline, minocycline)	AM alternate topical antimicrobial +/-benzoyl peroxide or topical sodium sulfacetamide wash or topical PM alternate topical retinoid or topical azelaic acid PLUS alternate oral antibiotic (TMP-SMZ)
Severe acne (nodular cystic)	Oral antibiotics (doxycycline, minocycline)	Consider oral isotretinoin soon if no response to oral antibiotics and referral to dermatologist if high risk for scarring

FIGURE 18. First- and second-line treatment for mild, moderate, and severe acne.

TMP-SMZ = trimethoprim-sulfamethoxazole.

[a]Consider oral contraceptives/antiandrogens in female patients. If refractory to treatment, consider gram-negative folliculitis.

treatment with an oral or topical antibiotic, as it reduces the development of bacterial resistance. Salicylic acid is also available over the counter and primarily works by removing and preventing comedones. The most frequent adverse effect of topical acne treatments is irritation. Lower concentrations of benzoyl peroxide (2.5%) are therefore recommended, as the efficacy is similar irritation is less than when formulations with benzoyl peroxide 10% concentration are used.

Topical retinoids are effective for comedonal as well as inflammatory acne. Topical retinoids can prevent acne by reducing follicular plugging and may also have anti-inflammatory effects. Because retinoids are preventive, they need to be applied to the entire acne-prone area and not used as a spot treatment. The most common adverse effects are dryness and irritation.

Antibiotics have been used for decades to treat acne vulgaris. Numerous studies have demonstrated the efficacy of oral antibiotics. Guidelines recommend that the duration of oral antibiotic therapy be limited, specifically that oral antibiotics be used for 3 months and then discontinued for patients with good clinical improvement. The same antibiotic can be used again for patients with good clinical improvement who have a subsequent relapse.

Isotretinoin is an oral retinoid. It is used as a first-line treatment for severe, nodulocystic acne (**Figure 19**) and for inflammatory acne that is recalcitrant to multimodality therapy with topical retinoids and oral antibiotics. The iPLEDGE program is an FDA-approved regulatory program to prevent birth defects from isotretinoin. Providers, patients, and pharmacies must be registered in the iPLEDGE program and complete monthly reports.

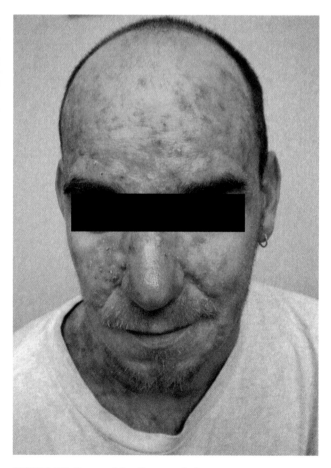

FIGURE 19. Severe nodulocystic acne on the face.

TABLE 10. Treatment of Acne

Medication[a]	Indication	Side Effects and Comments	FDA Pregnancy Category[b]
Topical retinoids (tretinoin, adapalene, tazarotene)	Mild comedonal acne; use singly or in combination with other treatments	Local irritation; superficial desquamation; may be combined with topical antibiotics	Tazarotene is pregnancy category X and requires pregnancy testing prior to prescription
Topical salicylic acid	Mild comedonal acne; use singly or in combination with other treatments	Mainly in patients with retinoid-intolerant skin	C
Topical azelaic acid	Adjunctive therapy for mild to moderate acne	Local irritation	B
Topical benzoyl peroxide	First-line therapy for mild to moderate acne; use singly or in combination with other treatments	Local irritation and, rarely, contact sensitivity	C
Topical antibiotics (clindamycin, erythromycin)	Therapy for mild to moderate inflammatory acne	Local irritation; promotion of antibiotic-resistant bacteria when used singly, therefore combination therapy with benzoyl peroxide is suggested	B
Topical dapsone	Moderate to severe inflammatory acne; can be part of a regimen with other treatments	Local irritation; G6PD testing is not necessary	C
Oral doxycycline	Moderate to severe inflammatory acne; can be combined with topical agents	Dose-related phototoxicity, vaginal yeast infection, dyspepsia; not for use in children <12 years of age or pregnant women	D
Oral minocycline	Moderate to severe inflammatory acne; can be combined with topical agents	Dizziness, vertigo, discolored teeth, blue-gray skin staining, rare hepatotoxicity and lupus-like syndrome, mild phototoxicity; not for use in children <12 years of age or pregnant women	D
Oral erythromycin	Moderate to severe inflammatory acne; can be combined with topical agents	Gastric upset, diarrhea; can be used in children <12 years of age	B
Oral contraceptives (norethindrone acetate-ethinyl estradiol, norgestimate-ethinyl estradiol)	First-line treatment of moderate to severe acne in adult women or with laboratory evidence of hyperandrogenism	Requires an average of 5 cycles to achieve 50% improvement; adjunctive topical therapy is usually needed	X
Spironolactone	Useful for moderate to severe acne in adult women	Concurrent oral contraceptives recommended	D
Isotretinoin	Treatment of choice for severe, recalcitrant nodular acne; prolonged remissions (1-3 years) in 40% of patients	All prescribers, patients, wholesalers, and dispensing pharmacies must be registered in the FDA-approved iPLEDGE program; cheilitis, dry skin and mucous membranes, hypertriglyceridemia; possible increased incidence of inflammatory bowel disease; depression	X

G6PD = glucose-6-phosphate dehydrogenase.

[a]For specific indications and precautions, please refer to the labeling information of the medications listed.

[b]See MKSAP17 General Internal Medicine for description of FDA Pregnancy Categories.

Acne can occur in adulthood, although the prevalence decreases with increasing age. Adult acne is more common in women and most commonly affects the lower half of the face or jawline. Androgens are believed to play a significant role in adult female acne; however, most women have normal androgen levels. Combination oral contraceptives and antiandrogens (such as spironolactone) can be useful therapies for adolescent as well as adult women, especially those with perimenstrual acne flares.

KEY POINTS

- Acne manifests as papules, pustules, and in severe cases, deep cysts, nodules, and interconnecting sinus tracts.
- First-line treatment for most patients with acne includes topical retinoid and topical antimicrobial therapy.

Rosacea

Rosacea is a common chronic condition of the facial skin characterized by pink papules, pustules, erythema, and telangiectasias. It is typically found in a bilaterally symmetric distribution on the convexities of the face, namely the forehead, cheeks, nose, and chin. Rosacea is sometimes called "adult acne." Both acne and rosacea have inflammatory papules and pustules, but comedones are *not* seen in rosacea. Rosacea more commonly affects women, especially those 30 to 60 years old.

The pathogenesis of rosacea is unknown. Multiple studies have demonstrated cutaneous inflammation; however, the trigger is highly debated. Alcohol, sun exposure, and other triggers can cause a transient increase in facial erythema but do not cause rosacea.

There are three cutaneous forms of rosacea (erythrotelangiectatic, papulopustular, and phymatous) and an ocular form. All three types of cutaneous rosacea cause some erythema and telangiectasia; however, they differ in the amount and severity of papulopustular lesions and phymatous changes. There is considerable overlap among the three main types, and while progression from one form to another is possible, it is uncommon and often slow.

Erythrotelangiectatic rosacea causes flushing and persistent erythema on the central portion of the face and few inflammatory papules (**Figure 20**). Patients may have swelling, stinging, burning, roughness, scaling, and a history of flushing. Flushing can be triggered by sun, stress, hot weather, alcohol, and warm or spicy foods. Caffeine has not been shown to be a consistent trigger.

Papulopustular rosacea causes central facial erythema with more frequent and numerous papules or pustules; burning and stinging may be present (**Figure 21**).

Phymatous rosacea is characterized by oily thickened skin with prominent pores and telangiectasias, and nodules of thickened skin can accumulate over years. The nose is most commonly affected (rhinophyma) (**Figure 22**), but

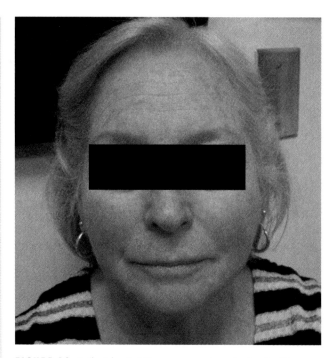

FIGURE 20. Erythrotelangiectatic rosacea presents predominantly with patches of erythema and telangiectasia.

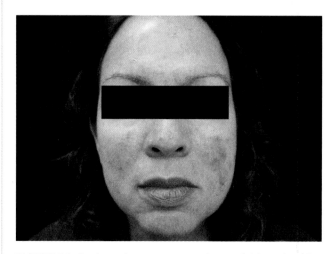

FIGURE 21. Papulopustular rosacea causes erythema and pink papules of the convexities of the face, namely, the forehead, nose, cheeks, and chin.

phymatous rosacea can also occur on the cheeks, forehead, chin, and ears.

Ocular rosacea reportedly affects 6% to 18% of patients with cutaneous rosacea. Symptoms of ocular rosacea are watery eyes, foreign body sensations, burning, and dryness. Conjunctivitis and styes are common.

The differential diagnosis for rosacea includes disorders that cause central facial erythema or inflammatory papules, such as periorificial dermatitis, cutaneous lupus erythematosus, sarcoidosis, contact dermatitis (eczema), seborrheic dermatitis, actinic damage, and folliculitis due to *Pityrosporum*

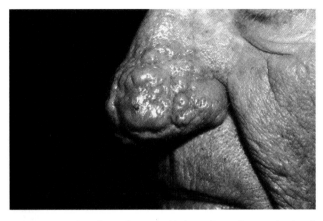

FIGURE 22. Rhinophyma, characterized by hyperplastic sebaceous glands and enlargement of the nose, in a patient with long-standing, uncontrolled rosacea.

or *Demodex* spp. Flushing is a common characteristic of rosacea; the differential diagnosis of this includes carcinoid syndrome, mastocytosis, and pheochromocytoma.

As with most chronic skin diseases, rosacea requires long-term treatment. Treatment is often tailored to target the most prominent manifestations in each patient (**Table 11**). Topical agents are often the first step in treatment. The most frequent side effect of any medication is dryness or irritation. Oral antibiotics are especially effective for ocular rosacea and the papules and pustules of papulopustular rosacea. Oral doxycycline is recommended; a dose of 40 mg twice daily is as effective as 100 mg twice daily but has fewer adverse effects. Topical or oral therapies are less effective for facial erythema and telangiectasia; laser and intense pulsed light are more effective. Laser and surgical debulking can be used to remove excess tissue for those with phymatous rosacea.

KEY POINTS

- Rosacea is a common chronic condition of the facial skin characterized by pink papules, pustules, erythema, and telangiectasias and is typically found on the forehead, cheeks, nose, and chin.
- First-line treatments for rosacea include avoidance of triggers (sun exposure, spicy or warm foods, hot drinks, and alcohol), topical metronidazole, topical sodium sulfacetamide/sulfur, topical azelaic acid and for papulopustular rosacea oral antibiotics.

Hidradenitis Suppurativa

Hidradenitis suppurativa (HS) or "acne inversa" is a chronic inflammatory disease that predominantly affects the apocrine-gland–bearing areas of the skin. The common sites are the axillae, breasts and inframammary creases, inguinal folds, and gluteal cleft (**Figure 23**). It is characterized by comedones, inflammatory papules, nodules, cysts, and scarring. The lesions are painful, and the drainage is often foul smelling. The distribution and severity of disease can range from minor to debilitating.

HS is estimated to affect 1% to 4% of the general population and frequently begins in the second to third decade. It is more common in women. Almost 40% of HS patients report a family history of the disease. About half of patients with HS have breast and armpit involvement and hypertrophic scars. Some also have a high incidence of acne, cysts, and folliculitis. Smoking, depression, obesity, and metabolic syndrome are more common in patients with HS than in the general population. It is therefore important to perform a complete history and physical examination to identify these factors and to determine the full extent and severity of disease.

TABLE 11. Management of Rosacea		
	Interventions	**FDA Pregnancy Category**
Avoidance	Sun-protection (sunscreen or sun-protective clothing)	N/A
	Triggers: Foods (spicy, warm), alcohol, warm environments	N/A
Topical	Metronidazole, 0.75% or 1%	B
	Sodium sulfacetamide/sulfur	C
	Azelaic acid , 15%-20%	B
	Topical calcineurin inhibitors (pimecrolimus, tacrolimus)	C
	Permethrin	B
Systemic	Tetracycline antibiotics (doxycycline, 40 mg)	D
	Macrolide antibiotics	B
	Erythromycin, azithromycin	C
	Clarithromycin	
Laser, light, and surgical	Lasers (PDL, Nd:YAG, CO_2, and others)	Avoided
	Intense pulsed light	
	Electrosurgery	
Nd:YAG = neodymium-doped yttrium aluminium garnet; PDL = pulsed dye laser.		

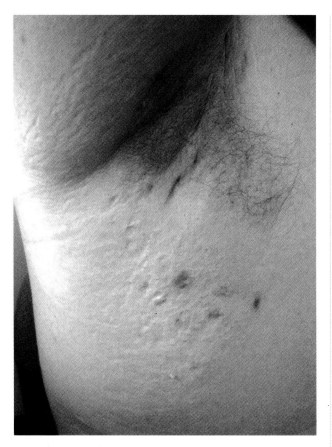

FIGURE 23. Hidradenitis suppurativa in the axilla demonstrating comedones and scars.

ifestations of Crohn disease, and sexually transmitted infections such as granuloma inguinale or lymphogranuloma venereum. HS can be distinguished by the presence of open comedones ("blackheads"), chronic relapses, predisposition for the folds of the body, and recurrence after both antibiotic and surgical therapy.

Many options are available for therapy, although there is little scientific evidence to support their effectiveness, and no treatment is effective for all patients (**Table 12**). Topical and oral antibiotics, topical and oral retinoids, intralesional glucocorticoids, incision and drainage, surgical excision, radiation, laser therapy, and TNF-α inhibitors are all treatment options. Clindamycin-rifampin combination antibiotics, infliximab, and surgical excision have the greatest evidence of effectiveness. Many patients require combination therapy. Potential complications of HS include scarring and contraction resulting in functional limitation, secondary infection, malignant degeneration into squamous cell carcinoma, lymphedema due to chronic inflammation and scarring, and rectal or urethral fistulas.

Common Skin Infections

The skin serves as an external barrier and is colonized with microorganisms that provide an opportunity for infections. Skin infections often are categorized by type of causative microorganism (bacteria, fungus, virus) and by the part of the skin infected.

Bacterial Skin Infections

Normal skin contains numerous microorganisms that comprise the natural microbiome, which helps keep the skin healthy and protects against pathogenic organisms. Although staphylococci or streptococci are commonly involved in skin infections, they are also a part of natural skin flora. Therefore, it is important to perform an appropriate culture to confirm that these microorganisms are the cause of infection with complicated skin and soft-tissue infections including abscesses, extensive areas of involvement, or non-response to antibiotics. It is important to obtain cultures before instituting systemic antibiotics to help with appropriate growth and appropriate

Acne inversa is an apt name because the pathogenesis of HS begins with follicular occlusion but not infection or inflammation of the apocrine glands. Following occlusion, secretions build up in the follicular duct and result in rupture and a subsequent inflammatory reaction that resembles a bacterial abscess. Following this, an acute inflammatory reaction is triggered in the surrounding tissue. The role of bacteria is controversial and is likely a secondary colonization since lesions are initially sterile and antibiotics are not entirely effective in preventing new lesions. In addition to their effects on bacteria, antibiotics may also exert anti-inflammatory effects.

The differential diagnosis includes folliculitis, abscess or carbuncle, ruptured epidermal inclusion cyst, cutaneous man-

TABLE 12. Treatment Options for Hidradenitis Suppurativa	
Disease Severity	**Treatment Options/Considerations**
Mild Predominantly comedones, small papules or pustules, solitary nodules	Antibacterial washes, topical antibiotics, analgesics, warm compresses, smoking cessation, weight loss
Moderate Multiple nodules, abscesses or cysts, scarring	Oral antibiotics with antibacterial washes and/or topical antibiotics, analgesics, wide local excision Women: Oral contraceptives, spironolactone
Severe Multiple nodules, sinus tracts, scarring	Referral to dermatologist or surgeon for consideration of wide local excision, tumor necrosis factor-α inhibitors, or clinical trial

antibiotic stewardship. Whenever possible, a culture should be performed by cleaning the skin surface with alcohol and then obtaining a sample from purulent material, yellow-crusted material, or a moist or broken down area of skin. With folliculitis or a collection such as an abscess, unroofing the outer skin may be necessary to obtain the best sample. This is especially important because of increasing resistance to antibiotics, such as methicillin-resistant *Staphylococcus aureus* (MRSA).

Bacterial infections are frequently categorized based on the location and type of infection: folliculitis; abscesses, furuncles, or carbuncles; impetigo; and cellulitis and erysipelas.

Folliculitis

Folliculitis is inflammation of hair follicles characterized by erythematous papules and pustules that are centered around a follicle on the face, chest, back, or buttocks (**Figure 24**).

Folliculitis can be noninfectious or infectious. When infectious, folliculitis is most often caused by *Staphylococcus aureus*, although other bacteria can induce folliculitis. These include *Pseudomonas* (hot tub folliculitis) and gram-negative folliculitis that sometimes occurs as a complication of acne therapy. Folliculitis can also occur from fungi such as *Malassezia* or *Candida* species, or from viruses, including herpesviruses. In addition, folliculitis can be secondary to noninfectious causes including acne vulgaris, eosinophilic folliculitis (seen in patients with HIV infection), or as a reaction to shaving or topical medications.

Although a diagnosis of folliculitis can be made clinically, culture can determine the causative organism and provide antibiotic sensitivity information when there is a lack of response to treatment or when surrounding extensive erythema is present. Biopsy also may be necessary to diagnose the underlying cause and rule out noninfectious causes of folliculitis.

Treatment for bacterial folliculitis includes topical antibacterial agents such as baths with dilute bleach, chlorhexidine washes, or benzoyl peroxide wash as a broad-spectrum antimicrobial agent. Topical mupirocin or clindamycin lotion also can be used. Culture is not necessary when these topical agents are used. For severe cases with widespread involvement or background erythema, oral antibiotics against *Staphylococcus aureus* can be given as a short course. If persistent or recurrent, maintenance with topical washes and/or further evaluation for an alternate diagnosis or for carriers of MRSA may be necessary. Decontamination can be performed as well. Lifestyle changes including avoiding shaving or using shaving cream and a sharp razor and wearing loose clothing to prevent friction also can be incorporated.

KEY POINTS

- Folliculitis is most often caused by *Staphylococcus aureus*, although other bacteria, fungi, and herpesviruses can also induce folliculitis.
- Treatment of folliculitis includes topical antibacterial agents such as chlorhexidine, topical antibiotics, or oral antistaphylococcal antibiotics.

Abscesses/Furuncles/Carbuncles

A carbuncle is a superficial inflammatory mass consisting of several inflamed hair follicles and multiple sites of drainage. A furuncle is an infection centered on a hair follicle with pus extending into the dermis and forming a small abscess. An abscess consists of a collection of neutrophils and purulent material within the dermis or subcutaneous tissue. Most abscesses are infectious in origin, although sterile abscesses can occur in some inflammatory conditions. These all present similarly with an inflamed, tender, fluctuant dermal and subcutaneous nodule and associated warmth (**Figure 25**).

The erythema can be confined to the immediate area overriding the purulent collection or can expand and represent a surrounding cellulitis. Purulent drainage may be easily expressed, and a rim of scale can occasionally be seen. The differential diagnosis includes an inflamed epidermal inclusion or other cyst. Although inflamed cysts can have associated erythema, they often lack the fluctuance observed in abscesses.

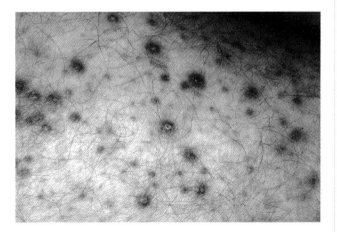

FIGURE 24. Pink papules and pustules centered around hair follicles, characteristic of folliculitis.

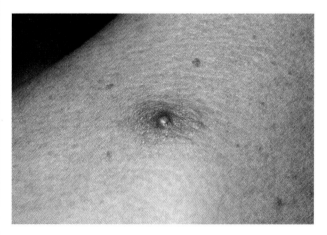

FIGURE 25. The abscess is characterized by a painful, inflamed nodule with some background erythema.

To diagnose an abscess, furuncle, or carbuncle, clinical appearance often is sufficient. Incision and drainage of the lesion is necessary. Culture from the purulent material is necessary to guide therapy and establish resistance patterns. For small, uncomplicated abscesses, furuncles, and carbuncles, local therapy with incision and drainage and warm compresses may be sufficient. Culture is still recommended when draining an abscess in case antibiotics are necessary. In immunosuppressed patients or those with associated cellulitis, fever, systemic symptoms, a large size (>5 cm), or multiple abscesses, systemic antibiotic therapy is also required. Hospitalization for initiating intravenous antibiotics may be required depending on the clinical findings. Because *S. aureus* is the most common pathogen in abscesses, antistaphylococcal antibiotics are generally indicated prior to obtaining culture results. The choice of antibiotics depends on the local antibiotic resistance patterns. Given the increased prevalence of MRSA, antibiotics effective against MRSA, including tetracycline-class antibiotics, clindamycin, and trimethoprim-sulfamethoxazole, are used as first-line therapy. **H**

When patients are colonized with MRSA or have close contacts with MRSA (such as daycare centers, prisons, military personnel, athletes, or persons who were recently hospitalized), recurrent abscesses can occur. Multiple recurrent abscesses also can be a sign of systemic immune disorders including HIV infection or underlying diabetes mellitus, and may trigger screening for these disorders. Stringent hygiene practices, such as frequent bathing, keeping any sores covered, and cleaning clothes, towels, and surfaces, are important. Although MRSA decolonization in the community is controversial, use of dilute bleach baths or chlorhexidine and topical mupirocin to the nares may be attempted when serious recurrent infections or repeated infections among a small cohort occur.

Methicillin-Resistant *Staphylococcus aureus* in Hospitalized Patients

Staphylococcus aureus is one of the most common causes of health care-associated infections, including catheter-associated skin and soft-tissue infections. An increasing number of these infections are from MRSA. MRSA carries potential for significant morbidity and mortality among infected hospitalized patients as well as an increased risk to other hospitalized patients because of its virulence, antibiotic resistance pattern, and increasing prevalence among hospitalized patients, especially ICU.

Hospitals mandate varied screening practices, with nares swabs being the most common method, although determining who needs to be screened is controversial. Evidence supporting MRSA screening and its ability to reduce MRSA infection or have an impact on morbidity and mortality is lacking. Some institutions require screening of every admitted patient, whereas others require it only for ICU admissions or those admitted with a prior colonization history. Contact isolation precautions in addition to universal precautions are often used with patients who screen positive for MRSA. Decolonization strategies for patients who screen positive also may be performed, especially for critically ill patients. Universal decolonization with twice daily intranasal mupirocin for 5 days and daily bathing with chlorhexidine in all ICU patients has recently been shown to be useful in preventing more infections.

Empiric antibiotic therapy against MRSA is often selected for most hospitalized patients with skin and soft-tissue infections until culture results are available. Knowledge of local resistance patterns can be helpful in selecting initial therapy. **H**

Impetigo

Impetigo is an acute, highly contagious, and superficial skin infection caused by gram-positive organisms, specifically *S. aureus* or *Streptococcus pyogenes*, or both. It is most common in young, healthy children but may occur in children or adults as superinfected dermatitis (impetiginized lesions) or infect a site of prior trauma such as an insect bite.

Impetigo can be either nonbullous or bullous impetigo. Nonbullous impetigo is the more common type and often affects the face or extremities. It presents as vesicles, pustules, and sharply demarcated areas with overlying honey-colored crust (**Figure 26**).

Bullous impetigo is a toxin-mediated process usually caused by production of an exfoliative toxin by *S. aureus*, which induces erythema and loss of the superficial layer of the epidermis (**Figure 27**).

The same toxin responsible for bullous impetigo can cause staphylococcal scalded skin syndrome, which results in erythroderma and skin peeling in children or occasionally in adults with acute kidney injury.

The diagnosis of impetigo often can be made based on clinical presentation; however, culture of the honey-colored crust can be used to confirm the pathologic organism and

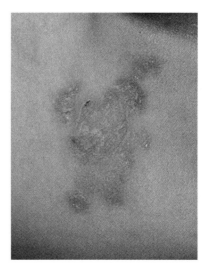

FIGURE 26. Nonbullous impetigo is a superficial infection characterized by a yellowish, crusted surface that may be caused by staphylococci or streptococci.

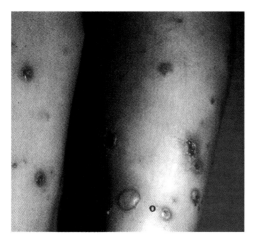

FIGURE 27. Clear, fluid-filled blisters with surrounding erythema on the legs of a patient with bullous impetigo.

obtain sensitivity testing, which is important when treating extensive disease or staphylococcal scalded skin syndrome.

Treatment for impetigo includes both topical and systemic therapies. Topical mupirocin often is first-line therapy, and washes with chlorhexidine and bleach baths also can be used. For more extensive infection, oral antistaphylococcal antibiotics are administered.

Systemic infection from impetigo is uncommon; however, ecthyma is a variant of impetigo characterized by an ulcerative lesion with an overlying eschar that extends into the dermis and may be associated with lymphadenitis. Ecthyma differs from cellulitis because of the presence of an overlying ulceration and eschar and involvement of the dermis. It is important to note that this differs from ecthyma gangrenosum, which is a highly

morbid infection caused by *Pseudomonas aeruginosa* that occurs in immunosuppressed patients and can be associated with high mortality rate.

Cellulitis/Erysipelas

Cellulitis is an acute, non-necrotizing infection of the skin that involves the deeper dermis and subcutaneous fat, most often caused by *Staphylococcus* or *Streptococcus* spp. This infection often results from superficial breaks or trauma in the skin. The trauma may be from an obvious source (arthropod bite, laceration, tinea pedis, onychomycosis) or may be a microscopic break in the skin with no visible inciting wound. The most common location in adults is an extremity, but in children includes the head and neck. Risk factors for the development of cellulitis include diabetes mellitus, older age, lymphedema, and peripheral vascular disease.

The diagnosis of cellulitis often is made based on the clinical presentation of a well-demarcated erythematous plaque. The four cardinal signs are erythema, pain, warmth, and swelling; associated lymphadenopathy can occur. Systemic symptoms including fever, chills, and malaise also may be present (**Table 13**). A useful clinical tool is to outline the erythema with a marker to monitor progression of the lesion (**Figure 28**).

The presentation of acute stasis dermatitis may mimic cellulitis, although the bilateral erythema and discoloration seen in stasis dermatitis would be atypical for cellulitis. The differential diagnosis of cellulitis also includes contact dermatitis, deep venous thrombosis, and panniculitis. If the diagnosis is in question, a skin biopsy can be performed. Tissue cultures and blood cultures are usually negative in the setting of cellulitis. The source of infection, including stasis dermatitis,

TABLE 13.	Differential Diagnosis of Cellulitis
Disease	**Clinical Characteristics**
Cellulitis	Well-demarcated erythematous plaque with erythema, pain, warmth, and swelling; associated lymphadenopathy can occur. Systemic symptoms including fever, chills, and malaise. Bilateral lower extremity cellulitis suggests an alternative diagnosis.
Stasis dermatitis	Erythematous, scaly, and eczematous patches most common on the lower extremities and affecting both legs with associated hyperpigmentation. Findings can persist for months to years. The medial ankle can be more severely involved, and ulcerations are common in this area. The erythema also can be striking, involving the ankle and extending to below the knee. Sharp demarcation often is less common in stasis dermatitis. Overlying cellulitis can develop in the setting of stasis dermatitis.
Contact dermatitis	Pruritic, geometric, and erythematous patches with superficial scale; differentiated from cellulitis by pruritus as opposed to pain.
Panniculitis (erythema nodosum)	Painful, erythematous subcutaneous, ill-defined nodules present bilaterally. Many panniculitides will resolve with hyperpigmentation. The acute onset of pain and erythema may be concerning for cellulitis, although distinct subcutaneous nodules would be unusual.
Deep venous thrombosis	Pain, swelling, and associated erythema and warmth in one leg, with changes often more prominent in the calf. A brightly erythematous, well-demarcated plaque is not often seen, although red, blue, or violaceous surface changes can be seen.
Herpes zoster	Grouped vesiculo-pustules on an erythematous patch or plaque localized to one area (dermatome). The erythema can be well defined. The presence of grouped, crusted vesiculo-pustules or punched out erosions is uncommon in cellulitis. Bacterial superinfection can occur.
For a complete list of potential entities on the differential diagnosis of cellulitis, please see the bibliography.	

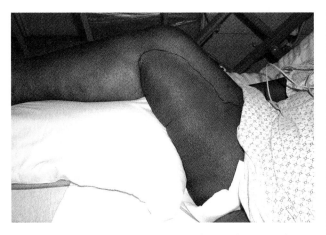

FIGURE 28. Cellulitis of the thigh. The cardinal features of cellulitis include erythema, swelling, warmth, and pain in the affected area.

trauma, abrasions, injection drug use, or tinea pedis, should be identified.

First-line therapy for cellulitis without a draining wound or abscess is an antibiotic with coverage against both *Streptococcus* spp. and *Staphylococcus* spp. with a β-lactam antibiotic such as cephalexin or dicloxacillin, clindamycin, or a macrolide antibiotic can be used. A 5-day course of antibiotics is as effective as a 10-day course. If the patient fails to respond to therapy, then expanding coverage for MRSA should be considered or parenteral antibiotics may be necessary. Noninfectious causes of erythema also should be considered in treatment failure cases. In patients with recurrent cellulitis, low-dose daily penicillin also can help prevent disease recurrence.

Erysipelas is a more superficial infection of the lymphatics that often presents as a violaceous-red, edematous, well-demarcated plaque on the face or lower extremities secondary to group A streptococci. Patients are extremely uncomfortable and often have systemic symptoms such as fever and malaise. Clinically, erysipelas may mimic allergic airborne contact dermatitis; however, contact dermatitis causes more diffuse erythema, and patients may be uncomfortable but not systemically ill. Because erysipelas is often due to streptococcal infection, first-line treatment is with penicillin. **H**

KEY POINTS

- Cellulitis is an acute, non-necrotizing infection of the skin, presenting as well-demarcated erythematous plaque with erythema, pain, warmth, swelling, and associated lymphadenopathy.

- **HVC** First-line therapy for cellulitis without a draining wound or abscess is a course of antibiotics against both *Streptococcus* spp. and *Staphylococcus* spp. (cephalexin or dicloxacillin, clindamycin, or a macrolide); a 5-day course of antibiotics is as effective as a 10-day course.

- Erysipelas is an infection of the upper dermis and superficial lymphatics that often presents as a violaceous-red, edematous, well-demarcated plaque on the face.

Erythrasma

Erythrasma is a benign condition caused by a superficial infection with *Corynebacterium minutissimum*. The infection can be asymptomatic or mildly pruritic and is characterized by symmetric, pink-to-brown patches with thin scale and an overlying wrinkled appearance and maceration in intertriginous areas such as the axillae, groin, inframammary areas, and interdigital spaces (**Figure 29**).

Erythrasma will fluoresce to a coral red color with a Wood lamp examination because of bacterial porphyrin production, which is a helpful feature in differentiating it from other causes of intertrigo. First-line treatment of erythrasma is a topical antibacterial agent such as erythromycin, clarithromycin, clindamycin, benzoyl peroxide, or fusidic acid. Oral agents including clarithromycin and erythromycin also could be considered in patients with extensive disease.

Pitted Keratolysis

Pitted keratolysis is a benign, superficial bacterial infection characterized by small pits primarily on the plantar aspects of the feet or palmar aspects of the hands in a setting of increased perspiration (**Figure 30**). This is most often caused by *Kytococcus sedentarius*, *Corynebacterium* spp., or *Actinomyces* spp. Although pitted keratolysis is mostly asymptomatic, an odor and scaling can be associated with this condition. Treatment requires decreasing perspiration by drying the feet with mechanical methods or antiperspirants. Topical clindamycin and erythromycin also are first-line antibacterial agents to clear the infection.

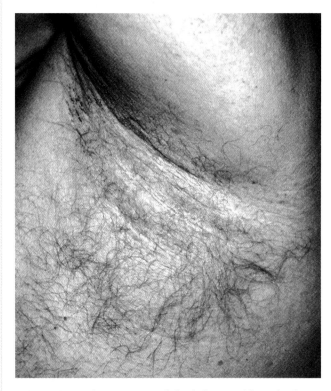

FIGURE 29. Erythrasma presents with sharply demarcated, fine pink-to-brown scaling patches that are typically found in skin fold areas.

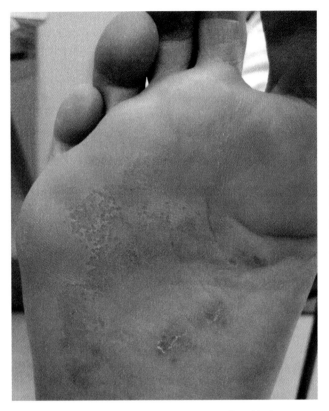

FIGURE 30. Multiple superficial pits on the plantar surface of the foot in a patient with keratolysis, a characteristic malodorous condition caused by *Kytococcus sedentarius, Corynebacterium* spp. or *Actinomyces* spp.

Superficial Fungal Infections

Superficial fungal infections are common and typically are caused by dermatophytes or *Candida* spp. The differentiation of superficial infections from deeper or angioinvasive fungal infections that can occur in immunocompromised patients is important, as the presentation, prognosis, and treatment are dramatically different. Superficial fungal infections by dermatophytes infect only the most superficial layers of the skin (stratum corneum, rarely epidermis and hair follicles). Angioinvasive fungal infections, in contrast, have a predilection for superficial and deep blood vessels and will present as violaceous to purple, necrotic patches or nodules, and deep fungal infections will often have both cutaneous changes, such as umbilicated or verrucous papules, and systemic involvement, often of the lungs.

Tinea

There are varied presentations of dermatophyte infections, ranging from mild to severe manifestations. Tinea is categorized according to the area of the body that is impacted, and different types of dermatophytes often are responsible for the respective infections.

Tinea capitis is infection of the hair follicles, typically of the scalp, although eyebrows and eyelashes can be infected. This is most common in children and can present with alo-

pecic areas, broken hair shafts, and scaling. A kerion can result from a tinea capitis infection and is manifested by a boggy, edematous scalp with overlying pustules (**Figure 31**). Associated cervical lymphadenopathy is common and is a useful clinical manifestation to differentiate from seborrheic dermatitis or other causes of alopecia. In children, washing or disposal of items in contact with the scalp (combs, hats, razors) is essential to prevent reinfection.

Tinea corporis classically presents as pruritic, annular erythematous patches with a rim of scale ("ring worm"). Risk factors include close contact in athletes, contact with animals, and immunosuppression. Majocchi granuloma, an erythematous plaque with overlying pustules and papules, is a granulomatous response to dermatophyte infection in the dermis and hair follicles (**Figure 32**). Risk factors include topical glucocorticoid use and shaving of legs in women, which causes spread of the organism. In immunocompromised patients, widespread involvement with varied presentations may occur.

Tinea cruris (jock itch) is dermatophyte infection of the inguinal folds (**Figure 33**). It presents as erythematous patches with a rim of scale and characteristically does not involve the scrotum, in contrast to candidal intertrigo, which can involve the scrotum.

Although tinea cruris is more commonly seen in men, both men and women can develop this infection. The presence of tinea cruris also necessitates examination of the feet as concomitant tinea pedis infection is not uncommon.

Tinea pedis is dermatophyte infection that presents with a flaky scale involving the plantar aspect of the feet

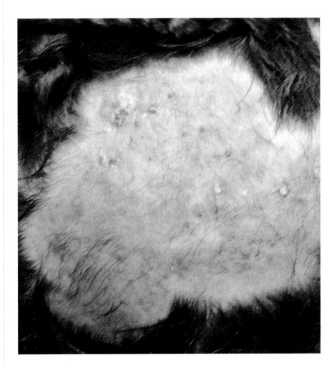

FIGURE 31. Kerion is a result of tinea capitis infection of the hair follicles of the scalp. It is a severe, painful inflammation that appears as raised, pus-filled abscesses.

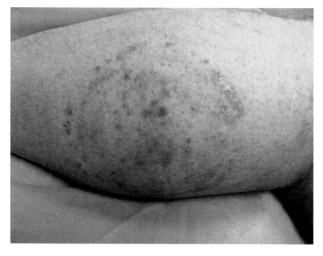

FIGURE 32. Majocchi granuloma presents as an annular plaque with erythema that is studded with pustules and papules and is a reaction to a dermatophyte infection in the dermis and hair follicle.

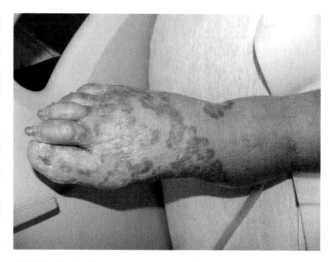

FIGURE 34. Erythematous patches with a scaling rim and associated onychomycosis (thickening of the nails) is seen in tinea pedis.

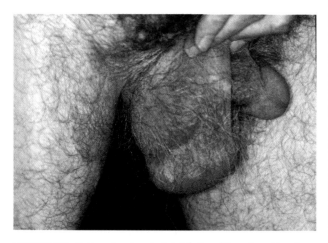

FIGURE 33. Tinea cruris, a dermatophyte infection of the groin, pubic region, and thighs, manifests with an annular lesion with slight scale, an erythematous, advancing edge, and central clearing.

and extending to the sides in a "moccasin" distribution (**Figure 34**). Interdigital involvement with scaling, maceration, and fissuring also is characteristic. Associated onychomycosis caused by the same organism is common. Tinea manuum is a fungal infection of the hands. "Two feet, one hand" tinea is a common presentation of concomitant tinea pedis and tinea manuum. Variants of dermatophyte infection also can occur. Bullous tinea presents with tense bullae, often on the extremities, and represents an exuberant reaction to dermatophyte infection. With extensive infections, an associated hypersensitivity reaction, a "dermatophytid" reaction, can occur away from the site of infection. For example, hand dermatitis also can occur in patients with extensive tinea pedis.

Tinea nigra is another dermatophyte infection presenting as a hyperpigmented, scaly patch, often on the palmar aspect of the hands.

Diagnosis of dermatophyte infection can be performed by examination of the scale, nail plate, or hair follicle using a potassium hydroxide (KOH) or chlorazol black solution. The presence of branching hyphae is diagnostic. Dermatophyte culture or biopsy also can be performed if the clinical presentation is unusual, if confirmation of the diagnosis is needed, or if KOH examination is equivocal.

Treatment of most superficial dermatophyte infections includes topical antifungal agents such as miconazole, clotrimazole, ketoconazole, or terbinafine. Over-the-counter preparations are cost-effective options with good efficacy. Nystatin is not effective against dermatophytes and should not be used. Combination therapy with topical glucocorticoids and antifungal creams should be avoided because of an increased risk of treatment failures, development of skin atrophy with prolonged use, and increased cost without increased efficacy. Oral antifungal therapy with terbinafine or an azole antifungal agent may be necessary for treating tinea capitis, onychomycosis, Majocchi granuloma, or extensive infection. Oral ketoconazole should not generally be used because of the potential for severe liver toxicity and adrenal gland suppression. In children, oral griseofulvin for tinea capitis also may be used. Tinea pedis will respond to 2 to 4 weeks of topical antifungal therapy, but effective treatment of onychomycosis often requires 12 weeks of oral therapy. Most infections will resolve but may recur and require retreatment. In immunosuppressed patients, recognition and treatment of superficial skin fungal infections is essential, as fungal infections can lead to epidermal breakdown and create a portal of entry for invasive pathogens.

Tinea versicolor is another superficial fungal infection caused by *Malassezia furfur* (formerly *Pityrosporum*) and is most common in warm, humid environments. It presents as hypopigmented, hyperpigmented, or pink patches that are dry and slightly scaly. Although the patches can occur anywhere, the neck, upper back, and chest, with extension to the abdomen or extremities, are commonly affected (**Figure 35**). These areas often become more noticeable after exposure to the sun because the organism prevents the skin from tanning. This type of superficial infection is not contagious. A form of folliculitis also occurs (*Malassezia* folliculitis). Diagnosis can be made clinically; however, yeast spores and short hyphae can be easily observed with KOH examination ("spaghetti and meatballs" appearance). Differential diagnosis includes vitiligo, postinflammatory pigmentation, seborrheic dermatitis, and pityriasis alba. Treatment of tinea versicolor with topical antiseborrheic shampoos or lotions such as selenium sulfide or ketoconazole leads to resolution of erythema and scaling, but the pigmentation changes may persist for longer periods of time. Recurrence is common, and retreatment and prevention with topical therapy often is necessary. With widespread involvement, short courses of oral azole antifungal agents (with the exception of ketoconazole as noted earlier) may be necessary.

KEY POINTS

- Diagnosis of dermatophyte infection can be performed by examination of the scale, nail plate, or hair follicle after preparation with potassium hydroxide (KOH) or chlorazol black solution; the presence of branching hyphae is diagnostic.

HVC • Treatment of most superficial dermatophyte infections includes topical antifungal agents; however, over-the-counter preparations are cost-effective options with good efficacy.

Candidiasis

Cutaneous candidiasis can present in multiple ways: intertriginous areas (**Figure 36**), oral involvement as oral thrush or angular cheilitis, vulvovaginal candidiasis (**Figure 37**), and disseminated disease in immunocompromised, hospitalized patients (see MKSAP 17 Infectious Disease).

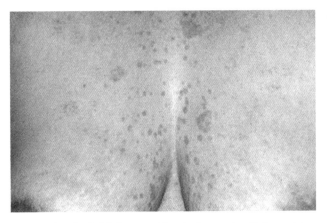

FIGURE 35. Small, light-brown to pink coalescing macules with fine overlying scale on the anterior chest characteristic of tinea versicolor.

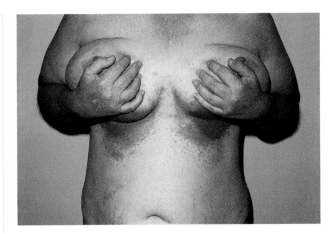

FIGURE 36. Bright red papules, vesicles, pustules, and patches with satellite papules in the intertriginous areas under the breasts characteristic of candidiasis.

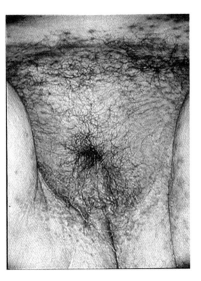

FIGURE 37. Acute vulvar candidiasis presents with erythema and edema of the vulva with satellite papules and pustules. Associated involvement of the vaginal mucosa is characterized by a discharge that may be thick, adherent, and "cottage cheese-like" or thin and loose, indistinguishable from the discharge of other types of vaginitis.

Cutaneous candidiasis clinically presents as bright red patches with satellite papules and pustules in intertriginous areas. Involvement of the vulva and scrotum is common. Associated vaginal involvement can be characterized by a discharge that may be thick, adherent, and "cottage cheese-like" or thin and loose, indistinguishable from the discharge of other types of vaginitis. Risk factors include chronic moisture and hyperhidrosis, and this may be more common in febrile, hospitalized patients. Diagnosis can be made clinically, and KOH examination showing pseudohyphae and spores can also be diagnostic. Reducing friction and moisture with barrier pastes and powders such as zinc oxide are important. Treatment with topical azole antifungal agents is the preferred first-line therapy. Although nystatin is effective against *Candida* spp., it is not effective for dermatophyte infection.

Topical azoles should also be used for superficial fungal infections in intertriginous areas. With concomitant vulvar and vaginal involvement (characterized by associated discharge), cutaneous candidiasis may be treated with oral antifungal agents or topical and intravaginal preparations.

Viral Skin Infections

Herpes Simplex Virus

The family of human herpes viruses causes numerous cutaneous infections including herpes simplex virus 1 (HSV1), herpes simplex virus 2 (HSV2), and varicella-zoster viral infections (VZV or human herpes virus 3 [HHV3]). Because they are closely related, the primary skin lesions are similar. The classic presentation is a group of painful, small vesicles on an erythematous base, transitioning to pustules and subsequent crusting of the lesions over time (**Figure 38**).

Because the viruses have a tropism for the nerve dorsal root ganglia, they migrate to this area after initial infection where they can remain latent and cause subsequent reinfection and recurrences. Phases of infection include primary infection (which often is most severe), latent infection in the ganglion when viral shedding can still occur, and viral reactivation leading to a clinical outbreak.

The primary lesions of HSV1 and HSV2 are clinically indistinguishable. HSV1 traditionally causes orofacial lesions, and HSV2 most often causes genital lesions; however, both viruses can lead to either oral or genital lesions. Herpes infection outside of these areas can occur, including infection on the fingers of children (herpetic whitlow) or in exposed skin as a result of skin-to-skin contact, such as in contact sports like wrestling (herpes gladiatorum). Diffuse infection can occur in the setting of an underlying skin disease, such as eczema (eczema herpeticum). The viruses are highly contagious, and transmission is by direct contact of salivary or genital secretions. Asymptomatic viral shedding can occur. Outbreaks can be triggered by stress, fever or other infection, and ultraviolet light exposure. Associated manifestations also can occur, including erythema multiforme.

Primary oral herpes simplex virus infection (herpes gingivostomatitis) can present as a mild or asymptomatic infection or can be severe with fever, malaise, lymphadenopathy, and widespread painful vesicles and erosions on the cutaneous and mucosal lips and gingiva (**Figure 39**). Secondary infection with *Candida* also can occur. Recurrent herpes labialis often causes prodromal pain and stinging, followed by solitary lesions on the vermilion border ("cold sores").

Most primary genital herpes infections are asymptomatic, with up to 70% to 80% of seropositive persons having no recollection of initial infection. Severe initial presentations also can occur with fever, malaise, tender lymphadenopathy, and painful erosions that can be secondarily infected and lead to an inability to urinate or defecate. Recurrent genital herpes is similar to oral herpes with a prodrome, followed by grouped vesicles on an erythematous base, erosions, and crusting. Involvement of the genitals and buttocks can occur. Immunocompromised patients can have severe presentations of both oral and genital herpes, including persistent verrucous nonhealing ulcers.

The differential diagnosis of genital ulcers is important because other sexually transmitted infections must be considered (including syphilis, chancroid, granuloma inguinale, lymphogranuloma venereum). HSV is the most common cause of painful genital ulcers, although chancroid also causes painful ulcers. Other infections often cause nonpainful ulcerations (see MKSAP 17 Infectious Disease). With any sexually transmitted infection, HIV testing also is important.

Diagnosis of HSV can be made clinically, but several tests also are available. Although the Tzanck smear was traditionally used to confirm the presence of a HIV, difficulties with reliable interpretation and its inability to distinguish between HSV1, HSV2, and varicella infections have led to the use of other diagnostic methods. Rapid tests are widely available such as direct-fluorescent antibody (DFA) and polymerase chain reaction (PCR) studies that can provide results in less than 24 hours and can differentiate between the viruses. To adequately perform

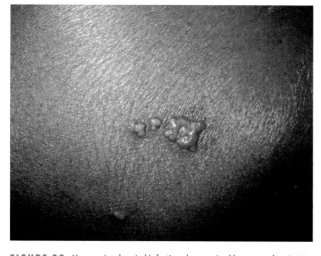

FIGURE 38. Herpes simplex viral infection characterized by grouped vesicopustules on an erythematous base that typically have associated tingling or pain.

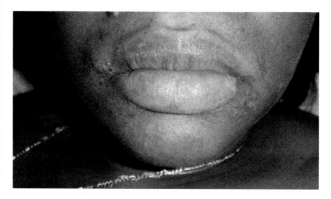

FIGURE 39. Primary herpes simplex virus on the sides of the mouth.

these tests, a vesicle needs to be unroofed, and material from the blister base (where the virus is present) is sent for examination. Viral culture has traditionally been the gold standard for diagnosis, but the culture can take 48 hours or longer to be interpreted. Culture is still valuable if resistance testing is necessary in patients with recalcitrant or chronic infections (typically immunocompromised patients). Serologic testing is not recommended for diagnosis because seroprevalence rates are high and do not correspond with active infection.

Oral antiviral agents are considered first-line therapies for herpes simplex virus infection and are most effective if instituted at presentation of the prodrome of an outbreak. Oral antiviral agents including acyclovir, valacyclovir, and famciclovir are considered first-line therapies, and dose and duration of treatment are dependent on the type and extent of infection (primary versus recurrent). Topical therapies are less effective in improving symptoms and reducing disease duration. With frequent outbreaks, daily suppressive therapy also can be instituted.

KEY POINTS

- The classic presentation of herpes simplex viral infections is a group of painful, small vesicles on an erythematous base, transitioning to pustules and subsequent crusting of the lesions over time.
- Oral antiviral agents are considered first-line therapies for herpes simplex virus infection and are most effective if instituted at presentation of the prodrome of an outbreak.

Varicella/Herpes Zoster

Varicella-zoster viral infections (VZV) can either be primary (chickenpox) or reactivation (herpes zoster). Primary varicella often is seen in children or young adults, but is now seen less frequently because of vaccination of young children.

Herpes zoster (shingles) is caused by the reactivation of latent VZV. Shingles typically presents with grouped vesicles on an erythematous base in a single dermatome (**Figure 40** and **Figure 41**). Elderly persons and immunocompromised patients are at increased risk, and recurrent outbreaks of herpes zoster should prompt an evaluation for possible malignancy or immunodeficiency. Lesions are infectious until they

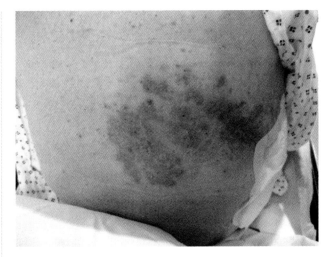

FIGURE 41. Herpes zoster infection on the flank with grouped vesicles and punched out erosions on an erythematous base.

become crusted over, and persons with herpes zoster should avoid contact with others who may be susceptible including pregnant women or immunocompromised persons.

The clinical presentation of herpes zoster is characteristic. Prodromal symptoms, such as burning, stinging, or tingling, often occur in a localized region, followed by an eruption of grouped vesicles or pustules on an erythematous base. The outbreak is unilateral and does not cross the body's midline. The most common dermatomes affected are in the thoracic region. Facial involvement may require further evaluation. With involvement of the first division of the trigeminal nerve (forehead extending over upper eyelid, or nasal tip involvement), ophthalmologic evaluation is mandatory as herpes zoster ophthalmicus and possible blindness can result. Evaluation by an otolaryngologist may be required if vesicles are noted in the external ear canal, as peripheral facial paralysis and auditory/vestibular symptoms can occur (Ramsay Hunt syndrome). Differentiation between genital herpes and herpes zoster in the sacral dermatomes also may be difficult. Diagnosis can be made clinically, or the tests previously outlined can be used.

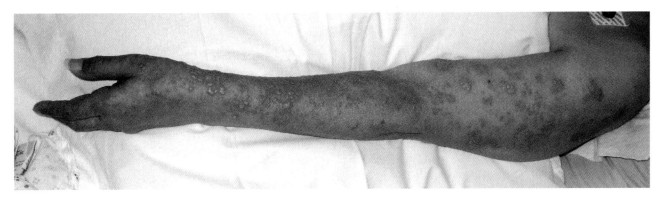

FIGURE 40. Herpes zoster infection characterized by vesicopustules on an erythematous base in a dermatomal distribution.

Disseminated VZV must be considered when more than three dermatomes are affected or more than 20 lesions outside of adjacent dermatomes are present. This is more common in immunocompromised persons who are at risk for associated hepatitis or pneumonia.

Oral acyclovir, valacyclovir, or famciclovir is effective for treating herpes zoster if initiated within 24 to 48 hours of presentation and can shorten the disease course as well as help prevent postherpetic neuralgia. If postherpetic neuralgia develops, gabapentin, pregabalin, tricyclic antidepressants, or topical anesthetics such as topical lidocaine and capsaicin can be helpful. Treatment with gabapentin at presentation of herpes zoster also may reduce the risk of postherpetic neuralgia. A shingles vaccine is available to decrease the incidence of herpes zoster reactivation and decrease the severity and duration of postherpetic neuralgia. The vaccine is indicated for persons 60 years of age and older. However, it is a live attenuated vaccine and is not recommended in immunosuppressed or pregnant persons (see MKSAP 17 General Internal Medicine).

KEY POINTS

- Herpes zoster (shingles) is caused by the reactivation of latent varicella-zoster virus and often presents with grouped vesicles on an erythematous base in a single dermatome.

- When herpes zoster involves first division of the trigeminal nerve (forehead extending over upper eyelid, or nasal tip involvement), ophthalmologic evaluation for eye involvement is mandatory as blindness can result; when more than three dermatomes are involved consider treatment for disseminated varicella-zoster viral infections.

- Oral acyclovir, valacyclovir, or famciclovir, if initiated within 24 to 48 hours of presentation, can shorten the course of herpes zoster and help prevent postherpetic neuralgia.

Warts

Warts are an infection of skin and mucosa caused by human papillomavirus (HPV). There are numerous different HPV subtypes, which may have a predilection for different anatomic sites. HPV is contagious and spread by direct skin contact or contact with infected surfaces, and self-inoculation within an individual can occur. There are many presentations of warts depending on the site and clinical appearance. Verruca vulgaris is an exophytic, hyperkeratotic papule that often develops on the hands but may be found anywhere (**Figure 42**). Verruca plantaris is characterized by larger, hyperkeratotic lesions on the plantar surface of the feet that can be difficult to treat. Differentiation from calluses is possible because warts cause dilated capillaries, which clinically present as black dots and obliteration of normal dermatoglyphics (ridges and furrows on the skin surface forming loops, whorls, and arches). Flat warts (verruca plana) are flat-topped papules that often are spread easily, especially from shaving.

Anogenital warts (condylomata acuminata) are the most common sexually transmitted infection and are most often caused by HPV types 6 and 11. They present as single or multiple papules on the penis, vulva, or perianal area and may be variably sized flat-topped or cauliflower-like papules (**Figure 43**). Lesions are diagnosed based on clinical appearance, but large, atypical lesions or those recalcitrant to therapy should be biopsied to rule out premalignant or malignant transformation.

Although warts may resolve spontaneously, treatment often is required. Over-the-counter preparations of salicylic acid or wart remover can be effective. If resolution does not occur, additional destructive techniques can include cryotherapy, topical application of prescription-strength salicylic acid, cantharidin, podophyllin, or laser therapy. Paring of the hyperkeratoses associated with a wart may be necessary to increase the therapeutic effect. Immune therapies, including

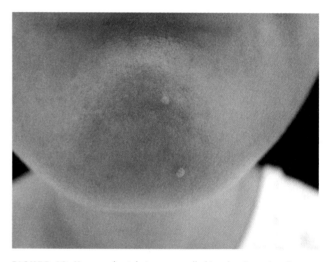

FIGURE 42. Verruca vulgaris lesions are small, skin-colored growths, often occurring in clusters, and are caused by the human papillomavirus.

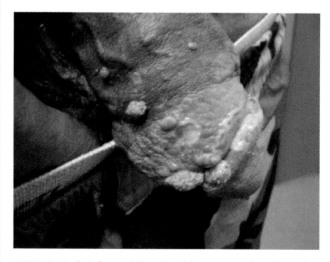

FIGURE 43. Typical anogenital warts (condyloma acuminata) over the penile shaft and foreskin with adjacent erosions after imiquimod therapy.

injection of *Candida* antigen and topical imiquimod, also can be effective. Surgical removal of large, bulky lesions also can be used. Numerous therapies have been reported to be effective, but controlled trials are lacking to compare modalities.

HPV vaccination is recommended for young persons (both female and male) ages 9 to 26 years to prevent cervical and anal carcinoma. Anogenital warts also can be prevented if the vaccine is effective against HPV 6 and 11 (see MKSAP 17 General Internal Medicine). It is unclear whether the vaccine confers protection against other strains of HPV.

Molluscum Contagiosum

Molluscum contagiosum is a common poxvirus infection among children, young adults, and immunosuppressed persons. In children, it presents as multiple small, flesh-colored umbilicated papules (**Figure 44**). Inflamed or large lesions and a surrounding eczematous dermatitis can be observed. In young adults, molluscum contagiosum is considered a sexually transmitted infection that also causes similar umbilicated papules in the genital area. Diagnosis can be made by the clinical appearance. Although lesions can self-resolve, this may take months to years. Because lesions are extremely contagious, treatment is recommended. Therapy includes destructive techniques including cryotherapy, salicylic acid, cantharidin, or physical removal with curettage.

Infestations

Scabies

Scabies (*Sarcoptes scabiei*) is transmitted by person-to-person contact. It typically presents as generalized and often intense pruritus with erythematous papulonodules and scaling patches, especially in web spaces, wrists, axillae, nipples, waistline, and genitals (**Figure 45**), with sparing of the head.

Burrows (serpiginous lines) may also be seen. Crusted (Norwegian) scabies is a highly contagious variant seen in elderly and immunocompromised persons that presents as hyperkeratotic plaques, especially on the extremities. Infestations occur in nursing homes, hospitals, or institutions, and a high clinical suspicion is necessary to avoid outbreaks, as pruritus often can be very minimal if present.

Diagnosis is suspected when multiple family members in close contact have generalized pruritus. Definitive diagnosis requires identification of the mite, eggs, or feces by microscopic examination (using potassium hydroxide [KOH] or mineral oil) after scraping several lesions (**Figure 46**).

Treatment of the patient and close contacts is required to eliminate the infestation (**Table 14**). Itching can persist for weeks after therapy. The resulting pruritus can be treated with antihistamines, topical glucocorticoids, and, if severe, oral

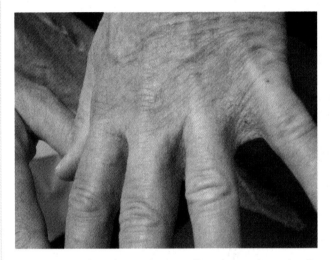

FIGURE 45. Scabies infestation characterized by erythema, scaling, and small crusted papules between web spaces.

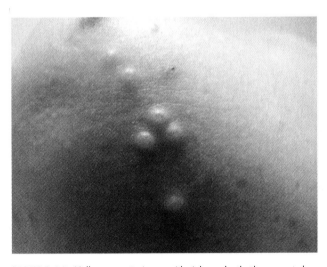

FIGURE 44. Molluscum contagiosum, with pink papules that have a central umbilication.

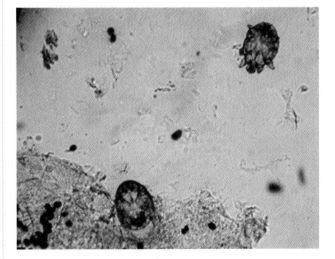

FIGURE 46. Microscopic examination of skin scrapings, showing mites and mite feces (scybala), diagnostic of scabies.

TABLE 14. Treatment of Scabies and Lice

Scabies		
Medication[a]	**Application/Dose**	**Notes**
Permethrin 5% lotion	Apply overnight from neck to feet, then rinse in the morning Repeat in 7-10 days	Considered first-line therapy
Oral ivermectin	Dose: 200 µg/kg Repeat in 7-10 days	Useful for persistent infestation, treatment failure, or intolerance to topical therapy Also may be important adjuvant therapy in crusted scabies Should not be used in pregnant/breastfeeding women or young children
Lindane 1% lotion	Apply overnight from neck to feet, then rinse in morning Repeat in 7-10 days	Not available in some countries because of neurotoxicity
Combination therapy with ivermectin and topical lotions		For treatment of crusted scabies
Lice		
Medication[a]	**Application/Dose**	**Notes**
Permethrin 1% lotion	Apply to affected areas (damp hair for 10 minutes), then rinse Repeat in 7-10 days	Considered first-line therapy unless there is known resistance Should perform nit combing
Pyrethrin 0.3% + piperonyl butoxide 4% shampoo	Apply to damp hair for 10 minutes), then rinse Repeat in 7-10 days	Useful therapy Should perform nit combing
Malathion 0.5% lotion	Apply to affected areas for 8-12 hours, then rinse Repeat in 7-10 days	Flammable Should perform nit combing
Benzyl alcohol 5% lotion	Apply to affected areas, leave on for 10 minutes Repeat in 7-10 days	Should perform nit combing
Spinosad 0.9% topical suspension	Apply to affected areas for 10 minutes, then rinse Repeat in 7 days if live lice are seen	Nit combing not necessary
Topical ivermectin 0.5% lotion	Apply to dry hair Rinse after 10 minutes	Nit combing not necessary
Oral ivermectin	Dose: 200 µg/kg Repeat in 7-10 days	Should not be used in pregnant/breastfeeding women or young children
Lindane 1% lotion	Apply overnight from neck to feet, then rinse in morning Repeat in 7-10 days	Not available in some countries because of neurotoxicity

[a]Treatment of the individual and close contacts at same time is essential for eradication. Washing of clothes, linens, and personal items in hot water should be performed to remove fomites.

glucocorticoids can be used. If new lesions (papules, changes in web spaces) occur, prompt evaluation for reinfestation or bacterial superinfection should occur.

Lice

Lice can be found on the head (*Pediculosis capitus*), body (*Pediculosis corporis*), or pubic area (*Phthirus pubis*) and often present with itching in the involved area. Pubic lice also can be found on eyebrows or eyelashes (**Figure 47**). Head lice often occur among children. Body lice typically live in clothing seams and can transmit infections such as typhus, trench fever, and relapsing fever. Persons living in close contact, including the homeless or refugee populations, are at increased risk.

Diagnosis requires visualization of the lice or the nits (adherent white egg casings) on the hair shafts.

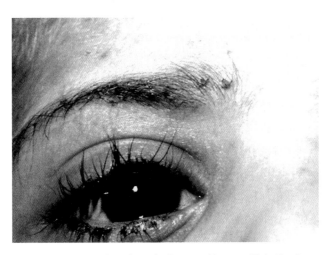

FIGURE 47. Lice on the eyebrow. The diagnosis of lice is established by identifying crawling lice in the scalp, eyebrows, or pubic hair.

Erythematous bite marks in the affected areas can be a clue to diagnosis. Even after successful treatment, nits can continue to persist.

Treatment of the patient and close contacts is required to eliminate the infestation (see Table 1). Clothes, linens, and personal items should be washed in hot water to remove fomites.

Bedbugs

Bedbug infestations (*Cimex lectularius*) are occurring at increasing rates and are a public health concern. Classic presentation is grouped, pruritic papules in close configuration ("breakfast, lunch, and dinner") on exposed body areas (**Figure 48**). Bites are typically noticed in the morning, as bedbugs feed at night (**Figure 49**). Diagnosis and eradication are difficult and often require a professional exterminator. Evaluation of hotel rooms when traveling for evidence of bedbugs (identifying blood spots under the mattress or identifying molted skin or bedbugs themselves in headboards, baseboards, under the mattress) may be helpful for prevention. Treatment is symptomatic, with topical glucocorticoids and oral antihistamines, as bedbugs do not live on humans.

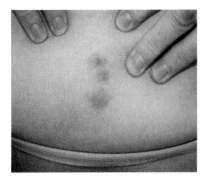

FIGURE 48. Bedbug bites usually occur in a series ("breakfast, lunch, and dinner"). The lesions are painless, pruritic, urticaria-like papules.

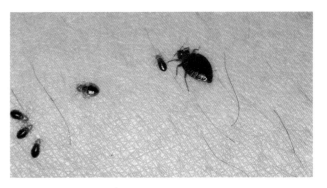

FIGURE 49. Bedbugs are nocturnal. They feed off human blood and tend to live near their food supply.

Bites and Stings

Arthropod bites and stings are common and often self-limited. Both mosquitoes and ticks can be potential vectors for systemic illnesses. Prevention using insect repellents that contain DEET, picaridin, or permethrin-impregnated clothes and wearing long-sleeved clothing is recommended.

Spider Bites

Most spider bites are unnoticed or may appear as pruritic red papules (**Figure 50**). Diagnosis is made upon clinical presentation, and treatment is symptomatic in most patients.

Severe spider bites that cause systemic symptoms are rare. The brown recluse spider, *Loxosceles recluse*, is found in southern and central United States (**Figure 51**) and can cause severe skin necrosis with significant pain and systemic symptoms, including nausea, vomiting, fever, muscle and joint pain, hemolysis, and acute kidney injury (**Figure 52** and **Figure 53**).

Brown recluse spider bites are uncommon because the spiders are timid insects and often are hiding. Most suspected

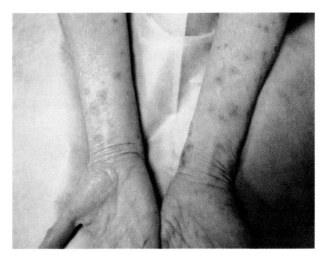

FIGURE 50. Spider bites presenting as red, pruritic, urticarial papules that are pruritic.

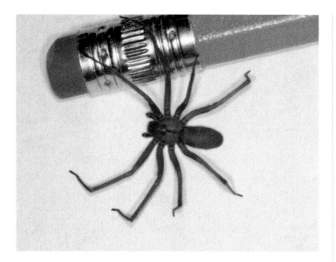

FIGURE 51. Brown recluse spiders are quite shy, and their bites are often misidentified and overdiagnosed.

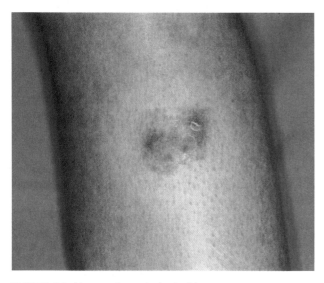

FIGURE 52. A brown recluse spider bite (early).

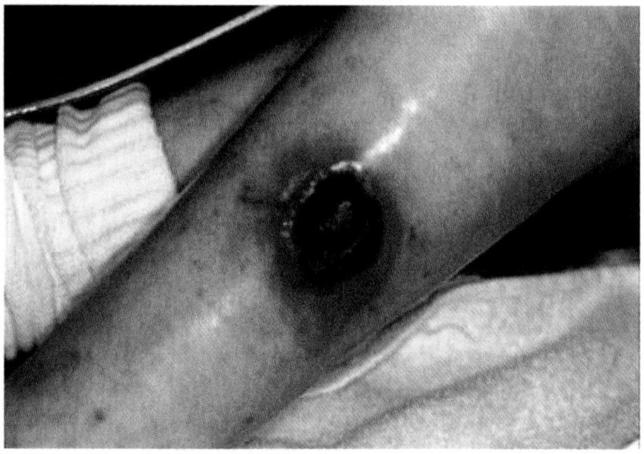

spider bites actually are misdiagnosed and are caused by other insect bites or infections, including bacterial abscesses. Although diagnosis is usually made clinically, serum enzyme-linked immunoabsorbent assays or biopsy can be performed to confirm a bite. Treatment includes analgesic agents, wound care, and debridement in some cases.

Hymenoptera

Wasp and bee stings are painful but often self-limited. Stingers should be removed rapidly, as venom can continue to be released. Localized reactions include pain, redness, and swelling. Systemic reactions including hives and anaphylaxis can occur in some persons, and such persons should carry an injectable epinephrine pen. Because massive wasp and bee stings can result in multiorgan failure, desensitization using allergy therapy can be performed in persons who have had systemic reactions.

Fire ants, found in the southern United States, can both bite and sting, causing a significant response. These bites cause an initial burning and itchy sensation followed by several pustules. The pustules can mimic other dermatologic diseases including infections. Topical glucocorticoids may be required for symptomatic relief. Persons with severe bites may require oral glucocorticoids.

Worms

Cutaneous larva migrans is an intensely pruritic skin eruption caused by hookworms as a result of walking barefoot in areas where animal feces may be present (such as on beaches). Wearing footwear is therefore recommended. The eruption is linear or serpiginous, and often occurs on the extremities (**Figure 54**). Oral antiparasitic agents (ivermectin as the preferred agent or albendazole as an alternative) can help resolve the eruption. Antihistamines or glucocorticoids can be used to relieve symptoms.

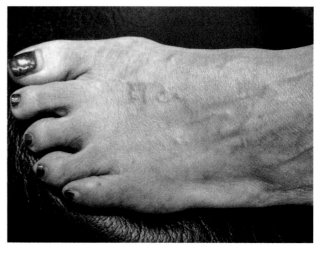

FIGURE 54. Serpiginous, linear red track marks that are pathognomonic for cutaneous larva migrans.

FIGURE 53. Ulceration from a brown recluse spider bite (late).

Cuts, Scrapes, and Burns

Minor cuts, scrapes, and burns often require only gentle cleansing with soap and water and local wound care using sterile petrolatum jelly and a nonadherent bandage over the wound. A contact layer is the first layer on top of the wound. The contact layer allows the wound to stay moist to aid in healing without sticking to it. Examples include petrolatum gauze or sterile petrolatum applied to a nonadherent dressing. Nonstick silicone sheets are an excellent first layer on top of a noninfected wound and can be placed over a topical antibiotic. This will aid in healing and may help lessen scarring, but silicone sheets are more expensive than petrolatum and their superiority has not been proved. The contact layer can be covered by a secondary nonadherent dressing that can be taped in place.

Cuts and Scrapes

For minor wounds that are not contaminated, thorough cleansing and application of topical sterile petrolatum is often sufficient. Topical antibiotics can be used for wounds that are contaminated or in locations such as around the perineum, major skin folds, or mouth that may be colonized with pathogenic bacteria, increasing the risk for secondary infection. Topical antibiotics such as neomycin and bacitracin are inexpensive over-the-counter agents with activity against gram-positive and selected gram-negative organisms but may lead to contact allergy. Mupirocin is effective against gram-positive organisms and has little risk of contact sensitivity, but bacterial resistance is emerging. Silver sulfadiazine is a broad-spectrum antibiotic with activity against gram-positive and gram-negative organisms including *Pseudomonas aeruginosa*. Silver sulfadiazine has been rarely associated with bone marrow suppression and severe drug reactions. Retapamulin is a newer topical antibiotic that covers gram-positive organisms but is more expensive. If pustules, drainage, or pain develops, wound culture is indicated to diagnose an infection. Red, itchy papules and increased drainage within a few days after application of a topical antibiotic may be caused by a topical antibiotic allergy.

The decision to suture or glue a laceration is based on the depth, likelihood of dehiscence, ability to cleanse the wound, and long-term cosmesis. Wound adhesives can be used for minor cuts that are not under tension, whereas sutures are indicated for larger, deeper cuts.

Burns

Patients with thermal burns can be triaged based on the amount of body surface area affected, specific body part involved (face or perineum may need more advanced care), and depth of the burn. Superficial burns affect only the epidermis and appear red. Superficial partial thickness burns involve the epidermis and superficial dermis, manifesting with clear fluid-filled blisters on a red base. Deep partial-thickness burns involve the deeper dermis, appear whiter, and are less blanchable. Full-thickness burns affect the deep dermis into the subcutaneous fat, are not blanchable, and appear white or yellow. Patients with severe or widespread burns should be referred to a burn unit. Estimating the body surface area affected can be done using the size of the patient's palm as 1% for small burns. The rule of 9s (each arm is 9%, each leg is 18%, anterior and posterior trunk are each 18%, the head is 9%, and the groin is 1%) can be used for more extensive burns.

Minor burns can often be treated in an outpatient setting. For burns that are in areas with high infection risk, such as perioral, perineal, or axillary locations, or the hands and feet, application of a topical antibiotic such as mupirocin or silver sulfadiazine is reasonable. Silver sulfadiazine has a sulfa moiety and therefore can cause severe allergic reactions or other sulfa medication effects. For clean, minor burns that can be easily covered and have a low risk of infection, applying sterile petrolatum and covering the area with a nonstick dressing are reasonable. Silicone-based dressings are available and may provide better healing but are more expensive than petrolatum and a nonstick dressing.

Patients with severe burns over broad body surfaces should be referred to an expert, and hospital admission should be considered to allow for advanced wound care, maintain fluid and electrolyte balance, and monitor for infection.

KEY POINTS

- Minor wounds and burns may be treated with thorough **HVC** cleansing, application of topical sterile petrolatum, and the application of a a nonadherent bandage; nonstick silicone dressings are a more expensive option.

- Thermal burns are characterized by the amount of body surface area affected, specific body part involved (face or perineum may need more advanced care), and depth of the burn; superficial burns appear red, deep burns appear white or yellow and are nonblanchable.

Common Neoplasms

Benign Neoplasm

Seborrheic Keratoses

Seborrheic keratoses are benign brown scaly papules and plaques commonly found in older adults (**Figure 55**). They have a wide range of shades and morphologies and vary in size from a few millimeters to several centimeters. Despite their brown color, they are of keratinocytic lineage rather than melanocytic lineage. Although harmless, they may occasionally resemble more worrisome pigmented lesions such as melanoma and are therefore often biopsied. They may become irritated when traumatized; if this occurs, they are often treated with cryotherapy.

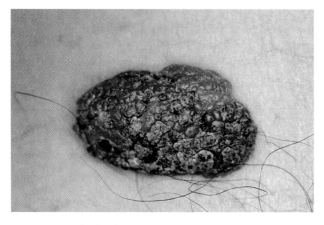

FIGURE 55. Seborrheic keratoses are brown, scaly, waxy papules that commonly occur in older persons. They frequently have a "stuck on" appearance and often are verrucous (warty) as well. Seborrheic keratoses typically demonstrate horned cysts (epidermal cysts filled with keratin) on the surface that can best be visualized with a magnifying glass.

Melanocytic Nevi

Melanocytic nevi, often referred to as "moles," are found in persons of all ages. They are benign collections of melanocytes and histologically consist of nests of melanocytes occurring at the dermal-epidermal junction (DEJ) and dermis. Although they occur most commonly in sun-exposed areas, they may arise anywhere on the skin or mucous membranes; they are also occasionally found on the iris, retina, or the lining of internal organs. Nevi most commonly start to appear in childhood and increase in number through adolescence and young adulthood. Junctional nevi are flat and often dark brown in color. Compound nevi are raised (papules) and may be irregularly pigmented. Dermal nevi are soft and flesh-colored and may resemble skin tags. The terms "junctional," "compound," and "dermal" refer to the location of the melanocytic nests: junctional nevi have nests located at the DEJ, compound nevi have nests at the DEJ and in the dermis, and dermal nevi have the nests in the dermis. Nevi undergo a benign maturation process from junctional to compound to dermal over a period of many years.

Dysplastic Nevi

Dysplastic nevi are melanocytic nevi that display one or more of the atypical clinical features seen in melanoma (the "ABCDEs") (see Malignant Melanoma), along with cytologic atypia and architectural disorder seen on histology. They are often asymmetric, irregularly bordered, and more than one shade of brown, and may be quite large in diameter (**Figure 56**). Although benign, they are important for several reasons. Patients with multiple dysplastic nevi are at risk for developing melanoma and should be monitored closely. Some of these patients have dysplastic nevus syndrome (DNS); criteria for this syndrome include a history of melanoma in one or more first- or second-degree relatives, the presence of a large number of nevi (>50), multiple nevi having atypical clinical features, and multiple nevi that have atypical histologic features. Many dys-

plastic nevi have a dark brown center and a surrounding ring of light brown, a pattern that is often referred to as a "fried egg" appearance. Histologically, dysplastic nevi are graded as having mild, moderate, or severe atypia. Although melanomas may arise within dysplastic nevi, the risk of this occurring within any given lesion is quite small. Removal is reserved for those lesions that display particularly worrisome features, are changing in size and color, are symptomatic, or stand out from the patient's other nevi.

Halo Nevi

Halo nevi are benign melanocytic nevi that are in the process of being attacked and eliminated by the immune system. Their name derives from the fact that the hallmark of this process is the formation of a white ring around the mole in question (**Figure 57**). The halo gradually enlarges, and the mole shrinks until all that is left is a depigmented area on the skin that resembles a small area of vitiligo. These lesions are particularly common in children. Halo nevi have sometimes, although not always, been observed at remote sites when patients have a melanoma, as the lymphocytes may be reacting to atypical melanocytes. Therefore, although most of these lesions occur in isolation, patients with halo nevi should have a thorough skin examination.

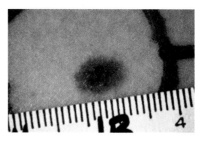

FIGURE 56. Dysplastic nevi are commonly larger than 6 mm with mottled pigment and irregular margins.

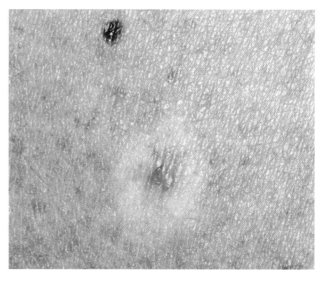

FIGURE 57. Halo nevus with white ring surrounding the lesion.

Sebaceous Hyperplasia

Sebaceous hyperplasia is a benign condition consisting of flesh-colored or yellow papules found on the face in patients with rosacea. These papules often have a central umbilication that is visible upon close inspection and may have telangiectasias on the surface as well (**Figure 58**). Although they are benign, they may be mistaken for basal cell carcinoma because of their shape, location, and presence of telangiectasias. Lesions caused by sebaceous hyperplasia differ from basal cell carcinomas in that they lack the translucency ("pearliness") that is often seen in the latter lesions. They are often removed for cosmetic reasons.

Neurofibromas

Neurofibromas are benign nerve sheath tumors that present as soft, flesh-colored papules on the trunk and extremities. Isolated lesions are common in the general population and are not associated with any underlying disease. They resemble skin tags and dermal nevi and are often confused with these lesions clinically; upon closer inspection, they are sometimes found to have a very faint violet or erythematous hue (**Figure 59**). The

presence of numerous neurofibromas suggests a diagnosis of neurofibromatosis type 1 (**Figure 60**). Additional findings that suggest this diagnosis include multiple café-au-lait macules, Lisch nodules (raised, pigmented hamartomas of the iris), and axillary freckling. Neurofibromas are benign and do not require treatment.

Acrochordons (Skin Tags)

Acrochordons (skin tags) are benign, flesh-colored papules that arise in areas of friction, such as the neck, axillae, and groin (**Figure 61**). They are harmless but often bothersome from a cosmetic standpoint. They may also occasionally become tender when traumatized. The presence of numerous lesions, particularly in the setting of obesity and acanthosis nigricans, is associated with insulin resistance and obesity.

Cherry Hemangiomas

Cherry hemangiomas are benign hereditary vascular papules composed of clusters of capillaries that commonly arise on the

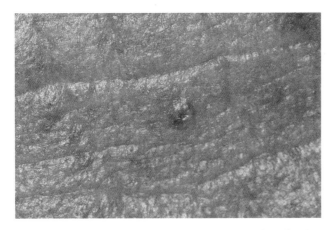

FIGURE 58. Sebaceous hyperplasia presents as a yellow-to-pink papule with a central dimple.

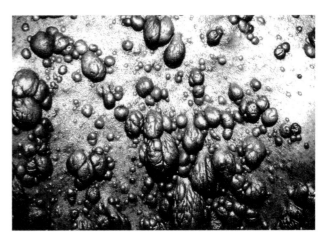

FIGURE 60. Multiple neurofibromas in a patient with neurofibromatosis type 1.

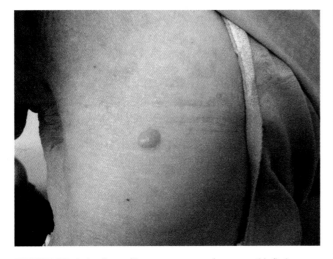

FIGURE 59. Isolated neurofibromas present as soft, compressible flesh-colored papules resembling skin tags or dermal nevi.

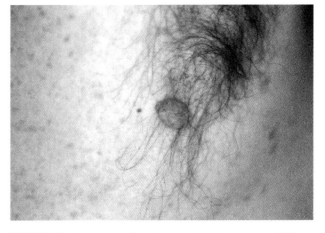

FIGURE 61. Acrochordon is a flesh-colored papule that arises in areas of friction, such as the neck, axillae, and groin. Multiple lesions are often present.

trunk of older persons. If traumatized, they will often bleed vigorously. Capillary hemangiomas are the most common type and are bright red in color (**Figure 62**). Lesions that consist of venules may be blue or violet. Neither variety is associated with other lesions or dieases, and treatment is not needed.

Dermatofibromas

Dermatofibromas are firm papules that arise after minor trauma, most commonly on the lower extremities. Histologically, they comprise dermal dendritic histiocytic cells with surrounding collagen bundles; the cause is unknown. They are typically flesh colored or slightly brown and often have a slightly darker brown ring encircling the main part of the lesion (**Figure 63**). When squeezed, they tend to pucker, a phenomenon known as the "dimple sign" (**Figure 64**). They do not require treatment.

Solar Lentigines

Solar lentigines are brown, well-demarcated macules and patches that occur on sun-exposed skin of older persons, particularly the face and dorsal hands (**Figure 65**). Previously, they

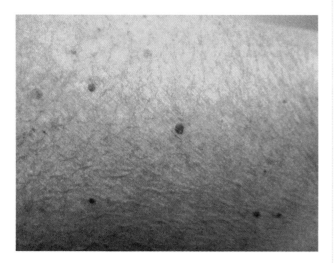

FIGURE 62. Cherry hemangiomas are bright red vascular papules commonly found in adults on the trunk and extremities.

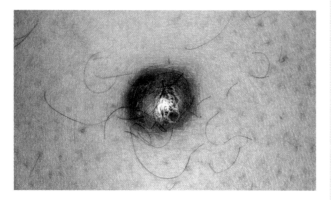

FIGURE 63. Dermatofibromas appear as firm nodules about the size of a pencil eraser. They are frequently hyperpigmented or may have pigmentation at the periphery.

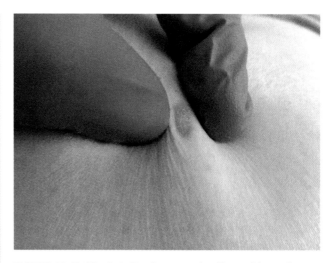

FIGURE 64. The "dimple sign" is a characteristic clinical feature of dermatofibromas.

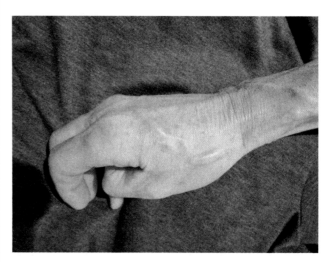

FIGURE 65. Solar lentigines are brown macules and patches that occur in sun-exposed areas in elderly fair-skinned persons. Although benign, they may occasionally be difficult to distinguish from lentigo maligna. Useful discriminating characteristics include more homogeneous pigmentation and lighter color.

were often referred to as "liver spots" because their color resembles that of liver. Although benign, they are a marker for someone who has relatively fair skin and has received a significant amount of sun exposure over the years. They frequently occur near more worrisome lesions such as actinic keratoses or skin cancers. Lentigines with atypical features or broad, growing lentigines (particularly on the face of older, light-skinned persons) should be biopsied to rule out lentigo maligna, a form of melanoma.

Hypertrophic Scars and Keloids

Hypertrophic scars are thick, firm, smooth papules and plaques that occur at sites of trauma; they represent excessive scar tissue formation beyond the normal healing process. They are more common in areas of tension such as the chest and the upper back and are also more common in persons with darker skin tones. They may be tender or pruritic and tend to resolve slowly over time. Unlike keloids, they are limited to the extent of the injury rather than extending beyond it. They are often treated with intralesional triamcinolone injections.

Keloids represent a more severe form of hypertrophic scarring in which the lesion extends beyond the borders of the original injury. They are firm, smooth, often tender nodules (**Figure 66**). Relatively minor trauma is often enough to trigger their formation. Ear piercing, for example, is a common inciting factor and can lead to the formation of a nodule many times larger than the injured area. Keloids may be treated with intralesional triamcinolone, excision, and laser surgery (see Dermatologic Problems of Special Populations).

Pyogenic Granulomas

Pyogenic granulomas are bright red vascular lesions that arise suddenly and grow rapidly; they often appear during pregnancy or in the setting of certain medications (such as antiretroviral therapy) (**Figure 67**). The name is misleading, as they are neither pyogenic nor granulomatous. They resemble cherry hemangiomas but are often more friable and tend to bleed more easily. They are treated with biopsy or electrocautery. They are benign lesions and do not have any negative implications.

Epidermal Inclusion Cysts

Epidermal inclusion cysts are benign nodules with a central punctum and a chamber containing keratinaceous material (**Figure 68**). They are often incorrectly referred to as "sebaceous cysts," a term that is erroneous because they possess keratin rather than sebum. When punctured, they often eject a copious amount of foul-smelling keratinaceous material; the odor is derived from the presence of anaerobic bacteria. The cyst wall may occasionally rupture, leading to the formation of a tender red swollen nodule that resembles a furuncle. They are benign but are frequently removed if they grow too large. Definitive treatment requires removal of the cyst wall; simple incision and drainage typically results in recurrence.

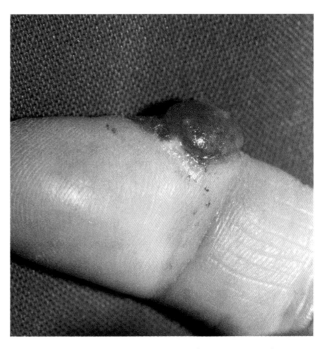

FIGURE 67. Pyogenic granulomas are red and friable benign vascular tumors that arise spontaneously and grow rapidly.

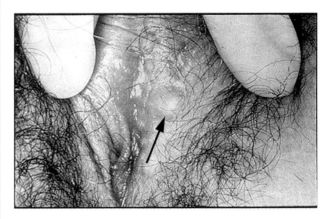

FIGURE 68. Epidermal inclusion cysts present as firm, nontender lumps. If they rupture, a local inflammatory response to the necrotic debris released can mimic infection. They often occur in the groin in both men and women.

Lipomas

Lipomas are benign collections of subcutaneous fat. They often occur as single lesions, but some patients may develop multiple lesions, particularly on the arms. Angiolipomas are a variant that may be tender. They are benign and do not require treatment but are often removed either for cosmetic reasons or to rule out a malignancy if atypical features are found.

KEY POINTS

- Dysplastic nevi removal should be reserved for those lesions that are changing, symptomatic, or stand out from the patient's other nevi.   **HVC**

(Continued)

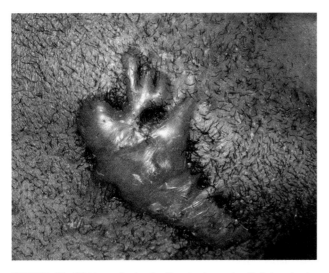

FIGURE 66. Keloids may develop claw-like extensions or dumbbell-shaped ends.

- Seborrheic keratoses, solar lentigines, acrochordons, melanocytic nevi, cherry angiomata, dermatofibromas, lipomas, and epidermal inclusion cysts are benign lesions that usually do not require biopsy or treatment.

Skin Cancers

Basal Cell Carcinoma

Basal cell carcinomas (BCCs) are the most common type of skin cancer. They arise from the basal layer of the epidermis and typically occur in sun-exposed areas on older persons with fair skin (**Figure 69**). BCCs may also be seen in younger persons who have an unusually high level of sun exposure or a genetic predisposition toward developing them. The risk of developing BCCs correlates strongly with cumulative sun exposure. Although they rarely metastasize, most have the ability to cause significant local tissue destruction if not removed. A skin biopsy is performed to confirm the diagnosis and the histologic subtype.

Most BCCs are of two histologic subtypes, nodular and superficial. Nodular BCCs are the most common. They typically present as "pearly" (translucent) telangiectatic papules (**Figure 70**); over time, they may develop a central area of erosion with rolled-up borders (sometimes referred to as a "rodent ulcer") (**Figure 71**). Superficial BCCs are well-demarcated, irregularly bordered, red patches; they tend to enlarge radially rather than invading into deeper structures (**Figure 72**). Several other subtypes of BCC may also be seen. Micronodular and infiltrative BCCs may resemble nodular BCCs clinically, but behave more aggressively, often with significant invasion of the surrounding dermis or subcutaneous tissue (**Figure 73**). Morpheaform BCCs often appear as flesh-colored or slightly erythematous plaques that resemble a scar. These are extremely infiltrative tumors and may extend much further into surrounding areas than their clinical appearance would suggest. Some BCCs are pigmented and may clinically resemble malignant melanoma.

Treatment of BCCs depends on many factors, including the histologic subtype, location, size, cosmetic considerations, and patient's age and comorbidities. Surgery is generally the mainstay of treatment. Mohs surgery, a form of margin-controlled

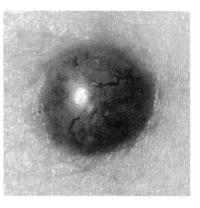

FIGURE 70. Nodular basal cell carcinoma. Note the prominent telangiectasias on the surface. Photo courtesy of Christopher J. Miller, MD.

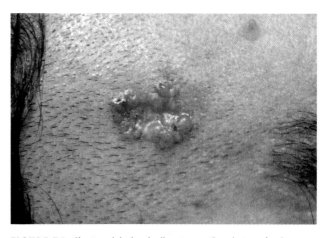

FIGURE 71. Classic nodular basal cell carcinoma. These lesions often have a rolled-up border and translucent appearance; ulceration may develop over time. Photo courtesy of Christopher J. Miller, MD.

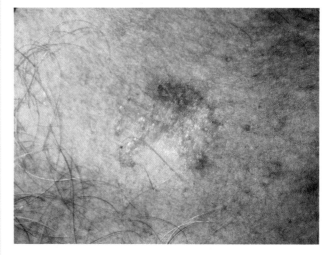

FIGURE 72. Superficial basal cell carcinoma. Note the reddish-violet color and relatively well-demarcated border. Photo courtesy of Christopher J. Miller, MD.

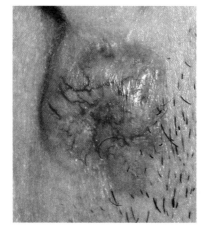

FIGURE 69. A pearly telangiectastic plaque characteristic of nodular basal cell carcinoma. Photo courtesy of Christopher J. Miller, MD.

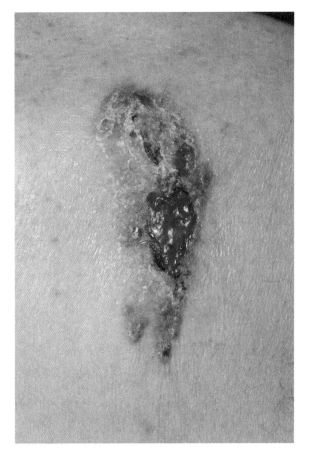

FIGURE 73. Over time, basal cell carcinomas can become quite large and ulcerate. They can cause significant local tissue damage. Photo courtesy of Christopher J. Miller, MD.

surgery that minimizes loss of normal tissue, is particularly useful for tumors in areas with limited surface area such as the head and neck, for large or recurrent tumors, or when cosmetic outcome is crucial. Superficial BCCs are often treated with cryotherapy, topical imiquimod, topical 5-fluorouracil, or photodynamic therapy. Nodular BCCs on the trunk and extremities are often treated with electrodesiccation and curettage. Radiation may be considered for patients with large tumors or those for whom surgery is not an option. Metastatic BCCs may be treated with vismodegib, which is a recently FDA-approved oral medication that interferes with the hedgehog signaling pathway; this signaling pathway is aberrant in most BCCs.

KEY POINTS

- Basal cell carcinomas typically occur in sun-exposed areas on older persons with fair skin, and although they rarely metastasize, most have the ability to cause significant local tissue destruction if not removed.

- Nodular basal cell carcinoma is the most common histologic subtype, typically presenting as "pearly" (translucent) telangiectatic papules that may develop a central area of erosion with rolled-up borders.

(Continued)

KEY POINTS *(continued)*

- Surgical excision is the mainstay of treatment for basal cell carcinoma; Mohs surgery should be reserved for head and neck lesions, large or recurrent tumors, or when cosmetic outcome is crucial; superficial lesions may be treated topically.

Actinic Keratoses and Squamous Cell Carcinoma in Situ

Actinic keratoses are red scaly macules and papules that occur in sun-exposed areas, generally in older persons (**Figure 74**). They have a "gritty" texture and are often easier to palpate than to see; they are typically diagnosed clinically rather than with biopsy (**Figure 75**). They are a precancerous condition; approximately 1% to 5% of these lesions will progress to invasive squamous cell carcinoma. Individual lesions are often treated with cryotherapy. In patients with a large number of actinic keratoses, treatment with topical preparations (such as 5-fluorouracil or imiquimod) or photodynamic therapy is often performed. Lesions that do not resolve with treatment require biopsy to rule out invasive squamous cell carcinoma.

Squamous cell carcinoma in situ (Bowen disease) is an advanced precancer or a noninvasive squamous cell carcinoma. It typically appears as reddish brown, well-demarcated, scaly patches on sun-exposed areas. Treatment is the same as for actinic keratoses, although surgery is occasionally required

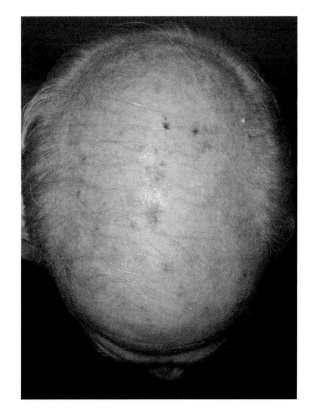

FIGURE 74. Multiple actinic keratoses on the scalp, a common location. Photo courtesy of Christopher J. Miller, MD.

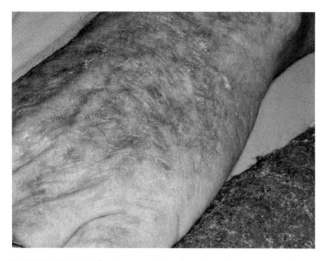

FIGURE 75. Actinic keratoses present as scaly red macules on sun-exposed areas; the dorsal hands are a common location. Photo courtesy of Christopher J. Miller, MD.

for lesions that are refractory to therapy. Lesions that develop exuberant scale or other atypical features should be biopsied to rule out invasive SCC (**Figure 76**).

Squamous Cell Carcinoma

Squamous cell carcinomas (SCCs) are the second most common type of skin cancer and the most common type of skin cancer seen in persons who are immunocompromised following solid organ transplant. They arise from epidermal squamous cells and typically present as red scaly papules and nodules on sun-exposed areas. Compared with BCCs, they tend to have more scale and lack the translucency seen in BCCs (**Figure 77**).

Although cumulative sun exposure remains the most important risk factor, additional factors are immunosuppression, arsenic exposure, human papillomavirus infection, and ionizing radiation exposure. SCCs may arise in chronic wounds or scars; a particularly aggressive form of SCC known as a Marjolin ulcer may arise in scars from burn injuries. Unlike most types of skin cancer, SCCs may occasionally be painful.

Although many tumors grow slowly and are relatively nonaggressive, certain subtypes may grow extremely rapidly and metastasize. High-risk features include tumor diameter greater than 2 cm, invasion beyond the subcutaneous fat, poor tumor differentiation, and perineural invasion (**Figure 78**). Tumors on the ear, lip, temple, and anogenital locations are also often associated with more aggressive growth for unknown reasons (**Figure 79** and **Figure 80**).

Because of their potential for aggressive behavior and metastasis, SCCs are generally treated surgically, with excision or Mohs surgery depending on the tumor size, location, and characteristics. High-risk lesions, particularly those with significant perineural invasion, may also be treated with adjuvant radiation therapy. Patients who are not candidates for surgery or in whom clear surgical margins are not achievable may be treated with radiation as the primary therapy.

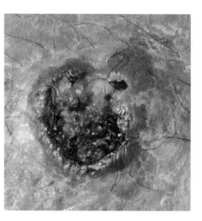

FIGURE 77. Squamous cell carcinomas typically appear as scaly red nodules on sun-exposed skin. They often ulcerate. Photo courtesy of Christopher J. Miller, MD.

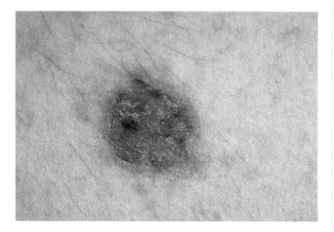

FIGURE 76. Squamous cell carcinoma in situ presents as a red or reddish-brown scaly flat plaque, typically in sun-exposed areas. It may be difficult to distinguish from superficial basal cell carcinoma. Photo courtesy of Christopher J. Miller, MD.

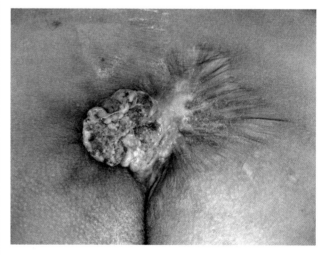

FIGURE 78. Squamous cell carcinomas arising in scars or chronic wounds can be particularly aggressive. Photo courtesy of Christopher J. Miller, MD.

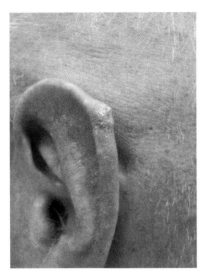

FIGURE 79. Scaly plaque typical of squamous cell carcinoma.

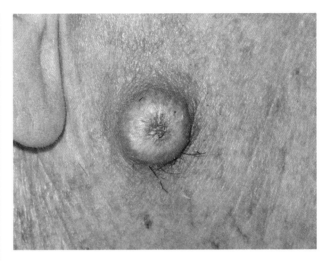

FIGURE 81. Red scaly "volcaniform" nodule with central crust typical of kerato-acanthoma. Photo courtesy of Christopher J. Miller, MD.

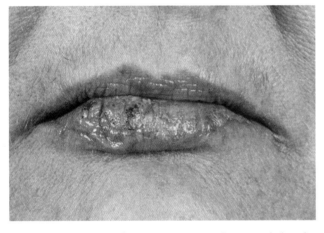

FIGURE 80. Squamous cell carcinoma more commonly occurs on the lower lip and may present as a nodule, ulcer, or indurated plaque. Photo courtesy of Christopher J. Miller, MD.

KEY POINTS

HVC

- Squamous cell carcinomas typically present as red scaly papules and nodules on sun-exposed skin and are treated with excision; Mohs surgery should be reserved for large tumors with high-risk characteristics in the head and neck region.

- Squamous cell carcinomas are the most common type of skin cancer seen in persons who are immunocompromised following solid organ transplant.

Keratoacanthomas

Keratoacanthomas generally appear as rapidly growing red nodules with a prominent central plug of scale and crust; their appearance is sometimes described as "volcaniform" since they resemble the cinder cone of a volcano (**Figure 81**). After a period of rapid growth, keratoacanthomas usually stabilize and then slowly involute, eventually resolving completely, even without treatment. Since some lesions fail to resolve completely and may persist and metastasize, they are usually treated with surgical excision.

Malignant Melanoma

Although malignant melanoma is the third most common type of skin cancer, it is responsible for the majority of deaths because of its tendency to metastasize. Malignant melanoma is now the most common type of cancer in young women. It is estimated that approximately 1 in 49 persons will develop melanoma in their lifetime. Risk factors include having fair skin, a history of blistering sunburns, a family history of melanoma, numerous nevi (50+), or atypical-appearing nevi (dysplastic nevus syndrome). Although it can arise anywhere in the skin or mucous membranes, it most commonly occurs in sun-exposed areas. The back is the most common location in men, and the legs are the most common location in women. Persons with darker skin types tend to develop melanoma most commonly on acral sites such as the hands or the feet.

The clinical features that suggest melanoma are represented by the mnemonic "ABCDE," where "A" stands for Asymmetry, "B" for irregular Border, "C" for multiple Colors, "D" for Diameter greater than 6 mm, and "E" for Evolution, meaning increasing size (**Figure 82**). The more of these features a pigmented lesion possesses, the more worrisome it is for melanoma. Unfortunately, melanomas do not always adhere to these criteria; they may be red or flesh colored, smaller than 6 mm, perfectly symmetric, or homogeneously colored. Thus, a low threshold for biopsy should be present for any atypical-appearing skin lesion, changing or symptomatic nevus, or any mole that stands out from the background nevi pattern of the particular patient.

Melanoma may be further classified into several different subtypes. Lentigo maligna often arises on the face of elderly

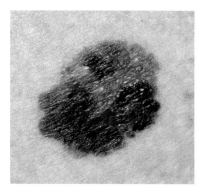

FIGURE 82. Classic malignant melanoma with asymmetry, an irregular border, multiple colors, and large size. Photo courtesy of Christopher J. Miller, MD.

persons. It tends to follow a more indolent course than other types of melanoma and may be present for many years before developing an invasive component. As the name would imply, it clinically often resembles a solar lentigo.

Superficial spreading melanoma is the most common type of melanoma and the most likely form to exhibit the atypical features identified by the "ABCDEs." It grows radially for a period of time, but ultimately develops an invasive component (**Figure 83**). Nodular melanomas are the most aggressive form and have an invasive component from the beginning; they are responsible for the majority of deaths from melanoma

(**Figure 84**). Acral lentiginous melanomas are the most common type of melanoma seen in patients with darker skin tones and usually occur on the hands and feet (see Dermatologic Problems of Special Populations).

There are several prognostic features that predict how likely a melanoma will spread. The most important of these is the depth of invasion of the lesion, also known as the Breslow depth. The presence of ulceration and a mitotic rate greater than $1/mm^2$ are additional negative prognostic indicators (**Figure 85**). Patients with melanomas are staged based on a tumor, nodal, and metastasis (TNM) system. Melanomas that are stage IB or higher are often candidates for sentinel node biopsy; patients with a negative sentinel node biopsy may not require complete lymph node dissection.

The skin biopsy is an important part of the diagnostic work-up for melanoma. Ideally, an atypical pigmented lesion should be removed using an excisional biopsy, in which the entire lesion is removed. Since this is not always practical or possible, additional options are sometimes used. These include

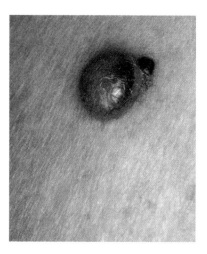

FIGURE 84. Nodular melanomas often present as uniformly dark blue or black, "berrylike" lesions that most commonly originate from normal skin. They can also arise from a preexisting nevus.

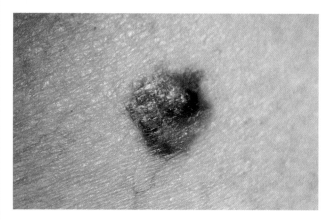

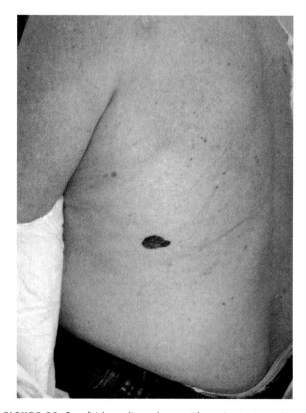

FIGURE 83. Superficial spreading melanoma with prominent asymmetric shape. Photo courtesy of Christopher J. Miller, MD.

FIGURE 85. The papular areas within a melanoma tend to correlate with the deepest depth of invasion. Photo courtesy of Christopher J. Miller, MD.

punch biopsy, in which a sample of the lesion is removed using a cylindrical blade and sent for analysis. Although this type of biopsy generally provides a sample of adequate depth, there is concern about sampling error given that the area removed may not necessarily be representative of the remainder of the lesion. Similarly, although shave biopsies are often readily available and easy to perform, this technique carries the risk of transecting the melanoma if a deep enough sample is not taken. This would result in an underestimate of the true depth of the lesion, which could have implications regarding further work-up and management. A modified version of this technique, a "scoop" biopsy, is often employed; this technique is characterized by extension of the shave into the deep dermis or subcutaneous tissue to reduce the risk of transecting the specimen. If lentigo maligna is suspected, a broad shallow shave biopsy is often the preferred technique for two reasons: (1) the atypical cells are found at the dermal-epidermal junction, so transection is less of a concern; and (2) punch biopsies are prone to sampling error with this type of melanoma because of the occasionally subtle appearance and inconsistent distribution of the atypical cells.

Treatment of melanoma depends on the stage. Stage I and stage II lesions are treated surgically, with the margin of excision dependent on the depth of invasion of the lesion. Stage III melanoma is treated with a wide local excision, lymph node dissection, and occasionally adjuvant interferon alfa. Stage IV melanoma is treated with chemotherapy or immunotherapy; significant progress has been made recently in this area, and several new agents were recently FDA approved for the treatment of metastatic melanoma. Radiation plays a limited role in the management of melanoma and is generally used for palliation.

KEY POINTS

- The clinical features of malignant melanoma are Asymmetry, irregular Border, multiple Colors, Diameter greater than 6 mm, and Evolution or increasing size, or "ABCDE."

- The depth of invasion of the lesion (Breslow depth) is an important prognostic feature that predicts how likely a melanoma is to have spread.

- Stage I and stage II melanomas are treated surgically, with the margin of excision dependent on the depth of invasion of the lesion; stage III melanoma is treated with a wide local excision, lymph node dissection, and occasionally adjuvant interferon alfa; and stage IV melanoma is treated with chemotherapy or immunotherapy.

Pruritus

Pruritus, or the sensation of itch, can be severe and can reduce quality of life to the same extent as chronic pain. Pruritus is transmitted through C fibers in peripheral nerves and is a symptom of many skin and nonskin conditions. A history and physical examination can help narrow the likely possibilities (**Table 15**). All types of pruritus may result in scratching; therefore, findings of scratching on examination, such as excoriation, prurigo nodularis, and lichen simplex chronicus, may result from any of these causes.

Pruritus is a common problem for elderly persons. Xerosis (dry skin) is a common cause of itch in this age group. Itch without a rash may occur, and it is important to investigate for occult internal diseases (**Table 16**) and medications that may be contributing to the symptom. In patients taking multiple medications, it can be challenging to determine which drug(s) may be contributing to pruritus, as patients may develop medication-induced itch even after months or years on a drug. Opiates, calcium channel blockers, and, in some studies, statin medications are not uncommon causes.

When primary skin lesions are absent and pruritus is generalized, systemic causes of pruritus are suspected. An internal disease or medication is the cause in 14% to 24% of patients; the risk is less likely for younger patients, those with pruritus for less than 6 weeks, or persons with a recent history

TABLE 15. Classification of Pruritus

Classification	Examples
Dermatologic	Xerosis, eczema, psoriasis, urticaria, infestations
Neuropathic	Brachioradial pruritus, notalgia paraesthetica, postherpetic neuralgia, multiple sclerosis, trigeminal trophic syndrome
Psychogenic	Neurotic excoriations, prurigo nodularis, delusions of parasitosis
Systemic	Medications, liver disease (cholestatic or noncholestatic), HIV infection, chronic kidney disease, hematologic disorders (polycythemia vera, anemia), Hodgkin and non-Hodgkin lymphoma, internal parasite infection, and hyperthyroidism
Mixed	Combinations of two or more of the above

TABLE 16. Suggested Evaluation of Patients with Generalized Pruritus Without a Primary Rash

Complete blood count with differential

Serum iron, serum ferritin, total iron-binding capacity

Thyroid-stimulating hormone

Kidney function tests (blood urea nitrogen and serum creatinine levels)

Liver chemistry tests (serum total and direct bilirubin, alkaline phosphatase, γ-glutamyltransferase, aspartate aminotransferase, alanine aminotransferase)

Chest radiograph

Age- and sex-appropriate malignancy screening, with more advanced testing as indicated by symptoms (weight loss, early satiety)

of a sick contact or travel. Liver diseases, primarily disease processes that result in cholestasis, can cause significant pruritus without primary skin lesions, but examination may demonstrate jaundice. Kidney disease can cause pruritus and, similar to liver disease, it is the final common pathway of organ failure that is associated with itch rather than a specific disease. Patients with end-stage kidney disease are most likely to be affected by pruritus ("uremic pruritus"). The investigation begins with the history including medication history (**Table 17**). A review of systems should be performed to investigate for thyroid disorders, lymphoma, kidney and liver diseases, and diabetes mellitus. Initial laboratory evaluation for occult systemic disease is outlined in Table 2. HIV antibody assay and chest radiography for lymphoma should also be considered. Hodgkin lymphoma is the malignant disease most strongly associated with pruritus.

Neuropathic pruritus describes itch that is caused by dysfunction of a peripheral or central nerve(s). Neurogenic itch is often localized to the alteration of a small number of nerves often from nerve injury and impingement; examples include surgery, accidental trauma, arthritis, neuropathy, or infection (postherpetic neuralgia). Brachioradial pruritus is localized pruritus of the forearm; radiologic changes in the cervical spine have been reported and may be due to arthritis or trauma including repeated minor traumas from sports or work.

Psychogenic itch describes localized or generalized pruritus associated with a concomitant diagnosis (or symptoms of) depression, anxiety, or somatoform disorders (**Figure 86**). The pruritus is often accompanied by great concern or anxiety by the patient and may flare in association with periods of reported stress. Self-reported depression is present in about 40% of persons with psychogenic pruritus. Psychogenic itch is often more severe during periods of inactivity such as when the patient is resting or attempting to fall asleep. It is important to examine patients carefully and to avoid missing a dermatologic or systemic cause of itch in those with concomitant psychiatric disease. One clue to diagnosis is that patients with psychogenic itch often present with erosions or ulcerations only in areas that can be reached by the patient.

When a dermatologic cause is found, therapy is tailored to the dermatosis. Topical glucocorticoids have anti-inflammatory effects and are a frequent therapy for patients with a primary dermatosis or evidence of inflammation. Glucocorticoids used for treatment of neurogenic or psychogenic pruritus may

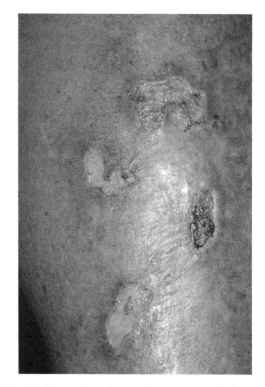

FIGURE 86. Patients with psychogenic itch often report nonhealing sores, such as those seen on this patient's arm. The lesions often have a linear or irregular shape from repeated manipulation. Scars from previous episodes are often seen among the active lesions.

not result in improvement but will cause cutaneous adverse effects such as atrophy, striae, or hypopigmentation. In addition to glucocorticoids, there are several topical and systemic treatment options (**Table 18**). These can be used as monotherapy for nondermatologic causes or as adjuncts to treatment of dermatologic causes.

Patient education is critical to the management of any pruritic condition. Patients should be taught that scratching causes skin damage and inflammation (**Figure 87**), which contribute to an "itch-scratch-itch" cycle. It is also important to discuss the feasibility of widespread topical therapy. Topical medications may be difficult to apply because of limited range of motion, and systemic therapies are limited by sedative side effects and the risk of drug interactions resulting from polypharmacy.

KEY POINTS

- When pruritus without a rash occurs, a review of systems, physical examination, and laboratory tests should be done to investigate for thyroid disorders, lymphoma, kidney and liver diseases, and diabetes mellitus.

- Patients may develop medication-induced pruritus even after months or years on a drug.

- Glucocorticoid treatment of neurogenic or psychogenic pruritus often will not result in improvement but will cause cutaneous adverse effects, such as atrophy, striae, or hypopigmentation.

TABLE 17. Medications Most Commonly Associated with Pruritus (>15% Frequency)
Opioids
BRAF inhibitors (vemurafenib)
CTLA-4 antagonist (ipilimumab)
EGFR inhibitors (cetuximab)
HMG-CoA reductase inhibitors
Hydroxyethyl starch (HES)

TABLE 18. Treatment of Pruritus

Skin Directed	Comments
Changes in skin care: decreased use of or change in soaps and increased use of moisturizers and emollients	Soaps can be drying and contribute to pruritus. Patients can be counseled to limit soap use to the underarms, groin, and buttocks and to apply a moisturizer immediately after bathing. These changes are especially helpful for any patient with dry skin.
Topical glucocorticoids and topical calcineurin inhibitors	Treat cutaneous inflammation.
Menthol (1%-3%)-containing creams	Antipruritic effects, sensation of cooling.
Topical anesthetics (pramoxine, lidocaine)	Act as a local anesthetic, reduce sensory nerve transmission of itch.
Ultraviolet light (UVB)	Can be effective for dermatoses such as psoriasis and eczema as well as pruritus of kidney or hepatic origin.
Systemic	**Comments**
Antihistamines (diphenhydramine, hydroxyzine, doxepin)	Most effective for urticaria, otherwise relief is likely due to sedative effects.
Antidepressants	May alter the perception of pruritus in the cerebral cortex.
Tricyclic (mirtazapine, amitriptyline)	
SSRI (fluoxetine, paroxetine)	
Neuroleptics (gabapentin, pregabalin)	May inhibit central or peripheral nerve processing of itch.
Opioid receptor effectors (naltrexone, naloxone, butorphanol)	May inhibit central nerve transmission of pruritus signals through μ- and κ-opioid receptors.

SSRI = selective serotonin reuptake inhibitor.

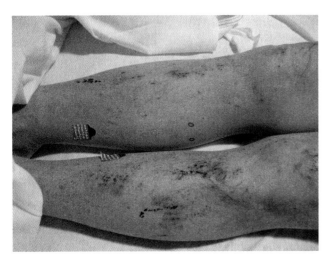

FIGURE 87. Linear excoriations in a patient with cholestatic liver disease.

Urticaria

Urticaria (hives) are localized areas of edema associated with pruritus caused by mast cell degranulation and release of inflammatory proteins, including histamine, leukotrienes, complement, and prostaglandins. Each individual area of edema characteristically lasts less than 24 hours, although the state of "erupting in hives" may persist for days or weeks. The lesions often flare in one area while resolving in another, giving the perception that they are "moving around." Individual lesions can be very large (many centimeters) and may appear annular or polycyclic. The center of a lesion of urticaria is blanchable pink or clear skin (**Figure 88**).

These features distinguish urticaria from erythema multiforme (see Dermatologic Urgencies and Emergencies) in which the lesions have a purple, dusky, or bullous center and are fixed and not blanchable. Physical maneuvers that can help with diagnosis include circling lesions and seeing if they have resolved within 24 hours, and gently scratching uninvolved skin with the wooden end of a cotton swab or tongue

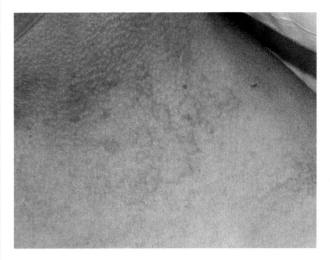

FIGURE 88. Edematous pink polymorphous papules and plaques on the neck caused by urticaria.

depressor to see if urticaria can be induced in the scratched area (dermatographism). If the skin just turns red, this is not a positive test. The scratching must cause an edematous, red plaque (wheal). Histopathology of urticaria is often very subtle, and biopsy is rarely useful unless attempting to diagnose or exclude urticarial vasculitis.

Urticaria is divided into acute (the total course <6 weeks) and chronic (the total course lasting >6 weeks). The most common causes of urticaria are infections (viral, bacterial, parasitic, mycobacterial, including chronic occult infections) and medications such as NSAIDs, aspirin, and intravenous contrast (**Figure 89**). Foods and environmental exposures (animal dander or dust mites) may also be implicated. Acute urticaria in adults is almost always due to a viral infection or medication reaction, generally a medication taken within hours of the development of hives. Food-induced allergic reactions can be severe. Urticaria has also infrequently been associated with autoimmune thyroid disease and malignancies, particularly lymphoma. Physical urticaria is induced by a physical stimulus such as the sun, sweating, physical pressure, or cold temperature.

The diagnosis of urticaria is clinical and is based on the evanescent nature of characteristic wheals, itching, and supportive features such as dermatographism. In patients who have a negative review of systems, no fevers, and no extracutaneous symptoms, an extensive evaluation is not needed; evaluation should focus on pertinent positive findings on review of systems.

Treatment of urticaria is most effective with long-acting antihistamines since they help treat active disease and prevent new flares of urticaria. Typical first-line therapy is a long-acting H_1 blocker. If this fails, the combination of H_1 and H_2 blockers is often more effective. Short-acting antihistamines such as diphenhydramine and hydroxyzine are effective in treating acute urticaria, but because they are short acting, they are often not dosed consistently enough to pre-

vent flaring. Systemic glucocorticoids and immunosuppressive agents have been used for urticaria, but in most patients, maximizing the dose of the long-acting antihistamines is equally effective and safer.

Angioedema is a deeper and more exuberant form of localized urticaria with severe soft-tissue swelling due to inflammatory mediator–induced vascular permeability, often caused by food or medication allergies or Hymenoptera stings. Angioedema can be life threatening when it involves the airway and compromises breathing. Treatment for severe or life-threatening angioedema is systemic epinephrine and glucocorticoids; patients should be counseled to carry emergency medications with them if they are at risk for angioedema.

Hereditary angioedema differs from mast cell–associated angioedema. It is caused by the unregulated activation of the complement cascade due to lack of or ineffective function of C1 esterase inhibitor, leading to increased vascular permeability. It may cause sporadic, localized swelling involving the head and neck and may be differentiated from mast cell–associated angioedema by the lack of pruritus and absence of typical urticarial lesions. Diagnosis is by testing for quantitative and functional levels of C1 esterase inhibitor and C4 complement levels, although this evaluation is indicated only in patients with a compatible clinical history and examination findings and is not required in individuals with the more common presentation of urticaria.

KEY POINTS

- The diagnosis of urticaria is clinical and based on the presence of pruritic wheals (skin edema with blanchable, pink, or clear skin in the center that come and go); there is no need for an extensive evaluation in patients with a negative review of systems, no fevers, and no extracutaneous symptoms. **HVC**

- Treatment of urticaria is most effective with long-acting antihistamines.

Autoimmune Blistering Diseases

The autoimmune blistering diseases result from autoantibodies to different antigens in the skin and have similar but distinct presentations. Clinically, they are characterized by persistent pruritic to painful blisters with erosions and variable mucosal and ocular involvement and scarring (**Table 19**). These diseases often arise in older persons.

Identification and diagnosis of these disorders are important because of the associated morbidity and mortality. Although most of these diseases are idiopathic, medications can also cause variants of almost all the disorders (**Table 20**, on page 51), and a thorough medication history and review are essential. Referral for evaluation and optimal management is important.

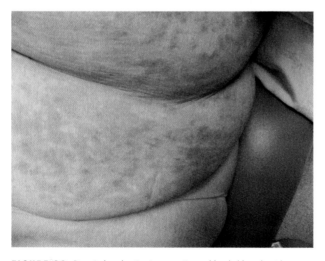

FIGURE 89. Drug-induced urticaria presenting as blanchable red patches on the flank.

TABLE 19. Characteristics of Autoimmune Blistering Diseases

Disease	Clinical Characteristics	Pathology	Comments
Pemphigus vulgaris	Tender, fragile blisters and erosions seen in oral mucosa and skin; mucous membrane lesions much more common than in bullous pemphigoid; Nikolsky sign (rubbing of the skin results in blister formation) is positive	Suprabasilar clefting compared with subepidermal clefting seen in bullous pemphigoid DIF/IIF: intercellular pattern within the epidermis	Incidence varies by country and ethnicity and is estimated to be 0.5 to 3.2 cases per 100,000 persons per year
Pemphigus foliaceus	Scaling and crusted lesions on face and upper trunk, and erythroderma with no mucosal involvement; Nikolsky sign is positive	High granular or subcorneal clefting compared with suprabasal clefting seen in PV DIF/IIF: intercellular pattern within the epidermis	Incidence varies by country with estimated occurrence of 0.5 to 6.6 cases per million persons per year. Endemic pemphigus foliaceus (fogo selvagem) occurs in central and southwestern Brazil and Columbia and has a higher incidence with up to 50 cases per million persons per year and up to 3.4% of the population affected.
Paraneoplastic pemphigus	Painful oral, conjunctival, esophageal, and laryngeal erosions occur more commonly than in pemphigus vulgaris; it is a polymorphous skin eruption marked by confluent erythema, bullae, erosions, and intractable stomatitis; patients also have respiratory problems that may be fatal	Mixed pattern of both suprabasal acantholysis and interface dermatitis DIF/IIF: IgG binds in intercellular pattern within the epidermis; reactants at the dermal-epidermal junction. The combination of intercellular and subepidermal deposition of immunoreactants is a clue to the diagnosis.	High mortality rate (up to 90%) and association with underlying neoplasms: non-Hodgkin lymphoma (42%), chronic lymphocytic leukemia (29%), Castleman disease (10%)
IgA pemphigus	A vesicopustular eruption with clear blisters that rapidly transform into pustules; trunk and proximal extremities are most commonly involved with relative sparing of the mucous membranes	Subcorneal collection of neutrophils DIF shows deposition of intercellular IgA at the epidermal surfaces	Newly described disease with unknown frequency
Bullous pemphigoid	Tense blisters preceded by intense pruritus or urticarial lesions most commonly seen in the elderly on the trunk, limbs, and flexures; does not usually present with oral lesions	Subepidermal bullae without acantholysis and with prominent eosinophils DIF shows linear IgG deposition at the basement membrane zone	One of most common autoimmune blistering diseases with up to 4.3 cases per 100,000 persons per year
Epidermolysis bullosa acquisita	Mechanically induced bullae and erosions mostly on extensor areas that heal with scarring and milia	Subepidermal cleavage without acantholysis DIF shows IgG deposition at the basement membrane zone that localizes to the base on salt-split skin	Rare disease with unknown frequency Can be associated with inflammatory bowel disease
Cicatricial pemphigoid	Presents with bullae, erosions, milia, and scarring seen on mucous membranes and conjunctivae of middle-aged to elderly persons; oral mucosa is almost always involved; conjunctival lesions are also common	Histology is similar to bullous pemphigoid DIF may reveal patterns similar to bullous pemphigoid, linear IgA bullous dermatosis, or epidermolysis bullosa acquisita	Rare disease with estimated incidence of 0.9 to 1.1 cases per million persons per year Increased risk for malignancy in some patients Prompt treatment should be initiated to avoid permanent ocular and oral scarring

(Continued on the next page)

TABLE 19. Characteristics of Autoimmune Blistering Diseases *(Continued)*

Disease	Clinical Characteristics	Pathology	Comments
Dermatitis herpetiformis	Severely pruritic grouped vesicles or erosions on elbows, knees, back, scalp, and buttocks; lesions occur in crops and are symmetrically distributed; often the vesicles are not seen because the process is so itchy that they are almost immediately broken	Histology shows neutrophilic infiltrate at the tips of the dermal papillae causing subepidermal separation DIF shows granular IgA deposition	Common blistering disease with 10-11 cases per 100,000 persons per year Nearly all patients with dermatitis herpetiformis will have celiac disease
Linear IgA bullous dermatosis	Pruritic, discrete, or clustered bullae in a herpetiform pattern ("cluster of jewels"); annular or polycyclic lesions with vesicles and bullae at the periphery are common	Subepidermal bullae with neutrophils Can be indistinguishable from DH, EBA, or bullous lupus DIF shows linear IgA deposition	In adults, the estimated incidence is 0.6 cases per 100,000 persons per year Ocular involvement can occur. A variant can occur in children called chronic bullous dermatosis of childhood
Porphyria cutanea tarda (and pseudoporphyria)	Erosions and bullae on hands and forearms, and occasionally face and feet that heal with milia, hyperpigmentation, hypopigmented scars. Porphyria cutanea tarda (but not pseudoporphyria) can also present with hypertrichosis on the face	Subepidermal bullae with little inflammation; dermal papillae protrude upward into the blister cavity and thickened upper dermal capillary walls DIF: deposition of immunoglobulins and complement around the dermal capillaries and linear at the basement membrane zone	Common disorder with estimated incidence of 1 case per 25,000 persons per year Not a true autoimmune blistering disorder but should be included in the differential diagnosis Can be associated with hepatitis C infection

DIF = direct immunofluorescence; IIF = indirect immunofluorescence; DH = dermatitis herpetiformis; EBA = epidermolysis bullosa acquisita; PV = pemphigus vulgaris.

Recognition and Diagnosis

Autoimmune blistering disorders should be suspected in any patient with persistent or recurrent blisters involving the skin, eyes, or oral and genital mucosa. The clinical presentation can vary depending on the underlying disorder, ranging from large urticarial plaques to flaccid blisters that may almost instantly rupture and appear as erosions to intact tense bullae. The extent of body surface area involved can vary in autoimmune blistering disorders. There may be minimal involvement of only localized blisters on the extremities to more extensive involvement of nearly the entire body surface area. As the blisters resolve, erosions, hyperpigmentation, and in some patients, scarring can occur. Pain can predominate when erosions and broken skin are present. In addition, some disorders (bullous pemphigoid) can present with significant pruritus. Thorough examination of the eyes, oral mucosa, and genital/perianal mucosa should be performed because permanent scarring can result leading to blindness and vaginal or oral contractures. Mucosal variants also can occur, and evaluation for an underlying autoimmune condition should be considered in patients with persistent mucosal erosions. In pemphigus, the blisters are flaccid and result in early blister erosion with subsequent superficial crusting (**Figure 90**), whereas in bullous pemphigoid, urticarial-like lesions, tense bullae, and a peripheral eosinophilia may be present (**Figure 91**). Cicatricial pemphi-

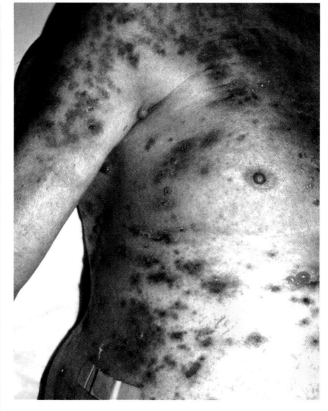

FIGURE 90. The flaccid intradermal blisters of pemphigus vulgaris are readily broken, leaving large weeping, denuded lesions and crusting.

TABLE 20.	Drug-Induced Autoimmune Blistering Disorders
Condition	**Medications**
Pemphigus	Thiol group (D-penicillamine, captopril, gold, pyritinol)
	Amoxicillin
	Ampicillin
	Cephalosporins
	Rifampin
Pemphigoid	Furosemide
	Amoxicillin
	Ampicillin
	Phenacetin
	Penicillin
	Penicillamine
	PUVA
	β-Blockers
	Terbinafine
Cicatricial pemphigoid	Penicillamine
	Indomethacin
	Practolol
	Clonidine
	Topical pilocarpine
Linear IgA bullous dermatosis	Vancomycin
	Captopril
	Amoxicillin
	Ampicillin
	Diclofenac
	Lithium
Pseudoporphyria	Furosemide
	Naproxen
	Oxaprozin
	Tetracycline
	Voriconazole

PUVA = psoralen-ultraviolet A light.

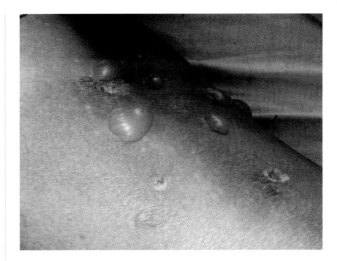

FIGURE 91. Tense bullae on erythematous base with some areas of eroded skin are seen in bullous pemphigoid.

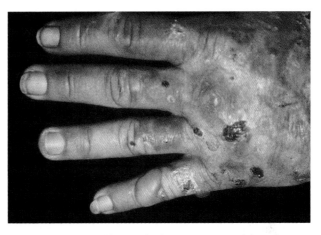

FIGURE 92. A chronic blistering skin disease on sun-exposed skin with erythema, bullae, erosions, and small milia, especially the back of the hands, consistent with porphyria cutanea tarda.

goid can be localized to the scalp and cause significant scarring. Epidermolysis bullosa acquisita and porphyria cutanea tarda (and pseudoporphyria, which presents the same as porphyria cutanea tarda but is medication induced) present with small blisters in areas of friction such as the dorsal hands, and scars and milia form with resolution of blisters (**Figure 92**).

Differentiation of the autoimmune blistering diseases can be made based on clinical features, but definitive diagnosis requires histopathologic examination and in some patients serologic testing for pathogenic antibodies. Depending on the location of the targeted antigen, flaccid or tense bullae will be present clinically, and the corresponding separation can be appreciated using histopathology. In pemphigus, flaccid blisters correspond with suprabasilar separation (**Figure 93**), whereas tense bullae correspond with subepidermal blisters in bullous pemphigoid and epidermolysis bullosa acquisita.

Two biopsies often are performed: one of lesional skin for histology and one of perilesional normal skin in order to perform direct immunofluorescence and identification of specific immunoglobulins that react with the skin. Both the type of immunoreactants (IgG, C3, IgA) and the pattern are helpful in diagnosis.

Serum from affected patients also can assist in diagnosis. The blood can be reacted with different substrates and will determine if circulating antibodies are present (indirect immunofluorescence). Tests such as serum enzyme-linked immunosorbent assays have been developed that detect the presence of specific antibodies in pemphigus vulgaris, pemphigus foliaceus, and bullous pemphigoid and may correlate with disease activity.

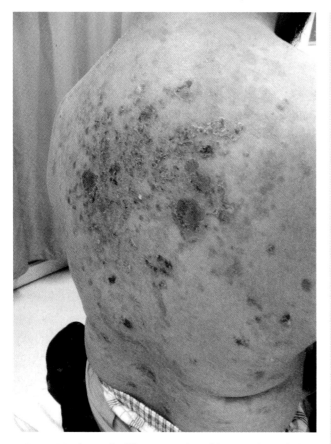

FIGURE 93. The superficial blisters in pemphigus foliaceus result in multiple erosions and crusting (similar to "corn flakes"). Intact vesicles are not seen regularly.

Although many of these disorders are idiopathic, they may be associated with other diseases that need to be considered. Pemphigus, bullous pemphigoid, and linear IgA bullous dermatosis have been reported in association with other autoimmune diseases including diabetes mellitus, rheumatoid arthritis, and thyroid disease.

Several of these disorders have also been associated with malignancy. Paraneoplastic pemphigus is highly associated with underlying leukemia, lymphoma, and Castleman disease. Cicatricial pemphigoid, and more rarely epidermolysis bullosa acquisita, may be seen in patients with an underlying cancer. Age-appropriate screening and a thorough review of systems are important in these patients. Patients with dermatitis herpetiformis almost uniformly have underlying celiac disease, although it may be asymptomatic in up to one third of patients, and this should be appropriately evaluated. Additionally, epidermolysis bullosa acquisita has been reported in association with inflammatory bowel disease.

Treatment

Management of autoimmune blistering disorders depends on the extent of skin and mucosal involvement, patient comorbidities, and the specific underlying blistering disorder. Medications that suppress the immune system are often required. In drug-induced cases, cessation of the causative medication is essential, but additional immunosuppressive therapy may still be required.

For limited disease, potent topical glucocorticoids may be sufficient. In most patients, systemic therapy is required, often with multiple therapies. Because of its quick onset of action, prednisone is usually the initial therapy. Additional medications, including immunosuppressants such as azathioprine, methotrexate, cyclophosphamide, and mycophenolate mofetil are often necessary to control the disease. Intravenous immune globulin and anti-inflammatory agents such as tetracycline class antibiotics also have been used. Recently, rituximab has been shown to be effective in pemphigus and could potentially be helpful in other autoimmune blistering diseases. Ocular cicatricial pemphigoid often requires rapid, aggressive therapy, or scarring can quickly develop. Dapsone is effective in conditions with a predominance of neutrophils in the inflammatory infiltrate including dermatitis herpetiformis, IgA pemphigus, and linear IgA bullous dermatosis. In dermatitis herpetiformis, a gluten-free diet is first-line treatment because of the association between dermatitis herpetiformis and celiac disease and an increased risk of bowel lymphoma, but additional therapy often is required.

Disease remissions can occur, but long-term immunosuppressive therapy often is required. Because of the erosions and breakdown in the skin barrier, secondary bacterial and viral infections can occur in these patients, and a high index of suspicion and cultures are often necessary for evaluation.

KEY POINTS

- The autoimmune blistering diseases are characterized by persistent pruritic to painful blisters with erosions and variable mucosal and ocular involvement and scarring.

- Medications that suppress the immune system are often required to treat autoimmune blistering diseases; in drug-induced cases, cessation of the causative medication is essential, but additional immunosuppressant therapy may still be required.

Cutaneous Manifestations of Internal Disease

Rheumatology

Lupus Erythematosus

The cutaneous manifestations of lupus erythematosus (LE) are essential for clinicians to recognize because skin findings are key diagnostic criteria. Because the subtypes of lupus are important to distinguish, the dermatologic examination is crucial. Skin lesions may be either specific or nonspecific. "Lupus-specific" skin lesions are cutaneous signs of lupus that are characteristic of the disease and when biopsied show diagnostic histologic findings ("interface reaction" of lymphocytes at the dermal–epidermal junction causing damage to the base of the epidermis). In addition, patients with lupus can also experience "lupus nonspecific" skin lesions representing cutaneous sequelae of the disease (**Table 21**).

The malar rash of acute cutaneous lupus consists of bright erythematous patches over both cheeks and the nasal bridge, almost always sparing the nasolabial folds (in contrast to the more violaceous facial erythema of dermatomyositis, which often involves that crease) (**Figure 94**). Other commonly mistaken entities include rosacea, which often has inflammatory papules and small pustules, as well as telangiectasias, both of which are rare to absent in lupus, and seborrheic dermatitis, which is often characterized by a greasy scale and tends to involve the nasolabial folds, eyebrows, and often the scalp as well.

The classic "discoid lupus" lesion is a dyspigmented patch or plaque that may be either atrophic or hyperkeratotic, with associated scarring within lesions. These occur in sun-exposed areas such as the face and scalp or within the conchal bowl of the ear (**Figure 95**).

A less widely known subtype of cutaneous lupus is subacute cutaneous LE (SCLE). The typical clinical eruption consists of circular or polycyclic scaly erythematous patches and

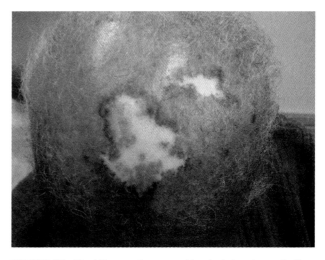

FIGURE 95. Discoid lupus erythematosus with active lesions characterized by erythematous-to-violaceous inflammatory patches and plaques with raised borders and scaling, and chronic areas of damage consisting of hyper- or hypopigmented-to-dyspigmented, scarred, atrophic, depressed plaques.

papulosquamous plaques over the forearms, chest, or especially the upper back, in a V-shaped configuration.

Less common variants of cutaneous lupus are lupus panniculitis, with inflammation confined to the fatty areas, which often presents with dell-like (shallow, smooth) depressions of the proximal extremities; bullous lupus erythematosus, which may present with blisters within or around the more classic lupus lesions; and tumid lupus, which presents with deeply indurated subcutaneous plaques.

Patients with the malar rash of acute LE should receive a thorough evaluation for systemic involvement. These patients are at high risk for lupus nephritis and severe internal disease. Diagnosis of SCLE should prompt evaluation of patients' medications, as this eruption is associated with a long list of potential causative medications, including hydrochlorothiazide, calcium channel blockers, ACE inhibitors, terbinafine, and the TNF-α inhibitors. Patients with SCLE are often photosensitive and frequently will be seropositive for antinuclear antibody (ANA), anti-Ro/SSA, or anti-La/SSB antibodies. Antihistone antibody positivity is nonspecific but may be a clue that the reaction is associated with a medication, although this is only present in about one third of patients (even if a medication may be the cause). A subset of patients with SCLE will have kidney involvement, and a thorough evaluation is warranted. Recognition of this entity is essential as patients may be inappropriately treated for systemic lupus erythematosus (SLE) when they have drug-induced SCLE, and discontinuation of the inciting causative medication is paramount. Patients with discoid lesions of chronic cutaneous lupus frequently develop irreversible scarring and may require early aggressive therapy even in the absence of significant systemic involvement.

Lupus, like many autoimmune skin diseases, is exacerbated by ultraviolet (UV) light. Patients with stable disease may experience severe disease flares when on trips to sunny

TABLE 21. Types of Lupus Lesions	
Lupus-Specific Skin Lesions	**Nonspecific Cutaneous Manifestations of Lupus**
Malar "butterfly" rash (acute lupus)	Livedo reticularis
Annular scaly patches (subacute lupus)	Vasculitis
Psoriasiform patches (subacute lupus)	Urticaria (generally atypical urticarial lesions lasting more than 24 hours and leaving bruising)
Discoid lesions (chronic cutaneous lupus)	Lobular panniculitis
	Oral ulcers
	Alopecia

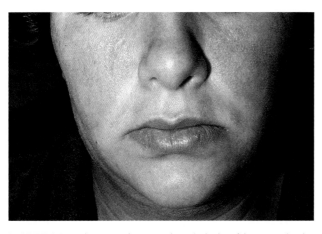

FIGURE 94. Erythematous plaques involving the bridge of the nose and malar areas with sparing of the nasolabial folds characteristic of acute cutaneous lupus erythematosus.

locations or as the seasons shift toward spring and summer. Photoprotection is an essential part of therapy. Patients should be counseled to avoid sun exposure, wear UV-blocking clothing, and apply and re-apply broad-spectrum sunblock (including extended-spectrum UVA-blocking chemical sunscreens, often in conjunction with physical blocking agents such as zinc oxide and titanium oxide). Most medications for cutaneous lupus are used "off label." Topical glucocorticoids, topical tacrolimus, topical retinoids, and injections of glucocorticoids may help improve individual lesions or limited skin disease. First-line systemic therapy is with antimalarial agents, usually hydroxychloroquine. Patients with refractory disease will sometimes respond to thalidomide; additional options include alternate or combination antimalarial drugs, methotrexate, mycophenolate mofetil, cyclosporine, dapsone, and combination immunosuppressant therapy. Patients who fail to respond to antimalarial agents, or those with extensive skin involvement or signs of scarring, should be referred to a specialist.

KEY POINTS

- Patients with the malar rash of acute lupus erythematosus should receive a thorough evaluation for systemic involvement; they are at high risk for lupus nephritis and severe internal disease.
- Subacute cutaneous lupus erythematosus is a drug-induced, photosensitive eruption of circular, scaly, erythematous patches over the forearms, chest, or upper back; potential causes such as hydrochlorothiazide, calcium channel blockers, ACE inhibitors, terbinafine, and the TNF-α inhibitors should be identified and discontinued immediately.
- Sun protection, topical glucocorticoids, and hydroxychloroquine are used to treat cutaneous lupus erythematosus.
- First-line systemic therapy for cutaneous lupus erythematosus is with antimalarial agents, usually hydroxychloroquine.

Dermatomyositis

Dermatomyositis can occur as the classic form, with skin involvement and muscle inflammation, or as amyopathic or hypomyopathic dermatomyositis, with either cutaneous disease only or with minimal muscle inflammation, respectively. Amyopathic dermatomyositis is almost as common as classic dermatomyositis, and recognition of the cutaneous features is essential (see MKSAP 17 Rheumatology).

The pathognomonic cutaneous features of dermatomyositis are the heliotrope rash and Gottron papules. The heliotrope rash is named after a purple flower, heliotrope, which moves to face the sun, an apt name that captures both the characteristic color of the cutaneous inflammation in dermatomyositis and the important role that ultraviolet light may play in exacerbating this disease. The heliotrope rash is a distinctive purple or lilac erythema of the eyelids that may be accompanied by edema (**Figure 96**).

Gottron papules are erythematous-to-slightly-violaceous, flat, atrophic-appearing papules concentrated over taut, stretched extensor surfaces, particularly the interphalangeal joints or elbows (**Figure 97**). Patients frequently exhibit inflammation of the proximal nail fold, which may be flat, atrophic, and pink, and often shows periungual telangiectasias or frayed cuticles.

Patients with dermatomyositis often exhibit cutaneous inflammation directly overlying the joints of the hands (namely, the proximal interphalangeal, distal interphalangeal, and metacarpophalangeal joints), whereas patients with lupus often exhibit cutaneous inflammation in the overlying space *between* the joints. Patients with dermatomyositis will frequently have areas of poikiloderma with ill-defined patchy erythema and "salt-and-pepper" dyspigmentation accompanied by telangiectasias on the chest or upper back. There may be slightly violaceous erythema over the "V" of the neck, chest, and the upper

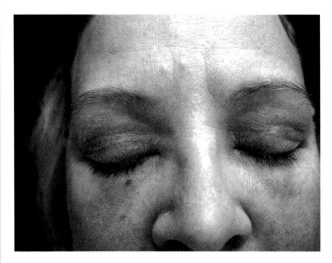

FIGURE 96. The heliotrope rash of dermatomyositis is a distinctive purple or lilac, symmetric erythema of the eyelids that may be accompanied by slight edema, generally focused around the orbits.

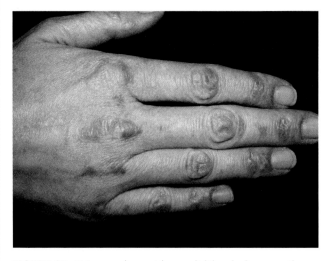

FIGURE 97. Gottron papules are violaceous slightly scaly plaques over the bony prominences on the hands.

back (the "Shawl sign") (**Figure 98**) or on the lateral hips (the "holster sign"). Patients may have violaceous erythema of the face, frequently involving the nasolabial fold, upper extremities, and trunk. Scalp erythema is very common in dermatomyositis. Patients with dermatomyositis frequently report lesional pruritus. These patients typically have normal serum creatine kinase and aldolase levels, but may have evidence of subclinical muscle inflammation on MRI or electromyogram. Notably, patients may have amyopathic dermatomyositis with no evidence of muscle involvement; recognition of this entity is absolutely essential as patients with amyopathic dermatomyositis are at the same risk of internal disease as patients with the classic form.

"Mechanic's hands," or thickened, scaly, hyperkeratotic skin on the tips of the fingers, is associated with interstitial lung disease, and physicians should consider baseline imaging and pulmonary function testing, including DLCO measurement in these patients.

Dermatomyositis is often difficult to treat. Similar to those with LE, patients with dermatomyositis should practice strict sun avoidance, wear protective clothing, and frequently apply broad-spectrum sunscreen. Topical glucocorticoids may be effective in some patients. Systemic therapy is limited to off-label treatment and usually consists of antimalarial agents (such as hydroxychloroquine, chloroquine, quinacrine), or methotrexate or mycophenolate mofetil; there are anecdotal reports describing the use of intravenous immune globulin, dapsone, and some of the newer biologic agents.

KEY POINTS

- The pathognomonic cutaneous features of dermatomyositis are the heliotrope rash and Gottron papules.

- Dermatomyositis may often be treated effectively with sun protection and topical glucocorticoids; systemic therapy usually consists of antimalarial agents.

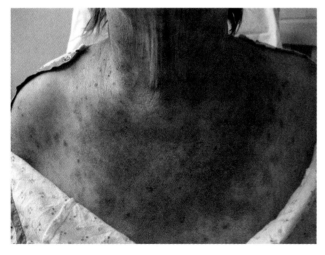

FIGURE 98. Dermatomyositis: erythema of the "V" of the neck and chest. There are photodistributed erythematous macules and patches with areas of poikiloderma on the sun-exposed part of the upper chest.

Vasculitis and Vasculopathy

Vasculitis, an inflammation of the blood vessels, can be caused by different types of inflammatory cells, and the inflammation may occur in different-sized blood vessels. The clinical manifestations, histology, serologies, organs affected, and treatment depend on the size of the blood vessel affected. Vasculopathy is an injury to the blood vessel from intravascular or luminal processes. This can be a depositional process, such as calciphylaxis, in which the vessel wall is infiltrated with calcium and subsequent thromboses, or a thromboembolic process, wherein clots form or embolize to damage the vasculature, such as in cryoglobulinemia or antiphospholipid antibody syndrome.

Livedo Reticularis

Livedo reticularis is a subtle, lacy network of faintly pink or bluish red vessels, usually seen on the lower legs (**Figure 99**). It is due to sluggish blood flow through the vessels, but

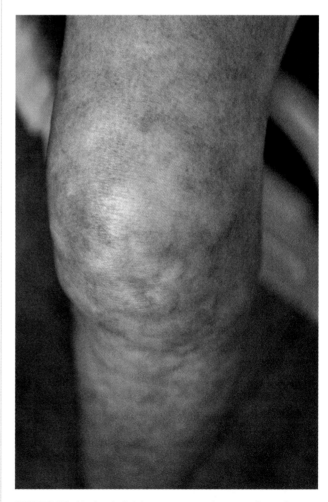

FIGURE 99. Livedo reticularis is a cutaneous reaction pattern that produces a pink or bluish-red, mottled, netlike pattern on the skin. It is caused by slow blood flow through the superficial cutaneous vasculature. It most commonly affects the lower extremities.

extravasation of blood does not occur, differentiating it from purpura or ecchymoses. Livedo reticularis can sometimes be elicited by keeping a leg in the dependent position; if this resolves when the leg is straightened horizontally, it is likely to be a normal or physiologic process rather than a pathologic process. Livedo reticularis is a nonspecific finding and may be seen in any condition in which there is altered blood flow through the superficial vasculature. Although typically transient, livedo reticularis may sometimes persist, and if advanced or long-standing, ulceration may rarely occur (**Table 22**).

Purpura

Purpura is the result of vascular compromise, either from vessel inflammation or plugging, causing subcutaneous microhemorrhage. The nonblanching red or purple skin lesions result from the presence of extravascular erythrocytes within the dermis. Purpuric lesions should be distinguished from ecchymoses, as ecchymotic lesions are typically small, superficial, nonpalpable, and display multiple colors ranging from red and purple to yellow and green from the breakdown of heme. The smallest purpuric macules are petechiae, which are pinpoint nonblanching red macules usually seen in the setting of low or abnormal platelet counts. Purpuric macules and flat patches may occur on sun-exposed areas (actinic or solar purpura) or in patients on chronic glucocorticoid therapy (due to thin, fragile skin and vasculature).

Small Vessel Vasculitis

A palpable area of the purpura, usually a small pinpoint barely perceptible papule within the purpuric macule, may be a clue to an active superficial skin or small vessel vasculitis. Small vessel vasculitis (also called leukocytoclastic vasculitis or cutaneous leukocytoclastic angiitis) is inflammation of the smallest blood vessels. This inflammation may affect the skin, but thorough evaluation of all other small vessels is essential. The palpable purpuric lesions tend to occur rapidly and simultaneously, often initially or more prominently in dependent areas and areas of pressure (including elastic waistbands and sock lines). Small vessel vasculitis symptoms may range from asymptomatic to mild itch to burning and tenderness (**Figure 100**). Rapid diagnosis is important, as small vessel vasculitis may affect internal organs. Diagnosis is made by skin biopsy. Any purpuric lesions with a palpable component require thorough investigation and may warrant a dermatology consultation.

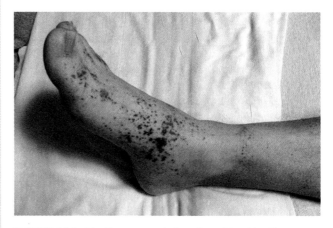

FIGURE 100. Palpable purpura on the lower leg and dorsal foot. The nonblanching red macules and small papules indicate areas of small vessel vasculitis and extravasated blood due to vessel injury.

TABLE 22. Selected Diseases and Conditions Associated with Livedo Reticularis	
Disease/Condition	**Example**
Neurohumoral diseases	Pheochromocytoma, carcinoid syndrome
Hematologic diseases	Polycythemia vera, leukemia, thrombocytosis
Hypercoagulable states	Antiphospholipid antibody syndrome
Paraproteinemias	Multiple myeloma and associated type 1 cryoglobulinemia
Autoimmune diseases	Systemic lupus erythematosus, dermatomyositis, scleroderma, Sjögren syndrome, Still disease, rheumatoid arthritis, Felty syndrome
Infections	Parvovirus B19, hepatitis C, syphilis, meningococcemia, pneumococcal sepsis, tuberculosis
Drug reactions	Amantadine, quinidine, warfarin, minocycline
Vasculitides	Polyarteritis nodosa, granulomatosis with polyangiitis, microscopic polyarteritis, eosinophilic granulomatosis with polyangiitis (formerly known as Churg-Strauss syndrome), Takayasu disease, temporal arteritis
Calciphylaxis	End-stage kidney disease with abnormal calcium-phosphorus product
Cholesterol emboli	Often following an intravascular procedure such as angiography
Endocarditis	—
Microvascular occlusion syndromes	Hemolytic uremic syndrome, thrombotic thrombocytopenic purpura, disseminated intravascular coagulation, heparin necrosis, paroxysmal nocturnal hemoglobinuria
Cryoglobulinemia	—

Another form of small vessel inflammation is urticarial vasculitis, which presents with either persistent urticarial plaques lasting longer than 24 hours or urticaria that presents with tingling pain rather than pruritus and resolves with bruise-like hyperpigmentation. Biopsy is important, as urticarial vasculitis is associated with underlying autoimmune disease, most commonly SLE, in 50% of patients.

Small vessel vasculitis is frequently idiopathic but may occur in the setting of infection or sepsis, underlying autoimmune disease, medication reactions, or, rarely, malignancy. Patients should be evaluated for extracutaneous manifestations, with particular attention to kidney involvement, and the laboratory evaluation may include a urinalysis, comprehensive metabolic panel, complete blood count, serum complement levels, antinuclear antibody titer, and evaluation for intravascular infection when appropriate. A thorough history and review of systems are necessary to assess for internal manifestations and to identify any potential triggers. Drug-induced vasculitis is not common, but there is a wide range of potential culprit medications to consider (antibiotics, particularly penicillins; NSAIDs; hydralazine; anti-TNF-α agents; and some targeted chemotherapeutic agents). In the inpatient setting, small vessel vasculitis is frequently seen in patients with infective bacterial endocarditis or antibiotic use. If endocarditis or antibiotics is a potential culprit, consultation with an experienced dermatologist is essential. For mild cases, it may be appropriate to continue antibiotics and monitor for progression; if the vasculitis improves, it may have been due to the endocarditis. If the vasculitis worsens or affects organs beyond the skin (that is, if there is kidney involvement), changing the antibiotic regimen should be considered. Depending on the severity of the eruption, skin-limited cutaneous small vessel vasculitis can be managed with rest and elevation, topical glucocorticoids, NSAIDs (unless implicated as a potential causative agent), or antihistamines. As the pathologic process is neutrophil-mediated, colchicine or dapsone may be effective in select patients. Patients with severe eruptions, including rare bullous eruptions or ulcerative lesions, or those with widespread disease may require systemic glucocorticoids. Most patients with small vessel vasculitis have resolution after a single episode or when the trigger is identified; approximately 10% of patients will have a chronic, intermittent course.

KEY POINTS

- Palpable purpura is a manifestation of small vessel vasculitis, and rapid diagnosis with skin biopsy is essential as the vasculitis may progressively affect internal organs (kidneys) and require systemic treatment.

- Skin-limited cutaneous small vessel vasculitis can be managed with rest and elevation, topical glucocorticoids, NSAIDs, or antihistamines.

Cryoglobulinemia

Cryoglobulins are cold-precipitating immunoglobulins that typically remain soluble at body temperature but may precipitate in the peripheral vasculature away from the warmer body core. This intravascular precipitation leads to small vessel fibrin thrombi and clotting, vascular injury that may include an active inflammatory vasculitis, and downstream tissue ischemia (**Figure 101**). Clinically, this presents as either palpable purpura (if there is an inflammatory small vessel vasculitis due to specific types of cryoglobulins that lead to complement fixation) or retiform, angulated purpura (see MKSAP 17 Rheumatology).

Rheumatoid Arthritis

The skin is involved in a subset of patients with rheumatoid arthritis (RA), either from cutaneous manifestations of the disease or complications of treatment. Rheumatoid nodules are the most common cutaneous manifestation of RA, occurring in up to one third of patients. These are typically firm subcutaneous nodules found over extensor joints or tendons (**Figure 102**). They may come and go in parallel with the underlying joint inflammation during treatment. The phenomenon of "accelerated nodulosis," or skin nodules developing rapidly while the

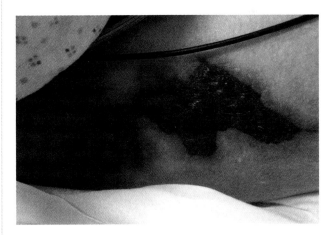

FIGURE 101. Large area of jaggedly branching, angulated retiform purpura consistent with a vascular injury process. In this patient, type 1 cryoglobulins precipitated in the small vessels of the skin, leading to intravascular clot formation and vessel injury, with overlying skin necrosis.

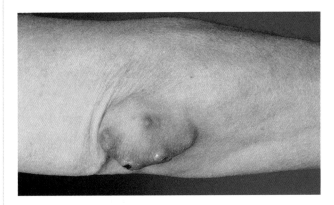

FIGURE 102. Firm, flesh-colored papules over the extensor elbow joint consistent with multiple rheumatoid nodules in a patient with rheumatoid arthritis.

arthritis is being treated and responding, has been noted as a side effect of many RA medications, particularly methotrexate. Other forms of granulomatous dermatitis seen in RA are palisaded neutrophilic and granulomatous dermatitis, characterized by symmetric, crusted, umbilicated, pink papules around the elbows, and interstitial granulomatous dermatitis, which classically manifests as a linear erythematous cord on the trunk. A rare skin manifestation of RA is rheumatoid vasculitis, which is generally seen in patients with chronic, severe RA. It may present as ulcerated purpura or severe livedo reticularis. Patients with RA who are treated with TNF-α inhibitors may develop a secondary psoriasiform eruption, including severe palmoplantar pustular dermatitis.

Sclerosing Disorders

Sclerosing disorders are discussed comprehensively in the MKSAP 17 Rheumatology section. Patients with all forms of sclerosing disorders may exhibit skin findings ranging from "puffy hands" of early diffuse systemic sclerosis (scleroderma), to diffuse skin tightening of advanced diffuse systemic sclerosis, to the characteristic calcinosis, Raynaud phenomenon, esophageal dysfunction syndrome, sclerodactyly, and telangiectasias of limited diffuse systemic sclerosis (CREST).

Morphea, or localized scleroderma, usually presents as a focal patch of skin thickening without internal manifestations. Morphea may occur as one or a few patches (circumscribed), widespread patches (generalized), linear or diffuse patches (pansclerotic). When morphea extends over joint spaces, it can impact the muscles, bones, and joint mobility. Recognition is important, as patients are at risk of being misclassified as having systemic sclerosis and thus are inappropriately treated. It is important to exclude scleroderma and CREST syndrome, and then management should be focused on symptom control, range of motion preservation (if a joint is affected), and prevention of new lesions with immunomodulatory or immunosuppressive agents. While there is limited evidence of efficacy, patients may be treated with glucocorticoids, hydroxychloroquine, methotrexate, phototherapy, and sometimes anti-TNF agents, or other immunomodulatory or immunosuppressive agents, depending on the severity and extent of the disease.

Nephrology

Both chronic kidney disease and advanced liver disease are commonly associated with intense, severe pruritus, attributed to the accumulation of toxins. Patients with end-stage kidney disease often exhibit dry, xerotic skin and commonly have secondary skin changes from chronic itching and scratching, including excoriations, prurigo nodules, and lichenified patches. Some patients may develop hyperpigmented umbilicated papules with a central keratin core, or Kyrle disease, in which collagen fibers are extruded through the epidermis. Pruritus from kidney disease should be man-

aged with lukewarm baths, gentle soaps, and thick, bland emollients; severe pruritus may require topical glucocorticoids or phototherapy. Two entities encountered in chronic kidney disease warrant particular mention, calciphylaxis and nephrogenic systemic fibrosis.

Calciphylaxis

Calciphylaxis typically occurs in patients with advanced kidney dysfunction and elevated calcium-phosphorus products (>60-70 mg^2/dL^2). Calciphylaxis occurs as a result of abnormal deposition of calcium within the lumen of arterial vasculature, which then compromises flow and leads to an increased risk of luminal thrombosis and downstream ischemia, resulting in subsequent painful tissue necrosis. Notably, a single measurement of normal calcium and phosphorus levels does not exclude the diagnosis. Patients receiving dialysis may have marked fluctuations in serum mineral levels, and the calcium-phosphorus levels may be normal at the time of calciphylaxis diagnosis but may have been markedly abnormal at the onset of disease that developed weeks before patient presentation. Calciphylaxis is rare, occurring in less than 5% of patients on dialysis, but is associated with a 60% to 80% 1-year mortality rate. Generally, patients have nonhealing skin ulcers that develop an eschar and secondary bacterial colonization and eventual infection and sepsis. Clinically, lesions of calciphylaxis are exquisitely painful subcutaneous nodules or plaques with overlying red-brown discoloration and often superimposed angulated purpuric patches, often with central necrosis. Patients with advanced calciphylaxis may have ulceration or large, thick, black eschar formation. Lesions usually occur in high-fat areas and are commonly seen on the lower extremities (especially the thighs) (**Figure 103**). Sodium thiosulfate may be helpful in treating the disease, possibly partially by causing the deposited calcium within the vessels to re-mineralize, mobilize, and be removed through dialysis. Other treatments are the use of a low-calcium dialysate and efforts to reduce overall serum calcium and phosphorous levels,

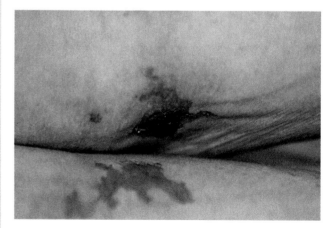

FIGURE 103. Calciphylaxis manifests as painful subcutaneous nodules or plaques with overlying red-brown discoloration and often superimposed angulated purpuric patches, often with central necrosis.

maintaining a normal parathyroid hormone level (by either chemical or surgical parathyroidectomy), cautious use of bis-phosphonates in select patients, and avoiding potential triggers (such as systemic glucocorticoids and warfarin). Meticulous wound care and surgical evaluation with limited debridement are also important; hyperbaric oxygen may also be beneficial. The use of thrombolytic agents may aid reperfusion but carries a high risk of severe bleeding complications.

KEY POINTS

- Calciphylaxis typically occurs in patients with advanced kidney dysfunction and elevated calcium-phosphorus products.
- Calciphylaxis lesions are painful subcutaneous nodules or plaques with overlying red-brown discoloration and angulated purpuric patches, often with central necrosis; patients with advanced disease may have ulceration or black eschar formation.

Nephrogenic Systemic Fibrosis

Nephrogenic systemic fibrosis (NSF) is a relatively recently described entity first recognized in the early 2000s. The first patients were described in the late 1990s as presenting with what was termed a "scleromyxedema-like" illness of kidney disease, with distal skin pain and thickening and loss of mobility (**Figure 104**). Epidemiologic studies implicated the use of gadolinium-based MRI contrast agents administered in the setting of acidemia from kidney disease as a key trigger; however, the limited numbers of affected patients compared with the number of contrast MRI studies performed in patients with end-stage kidney disease suggest that other important etiologic factors are required for NSF to occur. Since the recognition of the role of gadolinium and avoidance of this contrast agent in patients with kidney insufficiency, there has been a marked reduction in the number of new cases of NSF. NSF is gradually progressive, and whereas some case reports suggest possible benefit with a number of different therapeutic

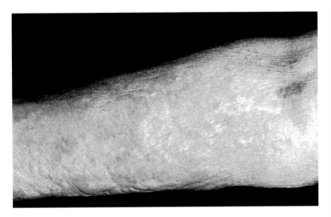

FIGURE 104. Nephrogenic systemic fibrosis presents with tightening and thickening of the skin, sometimes with clinically apparent fleshy or yellow papules and plaques, predominantly on the extremities.

modalities, including phototherapy (UVA therapy in particular), photopheresis, and antifibrotic agents, kidney transplantation seems to be the most effective treatment.

Kidney transplantation is associated with specific dermatologic risks. Patients who undergo solid-organ transplantation are at increased risk for the development of cutaneous malignancies, particularly nonmelanoma skin cancer. Kidney transplant recipients are up to 30 times more likely to develop squamous cell carcinoma than healthy hosts, possibly due in part to the oncogenic properties of human papillomavirus, which may be found within some squamous cell carcinomas in this patient population. The immunosuppressive regimen is a key factor as well, with specific medications having higher risks and some offering potential preventive benefits (OKT-3 and tacrolimus carry an increased risk and rapamycin offers a mild protective effect). All patients receiving an organ transplant should be counseled about sun protective measures and receive an annual skin check.

KEY POINTS

- The use of gadolinium-based contrast agents has been identified as a key trigger of nephrogenic systemic fibrosis.
- Patients who undergo solid-organ transplantation are at increased risk for the development of cutaneous malignancies, particularly nonmelanoma skin cancer.

Pulmonology

Sarcoidosis

Sarcoidosis is an inflammatory disease characterized by granuloma formation in multiple organs; approximately 30% of patients will have cutaneous involvement. Recognition of skin disease is essential, as it is much easier to obtain a tissue diagnosis by skin biopsy than by an internal surgical sampling. Sarcoidosis has been called "the great imitator," and a multitude of skin lesions have been described. Classic cutaneous sarcoidosis appears as violaceous papules around the nose including the ala, or periorbitally and periorificially (around the oropharynx and nasal openings) (**Figure 105**). Sarcoid lesions may also preferentially develop in sites of trauma, such as scars or tattoos. The term "lupus pernio" is a source of potential confusion. Lupus generally refers to systemic lupus erythematosus. Pernio generally refers to a condition of purple papules on the distal digits in some patients who live in cold, wet climates; and lupus vulgaris is a form of tuberculosis of the skin. Lupus pernio has little to do with these, however. Lupus pernio is sarcoidosis of the nose and central face, with violaceous subcutaneous plaques or nodules, often with some overlying scaling. This is more common in black persons and is important to recognize, as persons with lupus pernio frequently have a chronic, refractory course. Limited cutaneous sarcoidosis may be treated with topical glucocorticoids; more extensive disease warrants systemic therapy, with hydroxychloroquine the most appropriate first-line agent. Patients who fail to respond may be treated with thalidomide,

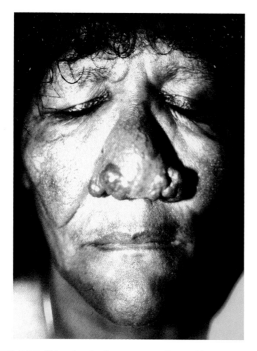

FIGURE 105. This patient has lupus pernio, with sarcoid lesions throughout the nose and cheeks, along with discrete sarcoid papules on the nasal tip and over the nasal ala.

methotrexate, or occasionally TNF-α inhibitors. Additional therapeutic options for some patients include tetracycline-class antibiotics, retinoids, phosphodiesterase inhibitors, and other immunosuppressive agents. Treatment depends on which organs are affected, with the more important or severely affected organ systems determining therapeutic consideration.

KEY POINT

- Classic cutaneous sarcoidosis appears as violaceous papules around the nose or periorbitally and periorificially; it may also develop in sites of trauma, such as scars or tattoos.

Erythema Nodosum

Erythema nodosum (EN) is the most common form of panniculitis, or inflammation of the fat, with most inflammation concentrated on the intralobular septae. Because the inflammation is deep under the skin, the clinical manifestation seen on the surface is often ill-defined erythema with some substance on palpation, which may fade from an active inflammatory red-pink to a more dull brown over time. The lesions are frequently tender when actively inflamed. Most commonly, EN occurs bilaterally and symmetrically on the anterior shins; however, it may also appear in any fatty areas (**Figure 106**). Although lesions will often come and go, most resolve over 4 to 6 weeks. EN is a nonspecific reaction pattern, with inflammation in the fat occurring in response to some systemic process. Multiple causes have been associated with EN, including systemic inflammatory diseases, reactions to medications or hormones, and occult or symptomatic infections. EN can also be idiopathic (**Table 23**).

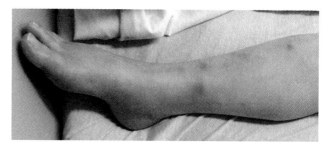

FIGURE 106. Erythema nodosum manifests as red, ill-defined, tender nodules of varying size typically on the anterior shins.

TABLE 23. Selected Causes of Erythema Nodosum
Infections
Streptococcal pharyngitis
Tuberculosis
Pulmonary fungal infections (coccidioidomycosis, blastomycosis, histoplasmosis)
Gastrointestinal bacterial infections (*Yersinia* enterocolitis, *Salmonella* gastroenteritis)
Psittacosis
Cat scratch fever
Leprosy
Drugs
Antibiotics (penicillin, sulfonamides)
Estrogen-containing medications (oral contraceptives, hormone replacement therapy)
Systemic Conditions
Inflammatory bowel disease
Pregnancy
Sarcoidosis
Connective tissue disorders (dermatomyositis, lupus erythematosus, scleroderma)
Malignancy (rare)
Sweet syndrome
Behçet syndrome

The most common associations are streptococcal infection, hormones (including oral contraceptives, hormone replacement therapy, or pregnancy), inflammatory bowel disease, sarcoidosis, and medication reactions. The appearance of EN in patients with sarcoidosis generally portends an acute presentation with a good long-term prognosis with lower risks of chronic disease. EN, arthritis, hilar lymphadenopathy, and fevers constitute Löfgren syndrome, which is more common in patients of Northern European descent (see Sarcoidosis).

Although EN itself is frequently self-limited, patients may be managed with NSAIDs, rest, elevation, and sometimes gentle compression. Patients with recalcitrant disease may require treatment with systemic immunomodulatory drugs; some patients may respond to saturated solution of potassium iodide, colchicine, or dapsone. **H**

Gastroenterology

Inflammatory bowel disease (IBD) may present with cutaneous manifestations. Erythema nodosum (EN) is one of the more common skin findings in patients with IBD, occurring in either Crohn disease or ulcerative colitis in up to 20% of patients. Crohn disease may also present with distinctive linear pustules and erosions of the oral mucosa and gingiva, termed "pyostomatitis vegetans," with cutaneous Crohn disease (typically granulating ulcers periorificially) or perianal skin tags. Patients with both ulcerative colitis and Crohn disease may develop inflammatory neutrophilic dermatitis, particularly pyoderma gangrenosum.

Pyoderma Gangrenosum

Pyoderma gangrenosum (PG) is an autoimmune neutrophilic dermatosis in which neutrophils invade and fill the dermis, leading to marked tissue edema and possible ulceration (**Figure 107**). PG may also present with bullous lesions, pustulonodules, and vegetative plaques. The typical history is a small pustule or red nodule that may develop after trauma and rapidly expands causing an edematous, infiltrated, actively inflamed border and a painful, exudative wet ulcer. Classically the border is described as violaceous and, because of the nature of the inflammation, the epidermis often overlies the ulcer, with a "hanging border" or residual thin anastomosing strands of epidermis remaining over the expanding ulcer (see Foot and Leg Ulcers).

As PG resolves, it tends to heal with atrophic scarring in a cross-like or cribriform pattern. One helpful clinical feature for diagnosing active PG may be the presence of "pathergy," or the occurrence of lesions at sites of trauma. Pathergy is seen in many neutrophilic dermatoses (PG, Sweet syndrome, and Behçet syndrome in particular), but only 20% to 30% of patients with PG will exhibit pathergy. Peristomal PG occurs around ostomy sites and may be a particular form of pathergy. The constant exposure of bowel contents to the skin and need for adhesives to bind the ostomy bags to the area can create a clinical challenge when ulcers develop.

Diagnosing PG is challenging, and all patients with suspected PG should be evaluated for potential underlying causes (**Table 24**). There are no definitive tests, and PG is a diagnosis of exclusion; excluding other causes almost always requires a skin biopsy and tissue culture. It is essential to rule out other diseases before making a diagnosis of PG and to reevaluate the diagnosis during treatment. PG is usually glucocorticoid responsive, and

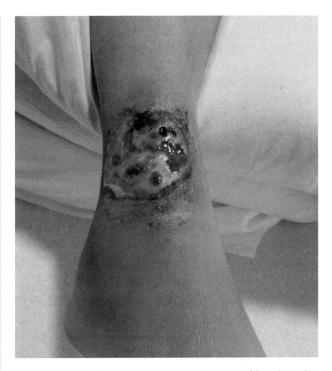

FIGURE 107. Pyoderma gangrenosum, presenting as a painful, exudative ulcer with a purulent base and ragged, edematous, violaceous, "overhanging" border.

failure to respond to therapy should prompt evaluation for an alternative diagnosis. PG may be idiopathic, but it is associated with an underlying disease in 50% of patients.

Management is threefold: evaluate for underlying disease, treat the PG inflammation, and manage the resulting wound. Treating PG can be a challenge, and if there is an associated underlying disease, therapy should be directed at controlling that process. PG is often responsive to topical or intralesional glucocorticoids. Cyclosporine and infliximab may also be effective, with infliximab having the highest quality evidence, although most clinicians use systemic glucocorticoids as first-line therapy. Second-line treatment includes other immunomodulatory drugs such as thalidomide, mycophenolate mofetil, azathioprine, methotrexate, intravenous immune globulin, and other biologic agents. Because the pathologic process is neutrophil-dependent, dapsone or colchicine therapy sometimes provides benefit, including potential dual benefit for dapsone as *Pneumocystis* pneumonia prophylaxis for patients requiring long-term glucocorticoids for disease control. Local supportive care is also essential to achieve ulcer resolution. Many patients will have PG inflammation controlled, and that is when systemic immunosuppressants should be tapered. Wound healing may take longer and require intensive local wound care. Important measures include achieving adequate pain control; maintaining a clean, noninfected ulcer base (potentially with antimicrobial soaks, topical antimicrobial agents, and absorptive dressings); and minimizing edema in the affected limb with compression as tolerated.

TABLE 24. Pyoderma Gangrenosum Evaluation

Diagnostic Criteria (2 major, 4 minor)

Major:

- History of rapidly progressing, painful ulcer with irregular, violaceous, undermined border

- Exclusion of other causes of ulcerations (typically vasculitis, neoplasm, infection)

Minor:

- Skin biopsy showing sterile neutrophilic inflammation

- Presence of pathergy or healing with cribriform scarring

- Presence of systemic diseases associated with pyoderma gangrenosum (inflammatory bowel disease, IgA paraproteinemia, internal malignancy, systemic lupus erythematosus, or other autoimmune disease)

- Response to systemic glucocorticoid therapy (1-2 mg/kg/d, anticipate 50% size decrease within 4 weeks)

Systemic Evaluation

All patients:

- Complete blood count, comprehensive metabolic profile

- Biopsy, often including a separate deep-tissue culture

Dictated by history, presentation, review of systems:

- Age- and sex-appropriate cancer evaluation

- Evaluation for inflammatory bowel disease with upper endoscopy and colonoscopy (almost always indicated)

- Chest radiography for lung pathology or malignancy

- Serum and urine protein electrophoresis for paraproteinemia (especially IgA)

- Hematologic studies for coagulation abnormalities (including antiphospholipid antibodies)

- Bone marrow aspiration and biopsy

- Extended serologic testing for alternative explanations or associated autoimmune diseases (RF/CCP, ANA, ANCA, cryoglobulins)

- Vascular flow studies (if on the leg) to exclude component of vascular insufficiency mimicking pyoderma gangrenosum or impacting wound healing

RF/CCP = rheumatoid factor/anti-cyclic citrullinated peptide; ANA = antinuclear antibody; ANCA = antineutrophil cytoplasmic antibody.

KEY POINTS

- Pyoderma gangrenosum presents as a painful, exudative ulcer with a purulent base and ragged, edematous, violaceous, "overhanging" border; it may be idiopathic but is associated with an underlying disease in some patients.

- Pyoderma gangrenosum is responsive to glucocorticoids, and cyclosporine and infliximab may also be effective.

Dermatitis Herpetiformis

Dermatitis herpetiformis (DH) is an eruption characterized by pruritic papules and transient, almost immediately excoriated blisters on the elbows, knees, and buttocks (**Figure 108**). Histologically, neutrophils are found in the papillary dermis, and direct immunofluorescence may reveal granular IgA depositions. Patients with DH have intense pruritus and almost immediately respond to treatment with dapsone. DH is strongly associated with gluten sensitivity and celiac disease, and patients should be evaluated for celiac disease and maintain a gluten-free diet, or they are at increased risk for small bowel lymphoma (see Autoimmune Blistering Diseases).

Patients with cirrhosis also frequently have skin involvement. These patients often have xerosis and develop diffuse, intense pruritus, potentially partially due to accumulation of bile salts in the skin. Chronic scratching leads to thickened, lichenified plaques and individual hypertrophic hyperpigmented, excoriated prurigo nodules. This form of pruritus is

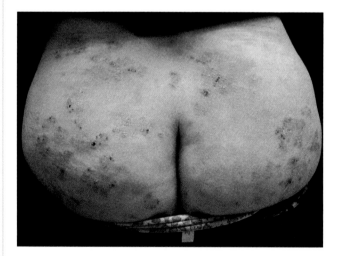

FIGURE 108. Group crusted, excoriated papules in a patient with dermatitis herpetiformis. The vesicles are so superficial and fragile and patients have such intense pruritus that the vesicles are rarely seen intact.

best managed with aggressive topical emollients, and patients with refractory disease may benefit from phototherapy. Patients with advanced liver disease may also develop spider telangiectasias (red papules with tiny networks of capillaries extending outward), jaundice, erythema of the thenar or hypothenar eminences, and changes to the nail plate such as Terry nails, in which the nail bed turns opaque.

Porphyria Cutanea Tarda

Porphyria cutanea tarda (PCT) is a rare skin disease associated with liver disease. It may develop from extensive alcohol use, hemochromatosis, or hepatitis C virus (HCV) infection. Only rarely is PCT a genetic disease caused by reduced activity of the enzyme uroporphyrinogen decarboxylase; however, 80% of cases are acquired, most of which are from chronic HCV infection. PCT presents with skin fragility and small, transient, easily ruptured vesicles in sun-exposed areas, mainly on the hands (**Figure 109**). When the lesions rupture, there is usually scarring, shallow erosions, and occasional white papules from pinpoint epidermal inclusion cysts from abnormal healing (milia). Excess hair growth, or hypertrichosis, may be seen on the tops of the hands or cheeks. Laboratory testing may show elevated uroporphyrin levels. A skin biopsy showing a pauci-inflammatory subepidermal bullae can confirm the diagnosis. Treatment is aimed at limiting iron overload by phlebotomy; antimalarial agents such as hydroxychloroquine may also be beneficial. PCT that develops in the setting of HCV may warrant treating the infection.

Treatment of HCV infection may result in secondary skin side effects that are important to consider. Interferon alfa treatment is associated with the development of granulomatous dermatitis and in some patients, sarcoidosis. A relatively new agent for treating HCV infection, telaprevir, has been associated with skin eruptions in a significant percentage of treated patients, with some reports indicating as many as 35%

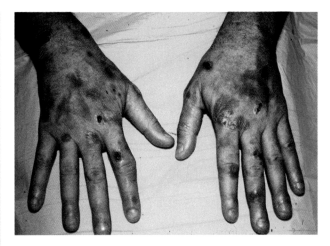

FIGURE 109. A chronic, blistering skin disease, with multiple scars and lesions of varying stages, on sun-exposed skin, especially on the back of the hands, consistent with porphyria cutanea tarda.

to 50% of these patients developing a cutaneous eruption. Some of the reported eruptions have been severe, with potentially life-threatening skin reactions developing in a few patients. Patients receiving telaprevir for HCV infection should be followed closely, and any skin eruption warrants a thorough evaluation.

Hematology/Oncology

Recognizing paraneoplastic dermatoses may lead to earlier diagnoses, and management of paraneoplastic eruptions is critical in the care of patients with internal malignancies. Cutaneous signs of malignancy include both features of hereditary syndromes with cutaneous manifestations and an associated increased lifetime risk of internal malignancy, and cutaneous inflammatory reaction patterns that develop in the setting of malignancy (**Table 25**). Paraneoplastic eruptions

TABLE 25. Genetic Diseases with Cancer Associations and Skin Findings[a]		
Condition	**Clinical Findings**	**Associated Malignancy/Comments**
Muir-Torre syndrome (Lynch syndrome)	Sebaceous neoplasms and keratoacanthomas (squamous cell carcinoma subtype)	Adenocarcinomas of the gastrointestinal tract or other tumors of the genitourinary tract. Lung, breast, and hematologic malignancies may occur.
Cowden syndrome	Tan facial papules (tricholemmomas) and oral papillomas or cobblestoning	Adenocarcinomas of the breast or thyroid and/or polyps of the gastrointestinal tract
Birt-Hogg-Dube syndrome	Fine white sclerotic facial papules (fibrofolliculomas or trichodiscomas); spontaneous pneumothoraces	Kidney cancer
Reed syndrome	Tender cutaneous papules (leiomyomas); uterine fibroids	Kidney cancer
Tuberous sclerosis complex	Multiple cutaneous lesions (facial angiofibromas, ash leaf spots, hypopigmented macules, subungual papules); cortical tubers and seizures; female patients may develop lymphangioleiomyomatosis	Kidney cancer

[a]This table is a brief review focused on genetic diseases that can present in adulthood; this is not a comprehensive list of genetic skin diseases with cancer associations.

may precede, parallel, or follow a diagnosis of cancer. Potential paraneoplastic skin eruptions warrant age- and sex-appropriate screening studies, with additional diagnostic testing depending on the specific skin reaction pattern (**Table 26**).

Sweet Syndrome

Sweet syndrome, or acute febrile neutrophilic dermatosis, is one of the classic "neutrophilic dermatoses," driven by

neutrophilic infiltration and cytokine inflammation. Other neutrophilic dermatoses include pyoderma gangrenosum; erythema elevatum diutinum (a vasculitis that predominantly affects the skin overlying extensor joint spaces); neutrophilic eccrine hidradenitis (typically seen following chemotherapy exposures); and subcorneal pustular dermatosis (which usually causes relapsing pustular plaques of the folds of skin in middle-aged and older women). Neutrophilic inflammation

TABLE 26. Paraneoplastic Disorders: Conditions That Are Strongly Linked to Internal Malignancy		
Condition	**Clinical Findings**	**Associated Malignancy/Comments**
Acanthosis nigricans	Velvety or verrucous hyperpigmentation of intertriginous areas, weight loss, glossitis	Adenocarcinoma, usually GI or GU, most commonly of stomach; occurs also in patients with endocrinopathy
Leser-Trélat sign	Rapid appearance or inflammation of multiple seborrheic keratoses; often occurs in conjunction with acanthosis nigricans	Same cancer association as acanthosis nigricans; seborrheic keratoses are common lesions; Leser-Trélat sign is very rare
Tripe palms	Rugose folds on the palms and soles; may occur with or without acanthosis nigricans	If occurring with acanthosis nigricans, same cancer association; if occurring without acanthosis nigricans, squamous cell carcinoma of the head and neck or lungs
Bazex syndrome (also known as acrokeratosis paraneoplastica)	Psoriasiform, violaceous scaling on the acral surfaces (fingers, toes, nose, and ears); keratoderma may also be present	Squamous cell carcinoma of the upper respiratory tract or upper GI tract; effective therapy of an associated cancer is followed by resolution of the dermatosis
Carcinoid syndrome	Episodic flushing, often accompanied by diarrhea and bronchospasm; can eventually result in telangiectasia or permanent ruddiness	Pulmonary carcinoid tumors or carcinoid tumors metastatic to the liver; tumor removal is followed by resolution of the skin and systemic findings
Ectopic ACTH syndrome	Generalized hyperpigmentation	Small cell lung cancer; tumor removal can result in improvement of the pigmentation
Necrolytic migratory erythema	Intertriginous erythema, scales, and erosions; glossitis and angular cheilitis are common	Glucagon-secreting tumor of the pancreas
Neutrophilic dermatoses	Sweet syndrome; atypical pyoderma gangrenosum (bullous lesions with a blue-gray border, often on the hands, arms, or face)	Myeloid leukemia, myelofibrosis, and refractory anemias; these disorders also occur without malignancy in 80% to 90% of patients
Paget disease of the breast	Erythematous, irregularly bordered plaque on the nipple	Represents an extension of a ductal adenocarcinoma of the breast
Extramammary Paget disease	Erythematous scaly patch or plaque on the perineal skin, scrotum, or perianal area	Cancer of the GI or GU tract is present in 25% of patients; it is not contiguous with the dermatosis; the dermatosis is a malignancy and needs appropriate excision or ablation
Paraneoplastic pemphigus	Severe mucosal erosions, tense and flaccid bullae that may be widespread	Non-Hodgkin B-cell lymphoma, Castleman disease, chronic lymphocytic leukemia
Dermatomyositis	Heliotrope rash, Gottron papules and sign, photodistributed violaceous erythema; scaly erythema of the scalp with diffuse alopecia; periungual telangiectasias and cuticular overgrowth	20% to 25% of patients with dermatomyositis had, have, or will have a malignancy; ovarian cancer is overrepresented; paraneoplastic course is possible but unusual
Necrobiotic xanthogranuloma	Purple-orange nodules and plaques, often on the upper eyelids, which frequently ulcerate	90% of patients have an associated paraproteinemia (generally IgG κ) and may develop multiple myeloma
Amyloidosis	"Pinch purpura" in sites of thin skin such as the periorbital area, usually accompanied by macroglossia and smoothing of the tongue	Seen in multiple myeloma or systemic amyloidosis
Scleromyxedema	Waxy fine papules over the face, neck, and upper trunk	Most patients have an associated paraproteinemia (generally IgG λ) and may develop overt multiple myeloma

ACTH = adrenocorticotropin hormone; GI = gastrointestinal; GU = genitourinary.

can predominate in other multiple skin eruptions, including Behçet syndrome, erythema nodosum, linear IgA bullous dermatosis, dermatitis herpetiformis, and more. Sweet syndrome may be idiopathic or occur in association with an underlying disease; the syndrome typically develops after an upper respiratory or gastrointestinal infection or in the setting of hematologic abnormalities, particularly myelodysplastic syndrome and myelodysplastic syndrome evolving into acute myeloid leukemia. Sweet syndrome has also been associated with solid malignancies and medications (particularly neutrophil-stimulating medications such as granulocyte-colony stimulating factor (G-CSF) and all-*trans* retinoic acid). Patients will have high fevers, leukocytosis with a left shift, elevated inflammatory markers, and often muscle or joint pain, along with the skin eruption. The skin lesions are described as "juicy" indurated edematous red-purple plaques and nodules, sharply demarcated from the adjacent skin. Biopsy will show a neutrophilic infiltrate with prominent superficial papillary dermal edema. This intense edema high up in the skin is what causes the characteristic "swollen, juicy" appearance clinically. Intensely inflamed lesions may ulcerate and resemble PG (**Figure 110**).

As with PG, pathergy may occur and offer a clue to the diagnosis. Unlike PG, lesions of Sweet syndrome resolve without scarring. All patients with Sweet syndrome should have a complete blood count and should be evaluated for potential underlying malignancy, particularly acute myeloid leukemia. Flares of Sweet syndrome can sometimes parallel the underlying disease, but Sweet syndrome may also develop as patients are being treated for the leukemia. Flares may be due to endogenous cytokine signaling, such as elevated levels of G-CSF in response to cytotoxic bone marrow ablative chemotherapy for leukemia. Sweet syndrome is dramatically glucocorticoid responsive, and patients often have immediate relief after just one dose, with resolution of fevers and dramatic reduction in skin lesions. Alternatives to glucocorticoids in patients who are unable to successfully taper off include saturated solution of potassium iodide, dapsone, colchicine, and NSAIDs. Select patients may require cyclosporine, mycophenolate mofetil, and TNF-α inhibitors or possibly targeted antineutrophilic biologic agents such as anti-interleukin-1 anakinra.

Skin findings in patients undergoing treatment for cancer are importatnt as well. Cutaneous eruptions can have severe impacts on patients undergoing chemotherapy, and failure to recognize or manage these side effects can lead to treatment interruptions or suboptimal dose reduction (**Table 27**). Almost all chemotherapeutic agents have been reported to cause the entire spectrum of classic cutaneous adverse drug reactions, such as morbilliform exanthems and urticarial eruptions. Multiple agents have also been associated with development of erythema multiforme, Stevens-Johnson syndrome, and toxic epidermal necrolysis.

Patients who are undergoing chemotherapy are often severely immunocompromised, and careful evaluation and management of the skin is essential to prevent and recognize infections. Violaceous nodules or areas of purpura, particularly if with necrosis, should be evaluated immediately to exclude rapidly progressive invasive infections. Careful skin examination for sites of breakdown or trauma, such as in the skin folds or web spaces, can help prevent superficial skin infections from serving as a portal of entry for systemic infection.

Patients who undergo bone marrow transplants have additional skin-specific issues. Graft-versus-host disease is one of the most common complications of bone marrow transplantation and may present initially or solely in the skin. Patients will classically develop erythema of the ears, upper back and neck, outer shoulders or outer arms, and dorsal feet or hands, and the erythema may be folliculocentric initially. Patients should be evaluated for signs of engraftment in the marrow (cell count recovery) and for liver or gastrointestinal involvement. Acute graft-versus-host disease rarely develops within the first 2 weeks following transplantation, but once count recovery has started, it is a common cause of significant morbidity and treatment-related mortality. Patients may have a morbilliform eruption, which can be clinically challenging to distinguish from cutaneous adverse drug reactions. The timing, morphology, distribution, and associated symptoms (such as diarrhea or liver chemistry abnormalities) can help differentiate these two entities; skin biopsy may be of use although there are not definitive features.

Chronic graft-versus-host disease generally occurs in the skin as either lichen planus–like lesions or scleroderma–like changes. Patients may develop chronic inflamed erythematous-to-violaceous papules or plaques with overlying scale, which may be accompanied by inflammation of the eyes, mouth, or genitals. **H**

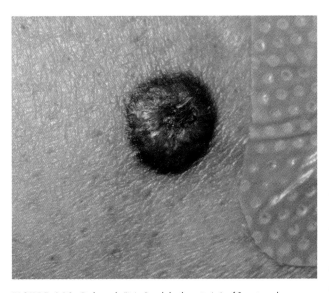

FIGURE 110. Red-purple "juicy" nodule characteristic of Sweet syndrome lesions. The marked edema is typical, leading to a "pseudovesicular" appearance.

KEY POINTS

- Lesions of Sweet syndrome can appear as "juicy" indurated edematous red-purple plaques and nodules, sharply demarcated from the adjacent skin.

(Continued)

TABLE 27. Select Dermatologic Chemotherapy Reactions

Reaction	Chemotherapeutic Agents
Dermatomyositis-like eruption	Hydroxyurea
Neutrophilic dermatoses (PG, Sweet syndrome)	G-CSF, GM-CSF, ATRA, thalidomide, lenalidomide, bortezomib
Acneiform eruption	EGFR inhibitors
Paronychia	EGFR inhibitors
Pseudoporphyria	5-Fluorouracil
Cutaneous lupus	5-Fluorouracil, capecitabine
Hand-foot syndrome/acral erythema	Cytarabine, 5-fluorouracil, capecitabine, methotrexate, docetaxel, paclitaxel, anthracyclines
Neutrophilic eccrine hidradenitis	Cytarabine, multiple other agents
Hand-foot skin reaction	Sorafenib, sunitinib
Serpentine supravenous hyperpigmentation	5-Fluorouracil
Flagellate hyperpigmentation	Bleomycin
Alopecia	Multiple agents
Morbilliform	Multiple agents
Urticarial	Multiple agents
SJS-TEN	Multiple agents
Erythema multiforme	Multiple agents
Vasculitis	Multiple agents

ATRA = all-trans *retinoic* acid; EGFR = epidermal growth factor; G-CSF = granulocyte colony-stimulating factor; GM-CSF = granulocyte-macrophage colony-stimulating factor; SJS = Stevens-Johnson syndrome; TEN = toxic epidermal necrolysis.

KEY POINTS *(continued)*

- Sweet syndrome has been associated with acute myeloid leukemia, solid tumors, chemotherapy, and infections.

Endocrinology

The skin is affected by a host of endocrinologic conditions, ranging from the association between autoimmune skin diseases such as vitiligo and alopecia areata with thyroid disease, to gynecomastia from hormonal imbalances, or the diffuse hyperpigmentation of Addison disease. This section will focus on diabetes mellitus and thyroid disease.

Diabetes Mellitus

Patients with diabetes mellitus can develop a wide range of skin findings such as the velvety hyperpigmentation of acanthosis nigricans, which tends to present in the intertriginous areas, particularly in the axillae, in obese persons with diabetes (**Figure 111**). This may be accompanied by skin tags, which are common in obese persons.

Some findings are connected to the underlying etiopathogenesis of the disease. For example, patients with type 1 diabetes are at increased risk for development of vitiligo (asymptomatic depigmented patches periorificially or in sites of trauma caused by autoimmunity against melanocytes).

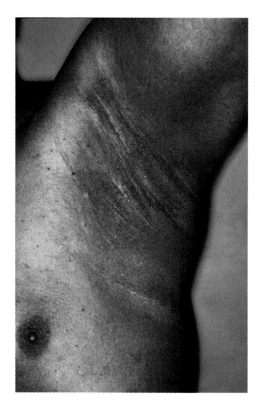

FIGURE 111. Acanthosis nigricans, characterized by a velvety brown plaque in an obese patient.

Patients with diabetes may develop orange, atrophic plaques on their anterior shins (necrobiosis lipoidica). Patients with necrobiosis lipoidica often have retinal or kidney damage as well. Other cutaneous findings associated with diabetes are bullous diabeticorum (large, asymptomatic, noninflammatory bullae on the lower extremities) and scleredema (an uncommon skin finding characterized by edematous induration of the upper back). Diabetic dermopathy (multiple hyperpigmented macules on the anterior shins) is one of the most common cutaneous findings.

Patients with diabetes are at an increased risk of skin infection, such as interdigital and intertriginous infection with *Candida* and dermatophytes. Early recognition is essential, as untreated cutaneous fungal infections may serve as a portal of entry for bacteria, resulting in cellulitis. Intertriginous erythematous eruptions with scale should be evaluated, and if due to tinea, the lesions should be treated with topical antifungal agents (such as ketoconazole), which often requires repeated use to clear and maintain normal skin.

KEY POINTS

- Acanthosis nigricans presents as skin thickening and darkening of the intertriginous areas, particularly the axillae.
- Necrobiosis lipoidica refers to orange, atrophic plaques on the anterior shins of patients with diabetes mellitus that are often associated with retinal or kidney damage.

Thyroid Disease

Hyperthyroidism can lead to warm, moist, smooth, thin skin, often with hyperhidrosis. The hair will grow thin and feel soft, and nail fragility may develop. Cutaneous myxedema can occur anywhere but typically is concentrated on the anterior shins, with the skin appearing indurated with compressible plaques that may have a "peau d'orange" appearance from intradermal mucin deposition.

Thyroid acropachy is a rare finding in some patients with Graves disease, characterized by swelling of the soft tissues of the hands and feet with associated digital clubbing due to periosteal bone formation (**Figure 112**). Patients with hypothyroidism develop cool, dry, pale skin, which may progress to ichthyosis or plate-like scaling resembling fish scales. The hair becomes dry and brittle and may fall out. Loss of the lateral third of the eyebrows is common. Generalized myxedema can lead to a waxy, swollen appearance with puffy lips and edematous and droopy eyelids.

Infectious Disease

HIV Infection

Patients with HIV infection (generally with CD4 cell counts <200/µL) may have a marked photosensitivity and develop a striking photodermatitis with thickening and lichenification

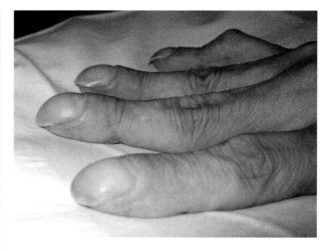

FIGURE 112. Clubbing is seen specifically in patients with Graves disease.

of sun-exposed areas. Patients presenting with new or worsening psoriasis should be evaluated for HIV risk factors, and HIV testing should be offered. Severe outbreaks of seborrheic dermatitis (erythema with greasy scale in the scalp or "T-zone" of the central face) may occur in patients with HIV infection as well, and patients with refractory or extensive seborrhea require prompt evaluation. Patients with other sexually transmitted infections, including genital warts, warrant evaluation for HIV infection as well.

The rash of acute HIV seroconversion is nonspecific, characterized by asymptomatic erythematous macules and small papules over the upper trunk, face, and proximal extremities, sometimes including the palms, and often accompanied by striking oral aphthous ulcers. HIV antibody testing may be negative in acute seroconversion, and viral load testing or delayed antibody testing is essential.

Patients with HIV infection frequently have pruritus. Chronic pruritus and subsequent lichenification and areas of thickened plaques of lichen simplex chronicus or papules of prurigo nodularis are common. Pruritus may be from skin superinfection and chronic bacterial folliculitis, HIV-related xerosis, or as a result of medications. Two specific pruritic eruptions are pruritic papular eruption of HIV (a common chronic papular rash seen in 10% to 45% of patients, which is characterized by symmetric skin-colored or hyperpigmented papules on the trunk and extremities) and eosinophilic pustular folliculitis (characterized by recurrent, extremely pruritic red or hyperpigmented papules on the face and upper chest) (**Figure 113**). Patients with HIV infection are at risk for secondary skin infection with molluscum, superficial bacterial infections, and superficial fungal infections and have a high rate of herpes simplex and herpes zoster virus infections and reactivation. These infections may present with more widespread disease and atypical clinical features in patients with advanced HIV infection. Patients with very low CD4 cell counts are also at risk for secondary cutaneous malignancies including cutaneous lymphoma and Kaposi sarcoma (caused

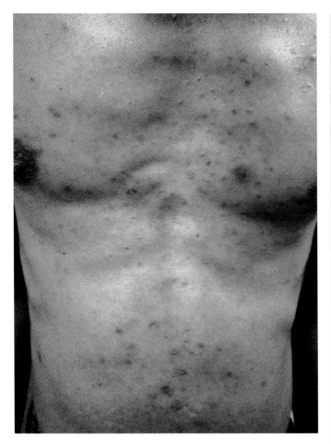

FIGURE 113. Pruritic papular eruption of HIV. The folliculocentric papules and excoriated, hyperpigmented remnants of previous lesions are clustered on the chest and trunk. Photo courtesy of Robert Micheletti, MD.

by human herpesvirus 8) (**Figure 114**). These patients often have an increased risk of squamous cell carcinoma (frequently HPV associated), including squamous cell carcinomas of the digital tips and under the nails and of the penis, perineum, and perianal region.

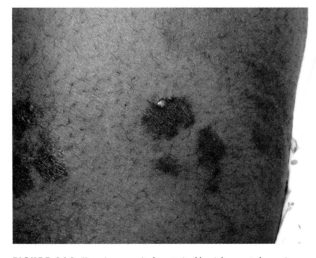

FIGURE 114. Kaposi sarcoma is characterized by violaceous to hyperpigmented plaques. The central plaque shown here has a vascular-appearing, violaceous papule within it.

Dermatologic Urgencies and Emergencies

Retiform Purpura

Purpura is characterized by nonblanchable, red-purple macules or papules that result from the leakage of erythrocytes into the skin. The term "retiform" describes the angulated or netlike configuration that reflects the vascular structure in the skin. The color is often a dark brick-red or purple (**Figure 115**). It is important to recognize these colors as they may indicate local skin ischemia due to occlusion or breakdown of vascular integrity that may lead to necrosis, which may become life-threatening if not aggressively treated. Various conditions can cause retiform purpura, many of which disrupt arterial blood flow (**Table 28**). Thrombotic and embolic causes should be considered first. Thrombotic causes include alterations to the coagulation cascade such as disseminated intravascular coagulation, thrombotic thrombocytopenic purpura, and drug-induced thrombosis (warfarin or heparin). Embolic causes include cardiac sources of emboli (bacterial or marantic endocarditis, atrial myxoma), as well as cholesterol emboli that may be dislodged after an intravascular procedure. Cholesterol emboli may cause multisystem changes such as eosinophilia, acute kidney injury, stroke, intestinal ischemia, and amaurosis fugax. Ecthyma gangrenosum and pyoderma gangrenosum are other diseases that can cause dark, dusky, or purple lesions but do not have a retiform configuration.

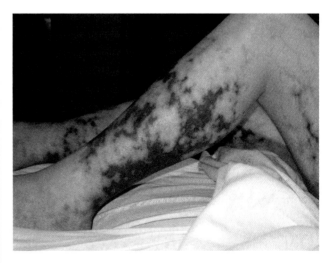

FIGURE 115. Retiform purpura on the lower legs due to vasculitis.

TABLE 28. Causes of Retiform Purpura and Associated Findings

Etiology	Associated Findings and Causes
Angioinvasive fungal infection	Infection caused by *Mucorales, Aspergillus, Fusarium, Pseudallescheria*
	Neutropenic, solid-organ transplant recipients, burn victims
	Infects locally but can become systemic
Necrotizing fasciitis	Pain out of proportion to examination
	History of preceding trauma
	Can be a mixed infection or due to *Streptococcus*
	Surgical emergency; imaging can be supportive but should not delay surgical exploration
Immune-mediated vasculitis	Polyarteritis nodosa
	ANCA-associated vasculitides:
	Eosinophilic granulomatosis with polyangiitis
	Granulomatosis with polyangiitis
	Microscopic polyangiitis
	Connective tissue disease-associated (systemic lupus erythematosus, rheumatoid arthritis, dermatomyositis)
	Evaluate for ANCA, signs of connective tissue disease, other end-organ damage (kidney, lung, eye, gastrointestinal, musculoskeletal)
Calciphylaxis	Associated with advanced kidney disease
	Extremely painful
	Extensive forms occur on central, adipose sites (breast, abdomen, hips)
	Limited forms often occur distally
Thromboembolism	DIC, purpura fulminans
	Systemic inflammation due to infection or other insult
	Evidence of organ ischemia and uncontrolled bleeding from multiple sites
Drugs	Levamisole-adulterated cocaine: tender purpura on the ears is prominent
	Warfarin skin necrosis: rare, occurs in first week of therapy, commonly involves adipose areas such as the breasts, abdomen, and hips
	Heparin necrosis: rare, onset in the first 5 to 10 days of therapy, can occur at the sites of injection or elsewhere, may or may not be associated with thrombocytopenia

ANCA = antineutrophil cytoplasmic antibody; DIC = disseminated intravascular coagulation.

The history can yield important clues to the cause such as infection, thrombotic disease, recent intravascular procedures, spontaneous abortion, solid organ or hematologic malignancy, or prescribed medication or illicit drug reactions. Laboratory tests, directed by the history and physical examination, are indicated to investigate the cause and assess for end-organ damage. In select patients, skin biopsy may be helpful in establishing the diagnosis. Large incisional biopsies, which include the dermis and subcutis, are preferred over punch biopsies. An additional specimen is sent for tissue culture if infection is suspected.

KEY POINT

- Retiform purpura often indicates infection, thrombotic disease, recent intravascular procedures, spontaneous abortion, solid organ or hematologic malignancy, or prescribed medication or illicit drug reactions.

Erythema Multiforme, Stevens-Johnson Syndrome, and Toxic Epidermal Necrolysis

Erythema multiforme (EM) can be recognized by the target lesions on the palms and soles as well as mucosal erosions, most frequently in the mouth (**Figure 116**). In contrast, typical target lesions are rare in Stevens-Johnson syndrome (SJS) and toxic epidermal necrolysis (TEN). SJS and TEN are distinguished by the amount of skin involved by blisters or erosions (**Table 29**). SJS is defined as affecting less than 10% body surface area (BSA), and TEN affects more than 30% BSA. When 10% to 30% BSA is involved, it is considered SJS-TEN overlap with a mortality rate between the two. SJS and TEN are rare, with a prevalence of 1:100,000 for SJS and 1:1,000,000 for TEN. The conditions on the SJS-TEN spectrum can cause significant pain and scarring of involved mucosal surfaces, although the mortality risk is associated with the more severe end of the

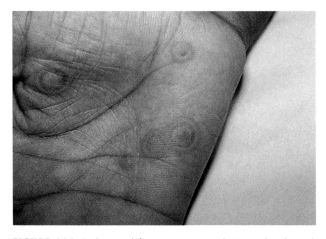

FIGURE 116. Erythema multiforme can cause target lesions on the palms and soles that can vary in size and may have a central erosion.

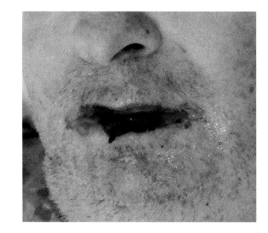

FIGURE 117. Hemorrhagic crusts and erosions of the lips and mouth are common in Stevens-Johnson syndrome and toxic epidermal necrolysis.

H
CONT.

spectrum. The causes of SJS and TEN are not definitely known; however, several cells and signaling pathways have been implicated in triggering keratinocyte death. Some of the possible apoptotic mechanisms include Fas-Fas ligand, damage by perforin or granzyme B, and granulysin. Cytokines and reactive oxygen species have also been linked to keratinocyte injury.

A drug or an infection can trigger EM. EM erupts 1 to 3 weeks following an infection such as herpes simplex virus or *Mycoplasma pneumoniae*. Children are affected equally by drugs and infections; however, drugs are a more frequent cause in adults. Most patients with EM are between 20 and 40 years of age. Target lesions on the palms and soles are often 1 to 6 cm in size. A central purpuric or dusky zone, surrounded by a pale ring and a peripheral red ring, forms the "target." The center often becomes vesicular or eroded. Target lesions are prominent on the palms and soles, whereas red macules and papules occur elsewhere on the body but favor the extremities. Mucosal erosions are painful, and intact vesicles or bullae on mucosa are rare.

SJS and TEN are potentially lethal because of widespread skin inflammation, necrosis, and erosion (**Figure 117** and **Figure 118**).

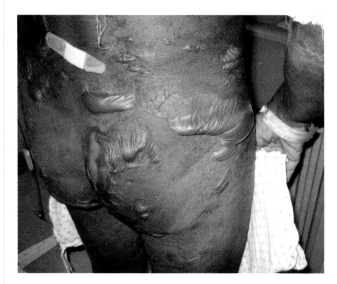

FIGURE 118. Toxic epidermal necrolysis can result in large areas of skin detachment, such as those seen here on the trunk.

TABLE 29. Comparison of Erythema Multiforme, Stevens-Johnson Syndrome, and Toxic Epidermal Necrolysis

	Erythema Multiforme (EM)	Stevens-Johnson Syndrome (SJS)	Toxic Epidermal Necrolysis (TEN)
Morphology	Typical 3-zoned target	Atypical targets and confluent erythema with sloughing	Extensive, confluent erythema with sloughing
Distribution	Favors extremities	Trunk and extremities; up to 10% body surface area involvement[a]	Trunk and extremities; at least 30% body surface area involvement[a]
Mucosal disease (oral, eye, genitourinary)	1 or 2 sites	2 or more sites	2 or more sites
Constitutional symptoms	+	++/+++	+++
Etiology: Infection (%)	50	26	6
Drugs implicated in (%)	50	74	94
Mortality rate (%)	0	5-13	25-39

[a]SJS-TEN Overlap: 10% to 30% body surface area involvement, remaining features the same as SJS.

H
CONT.

TEN is almost exclusively caused by medications (**Table 30**), whereas SJS is normally triggered by medications but may occasionally be caused by vaccines or infection. Patient factors such as HIV infection, kidney disease, active autoimmune disease, and human leukocyte antigen type (HLA-B*1502 and HLA-B*5801) also contribute to increased risk. Patients of Asian and South Asian ancestry who are positive for HLA-B*1502 have up to a 10% risk for SJS-TEN when exposed to aromatic anticonvulsants (carbamazepine, phenytoin, and phenobarbital). These patients should be tested for the presence of HLA-B*1502 antigen before these drugs are initiated. HLA-B*5801 positivity predicts risk of SJS-TEN upon exposure to allopurinol.

When due to drugs, SJS and TEN occur within 8 weeks of drug initiation, often between 4 and 28 days. Patients may report flulike symptoms for 1 to 3 days prior to the skin eruption. Initially, red-purple macules or papules develop on the trunk and extremities, which enlarge and coalesce. Skin pain is prominent. Vesicles, bullae, and erosions reflect the epidermal necrosis seen on biopsy. Nikolsky sign (the shearing off of the epidermis with lateral pressure, as by the examiner's thumb on the skin) is present. Two or more mucosal surfaces, such as the eyes, nasopharynx, mouth, and genitals, are involved in more than 80% of patients (**Figure 119**). Systemic inflammation can result in pneumonia, hepatitis, nephritis, arthralgia, and myocarditis.

Diagnosis and Treatment

Diagnosis of EM is usually made clinically. A biopsy is often performed when SJS or TEN is suspected. Frozen sections of fresh tissue can provide diagnostic information more rapidly than routine histology. The biopsy demonstrates acantholysis and epidermal necrosis, the degree of which depends on the age of the lesion. The biopsy can help to distinguish the spectrum of dermatoses from urticaria, urticarial vasculitis, drug hypersensitivity reaction, graft-versus-host disease, or autoimmune bullous diseases, but histopathology cannot distinguish among the entities in the SJS-TEN spectrum.

SCORTEN is a severity-of-illness score validated for TEN. It incorporates blood Sugar (plasma glucose >252 mg/dL), presence of Cancer, Older age (>40 years), heart Rate (>120/min), Ten percent or more BSA involvement on day 1, Electrolytes (serum bicarbonate <20 mEq/L), and blood urea Nitrogen (>28 mg/dL) (**Table 31**). If the diagnosis of TEN is made, the SCORTEN scale is a validated, severity-of-illness tool for TEN and SJS. The mortality rate is directly correlated with the number of SCORTEN variables that are fulfilled.

If *M. pneumoniae* is the trigger of EM or SJS, then antimicrobial therapy is helpful. Systemic glucocorticoids are highly effective for decreasing inflammation and pain even when patients have an infectious trigger for EM. For EM, short courses (3 to 4 weeks) of systemic glucocorticoids early in the course should be considered. EM can recur, and in approximately 70% of patients this is associated with herpes simplex virus infection. These patients may benefit from suppressive antiviral therapy.

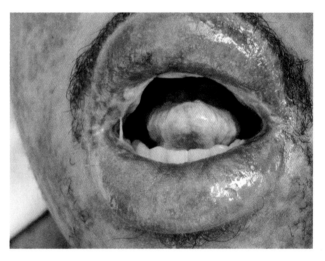

FIGURE 119. Stevens-Johnson syndrome causing erosions on the tongue, lips, and red-brown patches on the surrounding facial skin.

TABLE 30. Medication Classes Reported to Cause Stevens-Johnson Syndrome and Toxic Epidermal Necrolysis

Medication Class	Examples
Aromatic antiepileptic drugs	Carbamazepine, fosphenytoin, lamotrigine, oxcarbazepine, phenobarbital, phenytoin
Oxicam NSAIDs	Meloxicam, piroxicam, tenoxicam
Acetic acid NSAIDs	Diclofenac, indomethacin, lonazolac, etodolac, aceclofenac, sulindac, ketorolac
Antibiotics	Sulfonamides; fluoroquinolone; aminopenicillins, cephalosporins, macrolides, minocycline
Antiviral agents	Nevirapine, abacavir
Miscellaneous	Pantoprazole, sertraline, allopurinol

TABLE 31. SCORTEN Severity of Illness Scale

Plasma glucose	>252 mg/dL (14.0 mmol/L)
Cancer or associated malignancy	Yes
Older age	>40 years
Heart rate	>120/min
Detached or compromised body surface	>10%
Blood urea nitrogen	>28 mg/dL (10.0 mmol/L)
Electrolyte (serum bicarbonate)	<20 mEq/L (20 mmol/L)

CONT.

If a medication is implicated, the first step is cessation of the offending drug. Supportive therapy, such as avoiding dehydration and the use of topical analgesics for oral disease, is important for all patients. Skin findings commonly will worsen even if the trigger is removed. More aggressive supportive care, such as that received in a burn center or ICU, has consistently been shown to improve survival. Fluid, electrolyte, and nutritional support are critical. The role of glucocorticoids or intravenous immune globulin is controversial. Early intervention is essential, and many experts believe that intravenous immune globulin dosed appropriately may help arrest the process; however, firm data are lacking. Decisions regarding therapy should be multidisciplinary and include consultation with a dermatologist. Infection is a significant cause of mortality. A low threshold is recommended for performing cultures and initiation of empiric antibiotics. Use of prophylactic antibiotics is not recommended. Scarring is a complication, especially for mucosal surfaces such as the eyes and genitourinary tract. Ophthalmologic or urologic consultation should be obtained when involvement of these sites is suspected. ▣

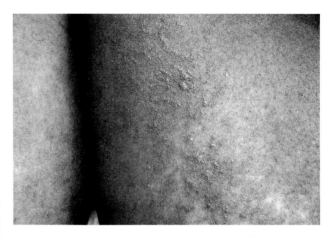

FIGURE 120. Generalized papular eruption in a patient with drug reaction with eosinophilia and systemic symptoms (DRESS).

KEY POINTS

- Erythema multiforme (EM) can be recognized by the target lesions; a drug or infection (herpes simplex virus or *Mycoplasma pneumoniae*) can trigger EM.
- Stevens-Johnson syndrome and toxic epidermal necrolysis are potentially lethal because of widespread skin inflammation, necrosis, and erosion; the two syndromes are distinguished by the amount of skin involved.

▣ DHS (or DRESS Syndrome)

Drug hypersensitivity syndrome (DHS) or drug reaction with eosinophilia and systemic symptoms (DRESS) is a severe, life-threatening, idiosyncratic medication reaction. The pathophysiology may involve drug-triggered viral replication and an exuberant host antiviral response with widespread inflammation. The most common culprit medications include sulfonamide antibiotics, allopurinol, and anticonvulsants, but many more medications have been implicated. DHS is unique in that the onset is usually 2 to 6 weeks after starting the causative medication. Because of this delayed onset, it is often underrecognized or misdiagnosed. The eruption is usually an exuberant morbilliform eruption with prominent facial edema, lymphadenopathy, fever, and, in severe cases, hypotension (**Figure 120**). DHS can be confused with lymphoma, viral eruptions, or hemophagocytic lymphohistiocytosis. Rarely, hemophagocytic lymphohistiocytosis can be due to a drug. Patients with suspected DHS should have a complete blood count with differential to evaluate for eosinophilia or atypical lymphocytosis. Liver chemistry tests, serum creatinine level, and urinalysis should be performed. Given the severity of DRESS-associated myocarditis, some experts suggest that baseline echocardiography should be performed on every patient. Because of the fever and lymphadenopathy, therapy for DHS is to stop the causative medication immediately. Systemic glucocorticoids are typically needed (often 1-2 mg/kg, tapered slowly over multiple weeks to months). Because there is a 10% mortality rate, any patient started on a high-risk medication who develops fever and a rash should be evaluated for DHS. There are reports of the widespread inflammation of DHS causing delayed autoimmune reactions, including thyroid disease and diabetes mellitus, which requires regular follow-up long after the eruption resolves.

DHS is often an underrecognized cause of fever of unknown origin, and if not properly diagnosed, can be fatal. The possibility of DHS must be kept in mind in patients in the ICUs who are on many medications. DHS caused by an aromatic antiepileptic agent can also pose a serious threat due to cross-reaction with other antiepileptics. For example, if phenytoin causes DHS but is appropriately stopped, neither phenobarbital nor carbamazepine should be substituted because of the risk of cross-reaction. ▣

Erythroderma

Erythroderma is characterized by erythema, indicating inflammation, of at least 80% to 90% of the skin surface (**Figure 121**). Peripheral edema, skin erosions, scaling, and lymphadenopathy are common findings. Dehydration, heat loss, and skin infections are potential complications and can compromise the skin barrier and lead to systemic infections and tissue damage. Erythroderma is more common in men than women; the average age of onset is 55 years. Erythroderma is a reaction pattern, and the specific cause can be elusive. The most common causes are medication reactions or an existing skin condition that has flared, most commonly atopic dermatitis or psoriasis following an abrupt

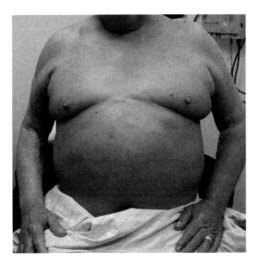

FIGURE 121. Erythroderma of the trunk and arms caused by mycosis fungoides, a form of cutaneous lymphoma.

CONT. discontinuation of systemic glucocorticoids. The cause is idiopathic in 25% to 40% of patients even after a rigorous evaluation. History and physical examination provide critical clues to the cause (**Table 32**). Alopecia, nail dystrophy, and thickening of the palms and soles are indicative of a long-standing cause such as cutaneous T-cell lymphoma, graft-versus-host disease, psoriasis, or pityriasis rubra pilaris. Pityriasis rubra pilaris is a chronic papulosquamous dermatosis that often begins on the scalp and with time becomes generalized. It can be distinguished from psoriasis by the prominent, firm, orange-red, follicle-based papules that coalesce with

TABLE 32.	Causes of Erythroderma
Existing dermatosis	
Psoriasis, atopic eczema, allergic contact dermatitis, lichen planus, pityriasis rubra pilaris	
Drug reaction	
Exanthem, drug hypersensitivity syndrome/drug rash with eosinophilia and systemic symptoms, acute generalized exanthematous pustulosis, TEN	
Infection	
Staphylococcal scalded skin syndrome, tinea corporis, scabies, viral infection	
Autoimmune disease	
Pemphigus foliaceus, pemphigus vulgaris, bullous pemphigoid, linear IgA disease, lupus erythematosus, dermatomyositis	
Malignancy	
Cutaneous T-cell lymphoma (mycosis fungoides), paraneoplastic syndrome with internal malignancy	
Sarcoidosis, graft-versus-host disease	
Idiopathic	

TEN = toxic epidermal necrolysis.

intervening "islands" of normal skin. Drug reactions, staphylococcal scalded skin syndrome, and autoimmune bullous diseases often have a more acute onset without a long-standing history of preceding dermatosis. Because erythroderma is acute, thick scaling of the palms and soles or nail changes do not occur.

Diagnosis and Management

Several diagnostic studies, guided by the clinical history and examination, are potentially helpful. A complete blood count with differential can assess for leukocytosis, which can be reactive or due to an occult hematologic malignancy. Eosinophilia can be a sign of a drug hypersensitivity reaction, scabies infestation, or cutaneous T-cell lymphoma. Imaging studies such as a chest radiograph can assess for lymphadenopathy (reactive or from lymphoma) or occult malignancy in other organs. A skin scraping can demonstrate dermatophytosis or the *Sarcoptes scabiei* mites that cause scabies. Immunofluorescence studies can distinguish possible autoimmune disease, and patch testing is done for a suspected contact allergy causing generalized eczema. Biopsy can be helpful in erythroderma, but nonspecific changes are common (30% to 40% of biopsies). It is not uncommon for patients to have multiple biopsies over time before a definitive diagnosis is made.

Management in conjunction with a dermatologist is frequently necessary. Treatment of infection, as well as management of fluid and electrolyte imbalance, is critical. Thick emollients help to restore skin barrier function. Topical glucocorticoids and systemic antihistamines can improve pruritus. Since drug hypersensitivity is a common cause, drug cessation is a frequent maneuver. Systemic therapy depends on the suspected cause and severity of symptoms. Additional therapies may include ultraviolet light therapy, systemic glucocorticoids, oral retinoids, and systemic immunosuppressants such as methotrexate, azathioprine, and mycophenolate mofetil. **H**

KEY POINTS

- Erythroderma is characterized by erythema of 80% to 90% of skin surface with peripheral edema, erosions of the skin, scaling, and lymphadenopathy.

- Treatment of infection, as well as management of fluid and electrolyte imbalance, is critical in managing erythroderma; thick emollients help to restore skin barrier function, and topical glucocorticoids and systemic antihistamines can improve pruritus.

Hair Disorders

Hirsutism

Hirsutism, or excessive hair growth in women, affects about 8% to 10% of women. In androgen-dependent sites, the fine vellus hairs are converted to thicker, coarser terminal hairs such as those on the underarms. The most to least common sites are the lower abdomen and areola, the chin and upper lip, and between the breasts and on the lower back (**Figure 122**). Polycystic ovary syndrome (PCOS) is the cause of 50% to 70% of cases of hirsutism. The differential diagnosis includes several conditions associated with elevated levels of androgens as well as idiopathic and familial causes (**Table 33**). The evaluation should begin by reviewing the menstrual and reproductive history, medication history, and family history, as well as performing a comprehensive physical examination and assessing for breast discharge, acne, clitoromegaly, weight gain, or striae. Therapeutic options include removal of surface hairs (shaving, depilatories, waxing, or tweezing), bleaching (camouflage), and medications (eflornithine cream,

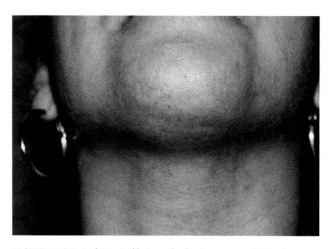

FIGURE 122. Dark, terminal hairs on the chin in a woman with hirsutism due to polycystic ovary syndrome.

TABLE 33. Diagnosing Excessive Hair Growth in Women		
Differential Diagnosis of Excess Hair Growth	**Associated Causes and Findings**	**Possible Testing/Assessments**
Hirsutism (androgen-dependent sites)	Polycystic ovary syndrome: chronic anovulation, hyperandrogenemia, menstrual irregularities, infertility, obesity	DHEAS
		Serum total and free testosterone
	Ovarian tumors (many types): persistent bloating, early satiety, abdominal pain	Pelvic examination, ultrasound
		CA-125 measurement
	Cushing syndrome: acne, striae, moon facies, abdominal obesity, muscle wasting	24-hour urine free cortisol
		Low-dose dexamethasone suppression test
	Adrenal adenoma	
	Congenital adrenal hyperplasia: salt-losing crisis, ambiguous genitals, precocious puberty, oligo- or amenorrhea	Imaging
		17-Hydroxyprogesterone level
	Prolactinoma: galactorrhea, visual changes, amenorrhea	ACTH stimulation test
	Drug-induced: testosterone, DHEAS, danazol, corticotropin, high-dose glucocorticoids, androgenic progestins, acetazolamide, anabolic steroids	Serum prolactin level
Idiopathic/Familial	Present since puberty	Testosterone, 17-hydroxyprogesterone, DHEAS levels
	Slow development/progression	
	Normal menses	
	Family history	
Hypertrichosis (non-androgen-responsive hair)	Porphyria: blistering, skin fragility, scarring	24-hour urine porphyrins, possibly stool or blood porphyrin levels
	Hyperthyroidism: weight loss, anxiety, tachycardia, increased sweating	Thyroid function testing, thyroid antibodies
	Drug-induced: cyclosporine, phenytoin, diazoxide, minoxidil, hexachlorobenzene, penicillamine, methyldopa, metoclopramide, reserpine	History
Acquired hypertrichosis lanuginosa (rare)	Excessive growth of fine lanugo hair (white or blonde, 1-2 cm long) on all hair-bearing surfaces including the face	Associated with malignancy, especially colorectal cancer
		Colonoscopy
		Age-appropriate and symptom-directed cancer screening

ACTH = adrenocorticotropic hormone; DHEAS = dehydroepiandrosterone.

spironolactone, finasteride). It is important to inform women that finasteride is an FDA pregnancy category X drug and that spironolactone (pregnancy category C) has demonstrated feminization of male rat fetuses. Electrolysis and laser hair removal are more durable methods but are expensive and not permanent (see MKSAP 17 Endocrinology and Metabolism).

KEY POINTS

- Polycystic ovary syndrome is the cause of 50% to 70% of cases of hirsutism.
- Therapeutic options for hirsutism are removal of surface hairs, bleaching, and medications such as eflornithine cream, spironolactone, or finasteride.

Alopecia

Alopecia or hair loss can manifest as either a reduced amount or complete loss of hair in a specific location on the scalp. Even mild alopecia can be associated with decreased quality of life and self-esteem. Diagnosis can be simplified by first determining if the alopecia affects localized or diffuse areas of the scalp and, second, if the process is scarring. Scarring alopecia results in the loss of hair and follicle openings (ostia) and appears as very smooth patches of skin (**Figure 123**). A 4-mm punch biopsy from an area of active alopecia (*not* from areas suspicious for scar) can yield useful information regarding diagnosis, therapy, and prognosis if the diagnosis is uncertain following the history and physical examination (**Table 34**). A biopsy should also be performed is there is a clinical suspicion for scarring or lack of response to or worsening with treatment.

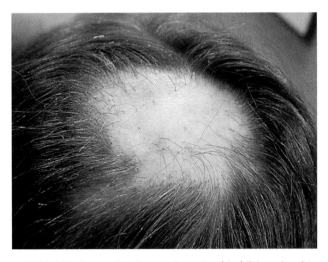

FIGURE 123. Scarring alopecias cause destruction of the follicles and result in a smooth patch of skin. Some follicles that were spared from the inflammation stud the surface of this patch of scarring alopecia.

KEY POINTS

- In diagnosing alopecia, first determine if the alopecia is localized or diffuse, and, second, if it is scarring or non-scarring.
- A 4-mm punch biopsy from an area of active alopecia can yield useful information regarding diagnosis, therapy, and prognosis of alopecia.

Localized/Limited Alopecia

Nonscarring

Alopecia areata (AA) is a chronic autoimmune disorder that results in smooth, hairless patches of skin (**Figure 124**, on page 77). The scalp is the most common site. In contrast to tinea capitis, there is no scale. At the periphery of the patch, there may be "exclamation point" hairs, which are characteristic of AA. The hair shaft of exclamation point hairs narrows the closer the shaft is to the skin surface. This tapering resembles the upper portion of an exclamation point and is thought to be due to inflammation around the hair follicle. Individual patches can spontaneously resolve within 12 months; however, new patches may develop. Onset is often before age 30 years but is rare before 3 years of age. An autoimmune mechanism is supported by the increased rate of other autoimmune diseases; for example, autoimmune thyroid disease is three times more common in those with AA.

Severe forms of AA can result in large patches of hair loss involving more than 50% of the scalp, complete loss of scalp hair (alopecia totalis), or loss of all body hair (alopecia universalis). These forms are uncommon and occur in about 10% to 15% of all persons with AA.

Syphilis is an uncommon cause of alopecia. On examination, there are patchy or "moth-eaten" areas of alopecia over the entire scalp. Other findings of secondary syphilis may be present.

Traumatic alopecia encompasses traction alopecia (from tension), trichotillomania (from compulsive twisting and pulling), and damage from chemicals or heat. Traumatic alopecia, regardless of the cause, is initially reversible but can progress to a scarring alopecia if the trauma continues. Patches of alopecia are rarely completely bald but have short, broken hairs mixed with longer hairs (**Figure 125**, on page 77). Traction alopecia develops at the peripheral edges of a hairstyle, such as the frontotemporal hairline with ponytails or buns and in geometric patterns across the scalp with braids. Traction alopecia can affect persons of any race or either sex. In contrast, the distribution of trichotillomania can be "bizarre" with linear, irregular, or asymmetric shapes. Treatment is directed at the source of the trauma (see Table 2). Rarely, internal malignancies may metastasize to the scalp and lead to alopecia at the metastatic site.

Scarring

Discoid lupus erythematosus (DLE) is the most common type of chronic cutaneous lupus. On the scalp, DLE manifests as

TABLE 34.	Management of Selected Types of Alopecia	
Type of Alopecia	**Treatment Options**	**Possible Systemic Associations**
Androgenetic alopecia	Men: Topical minoxidil 5%,[a] finasteride,[a] dutasteride Women: Topical minoxidil 2%,[a] spironolactone Both: Hair transplant, cosmetic camouflage	Men: Increased rate of prostate cancer (if onset in the 20s) Women: Polycystic ovary syndrome
Alopecia areata	<50% scalp involvement: watchful waiting, topical glucocorticoids ± topical minoxidil, anthralin, intralesional triamcinolone	Autoimmune disease (hyperthyroidism, hypothyroidism, vitiligo, pernicious anemia, diabetes mellitus)
	>50% scalp involvement: topical immunotherapy (squaric acid or DPCP, topical glucocorticoids, ± topical minoxidil, phototherapy, wigs or other cosmetic camouflage, intralesional triamcinolone for brows, latanoprost for eyelashes	Atopic eczema

Telogen effluvium	Remove or correct potential trigger
	
	Watchful waiting
		Anemia, thyroid disease, significant weight loss, eating disorders, parturition, high fever, major surgery, blood loss, mental stress
		
		Medications:
		
		    Anabolic steroids or supplemental androgens
		
		    Antithyroid medications
		
		    Antiepileptics
		
		    β-blockers
		
		    Oral retinoids
		
		    Warfarin

Tinea capitis	Oral therapy with terbinafine, fluconazole, or itraconazole for about 6 weeks Oral therapy with griseofulvin for ~12 weeks	Screen close contacts

Discoid lupus erythematosus	Sunscreen or other sun-protection
	
	Glucocorticoids:
	
	    Topical are first line
	
	    Intralesional for recalcitrant or thick lesions
	
	    Oral glucocorticoids are reserved for patients with rapid progression
	
	    Antimalarial agents
	
	Retinoids: topical or oral if severe
		Systemic lupus erythematosus (5%-10%)
		
		ROS for symptoms
		
		Examination for signs
		
		Urinalysis, ANA

Traumatic alopecia	Traction/styling alopecia: decrease tension from styling practices Trichotillomania: Cognitive behavioral therapy If severe or recalcitrant, antidepressants or anxiolytics may be helpful	Concomitant psychiatric disorder is more common in adults than children Consider referral to psychiatrist or psychologist
Lichen planopilaris	Topical, intralesional, or oral glucocorticoids, hydroxychloroquine, immunosuppressants	Check for concomitant lichen planus on the skin, nails, and oral and genital mucosa
Frontal fibrosing alopecia	Hydroxychloroquine, 5-α reductase inhibitors	
Central centrifugal cicatricial alopecia	Topical and intralesional glucocorticoids, oral tetracyclines, hydroxychloroquine, immunosuppressants, avoidance of associated styling practices	Use of hair straightener or relaxer Use (especially prolonged use) of styles with high tension on the hair

[a]FDA-approved treatment for that condition/indication.

DPCP = diphenylcyclopropenone; ROS = review of systems; ANA = antinuclear antibody.

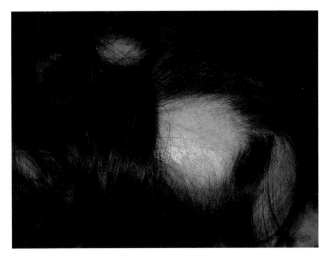

FIGURE 124. This patient with alopecia areata (AA) has patches of hair loss with preservation of the follicular ostia and "exclamation point" hairs at the peripheral edge, which are typical of AA.

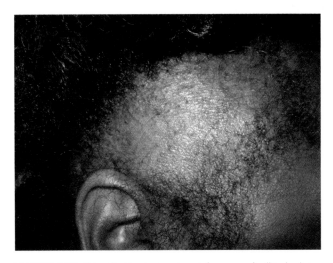

FIGURE 125. This patient has traction alopecia from years of pulling her hair back in a bun. She demonstrates a decreased density of hair at the periphery where the tension was the greatest.

scaling, erythematous, hyper- and hypopigmented patches with alopecia. Multiple lesions are more likely than a single lesion. DLE may be present on other sun-exposed areas or in the conchal bowl of the ear. Glucocorticoids (topical, intralesional, or oral) are the most common therapy. Sun protection is a critical part of management for DLE.

Acne keloidalis nuchae is a chronic, scarring folliculitis that causes hairless areas of scar on the nape of the neck. It mostly affects black men but can occur in other populations (see Special Populations).

Diffuse Alopecia

Nonscarring

Androgenetic alopecia (AGA) can affect both men and women. It is the most common alopecia in men. The prevalence varies by sex and ethnicity. The prevalence in white

men is 50% at age 50 and more than 70% at age 70. The prevalence is lower in women and Asian men. AGA is due to the effect of androgens on genetically susceptible hairs and results in shorter, thinner hairs that grow for shorter periods of time. The mechanism is not as clear for women. On examination, there are "miniaturized" hairs and in men, areas of complete hair loss. In men, the temples and vertex are often affected. In contrast, in women the top of the head is affected, and balding is not complete. A classic examination finding is "widening" of central part compared with the occipital part.

Telogen effluvium (TE) is the most common cause of diffuse alopecia in adult women. The differential diagnosis includes AGA and an uncommon and diffuse form of AA. TE is caused by a rapid shift of many hairs from a growing phase to a resting phase with a subsequent wave of increased "shedding." Patients often report sudden and excessive shedding from all over the scalp. History may reveal a triggering event 3 months prior to the start of the alopecia. In contrast to AGA, the frontal and occipital parts are similar in width and quality. TE often spontaneously resolves in about 6 to 12 months if the trigger is removed or treated.

Scarring

Lichen planopilaris (LPP) and frontal fibrosing alopecia (FFA) are variants of lichen planus that affect the hair (see Common Rashes). Patients may have significant pain, burning, or pruritus. On examination, there is mild scaling and erythema, which may be subtle and concentrated around follicular ostia. FFA predominates in postmenopausal women and causes alopecia at the frontotemporal hairline and eyebrows. LPP has a more scattered distribution around the entire scalp (**Figure 126**). Treatment of both LPP and FFA is challenging, and relapses are common.

Central centrifugal cicatricial alopecia is a scarring alopecia. It begins on the vertex (or crown) of the scalp and expands outwardly over time (**Figure 127**). The female to male ratio is about 3:1. The cause is unknown but is likely multifactorial

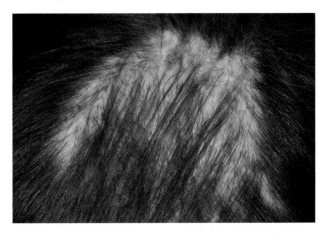

FIGURE 126. Lichen planopilaris is a cause of scarring alopecia and often demonstrates redness around the follicles.

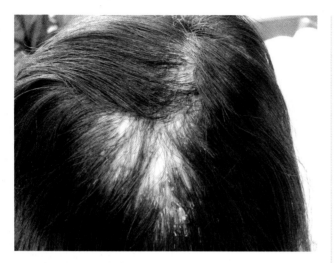

FIGURE 127. Hair loss due to central centrifugal cicatricial alopecia (scarring alopecia).

and may include styling practices. Treatment is challenging and often not curative.

Nail Disorders

The nail is a complex anatomic structure composed of the nail matrix, nail plate, nail bed, and nail folds. The nail folds comprise both the proximal and lateral folds. The nail plate originates from the matrix that is located under the proximal nail fold (cuticle). Thus, proximal nail fold inflammation of any etiology (hand eczema, psoriasis) can cause dystrophy of the nail plate. The nail plate grows over the nail bed. The finger- and toenails grow 3 and 1 mm per month, respectively. Starting in the third decade, the rate can slightly decrease with each year of age. Nail disorders can be caused by various diseases, and it is important that a correct diagnosis is made (**Table 35**). Nail problems are rare in children.

TABLE 35. Nail Changes Associated with Possible Systemic Diseases/Conditions	
Type of Nail Change	**Possible Causes**
Transverse indentations (Beau line, onychomadesis)	Description: Transverse linear depressions in the nail plate; at the same level of the nail in most or all of the nails
	Associated with: Local injury or any severe systemic insult such as infection, surgery, chemotherapy
Pitting	Description: Small, punctate indentations in nail plate
	Associated with: Psoriasis, lichen planus, alopecia areata
Splinter hemorrhages	Description: Red-brown, short, fine lines in the nail bed, due to injury in nail bed vessels
	Associated with: Trauma, psoriasis, lichen planus, infective endocarditis, chronic kidney failure, autoimmune connective tissue diseases
Color change:	
Brown/black	Subungual hematoma, nevus, melanoma, drug-induced (azidothymidine, minocycline)
Yellow	Aging, dermatophyte infection, yellow nail syndrome
White nails	
Punctate	Description: Nonuniform, small white macules on some nails, appear in different places on different nails, due to day-to-day trauma
Half-and-half nails (Lindsey nails)	Description: White change comprises proximal half of the nail and the distal half is pink, red, or brown.
	Associated with: chronic kidney failure
Terry nails	Description: Mostly white nail with a distal rim of normal color at the distal edge.
	Associated with: Liver disease, chronic heart failure, and normal aging
Clubbing	Description: Spongy thickening of distal digit due to hypervascularization
	Associated with: Pulmonary diseases, congenital heart disease, arteriovenous malformations, cirrhosis, inflammatory bowel disease, celiac disease, infective endocarditis, lung cancer, pachydermoperiostosis
Koilonychia (spoon nails)	Description: Upward curving of the periphery of nail to mimic the bowl of a spoon
	Associated with: Chronic occupational injury, iron deficiency anemia
Cuticle changes; ragged torn cuticles	Also known as Samitz sign
	Associated with: Dermatomyositis
Periungual (around nail) erythema with dilated, tortuous vessels	Increased number of visible vessels near the cuticle
	Associated with: Dermatomyositis and scleroderma
Periungual (around nail) erythema with numerous fine vessels	Increased number of visible vessels near the cuticle
	Associated with: Lupus erythematosus

Aging

With aging, the thickness, curvature, surface, and color of the nail plate can change. The underlying mechanisms are unknown. The nail plate may become thicker or thinner. The normal texture of the nail can become rougher and more friable, resulting in striations and splitting. The color of the nail may become paler or yellow. These changes may predispose to onychomycosis, pain, and subungual hemorrhage.

Connective Tissue Diseases

The proximal nail fold can demonstrate signs of systemic lupus erythematosus, dermatomyositis, or scleroderma. The proximal nail fold can appear erythematous and with magnification demonstrate irregular, twisted, and dilated vessels. The cuticle can become dry and ragged with dermatomyositis (Samitz sign) (**Figure 128**).

Infection

Onychomycosis

Onychomycosis is a fungal infection of the nails. It affects 10% to 20% of adults and is the most common nail infection. Infection is more common in older men with comorbidities such as diabetes mellitus, peripheral vascular disease, and immunosuppression. Dermatophytes cause more than 90% of fungal nail infections. Yeasts and molds are uncommon causes. The fungus may enter the nail from a tinea infection elsewhere in the body or from the environment. The most common pattern is distal subungual onychomycosis; the distal corner of the nail becomes yellow, lifted, and develops subungual debris. This can then spread proximally and laterally to involve the entire nail plate. Proximal subungual onychomycosis evolves similarly but begins at the proximal nail fold (the cuticle). This is a rare pattern and is associated with the effects of HIV infection and the severely immunocompromised patients. Treatment is rarely medically necessary and is often pursued for cosmetic reasons. Infection should be confirmed, especially if considering systemic therapy, by processing the nail or subungual debris with potassium hydroxide (KOH), staining with periodic acid–Schiff (PAS), or fungal culture. Topical therapies traditionally have been limited in their efficacy and require long treatment durations. Efinaconazole is a new topical agent with a better response rate then ciclopirox. These topical agents are available by prescription. Terbinafine cream is available over-the-counter and has slightly better efficacy then azole creams. Systemic terbinafine is the most effective oral therapy, whereas itraconazole is a second-line agent. Continuous terbinafine therapy is more effective than pulse therapy. Toenails are treated for 12 weeks, and fingernails are treated for 6 weeks. Topical agents can be an effective therapy for superficial white onychomycosis and early subungual onychomycosis.

Paronychia

Acute paronychia often presents as a painful swelling of the nail fold (**Figure 129**). It often follows minor trauma and affects only a single finger. *Staphylococcus aureus* is a frequent cause. Management consists of warm compresses or soaks, incision and drainage, or topical or systemic antibiotics. In contrast, chronic paronychia affects multiple fingers and manifests as red, swollen nail folds that lack a cuticle. It causes ridging and dystrophy of the nail plate. Chronic irritation from water or

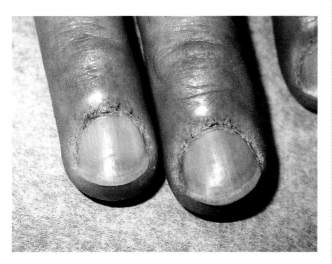

FIGURE 128. This patient has dermatomyositis and has redness of the periungual skin as well as tortuous, dilated, and thrombosed vessels in the proximal nail fold.

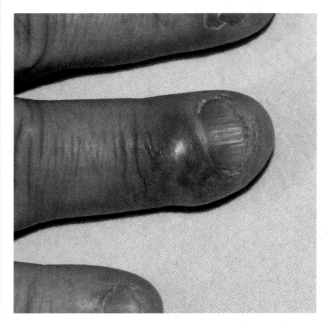

FIGURE 129. Bulbous focal swelling of the periungual skin of one finger due to acute bacterial paronychia.

chemical contact is the primary cause. *Candida* species or gram-negative bacteria can cause secondary infection. Management includes minimizing wet-work and the use topical glucocorticoids to minimize inflammation and topical antifungal or antiseptic agents.

KEY POINTS

- Onychomycosis, a fungal infection of the nails, is more common in older men with comorbidities such as diabetes mellitus, peripheral vascular disease, and immunosuppression.
- Acute paronychia often follows minor trauma and affects only a single finger; *Staphylococcus aureus* is a frequent cause.

Inflammatory Dermatoses

Lichen planus (LP) causes nail disease in about 10% of patients with generalized LP (see Common Rashes). The nail plate can become thinner or be completely destroyed (**Figure 130**). The cuticle may become attached to the nail plate (pterygium). Red streaking of the nail can also occur. It is important to examine the rest of the skin and mucosae for signs of LP.

Nail changes occur in about 75% of persons with psoriasis. The most common nail abnormality observed on both fingernails and toenails is subungual hyperkeratosis. Toenails more often demonstrate thickening and discoloration (whitening or yellowing), whereas pitting and ridging are more common on fingernails. Persons with psoriatic nail dystrophy are often older and are more often affected by psoriatic arthritis. Some of the nail damage can result from onychomycosis. About 20% of those with psoriatic nail dystrophy have positive fungal cultures.

Malignancy

Acral Lentiginous Melanoma

Acral lentiginous melanoma (ALM) is the most common form of melanoma in Asian, Hispanic, and black populations. It can originate in the nail and present as a longitudinal brown stripe that is either solitary or different from other brown lines (darker, broader, changing) (see Special Populations).

Squamous Cell Carcinoma

Squamous cell carcinoma of the nail unit often begins at the nail fold and is associated with a history of trauma, arsenic ingestion, radiation exposure, chronic paronychia, and human papillomavirus (HPV) infection (**Figure 131**). It manifests as an irregular pink keratotic patch or papule that can be mistaken for a wart. Warts, however, are discrete, skin-colored papules with punctate brown dots (thrombosed vessels). If a wart is not responding to therapy as expected, a biopsy or referral to a dermatologist is appropriate. Immunosuppressed patients with HPV/warts around the nail plate may be at higher risk of developing squamous cell carcinoma in those locations and should be monitored closely.

Disorders of Mucous Membranes

Evaluation of the mucous membranes is an important part of the skin examination because findings can be potentially harmful and a clue to systemic disease.

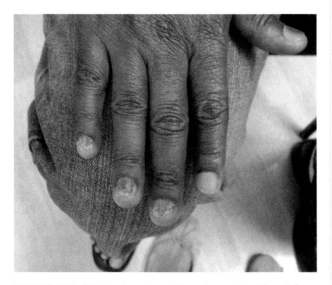

FIGURE 130. Thinning, shortening, and hyperpigmentation of the nails from lichen planus.

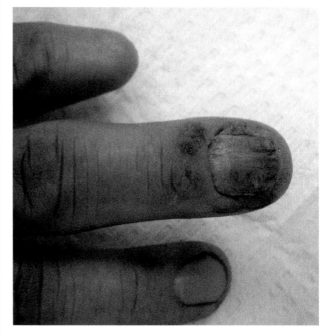

FIGURE 131. This pink plaque on the finger and dystrophic nail was treated as a wart, but a biopsy demonstrated squamous cell carcinoma.

Melanotic Macule

Melanotic macules are well-circumscribed, often round, evenly hyperpigmented lesions that can occur on oral or genital mucosa. In the oral cavity, they are most common on the lower lip, although they may be seen on the gingiva, buccal mucosa, or tongue. Single or multiple lesions can be observed. No treatment is necessary, but biopsy can be performed if there are irregular or changing spots (**Figure 132**).

Amalgam Tattoo

Amalgam tattoos are the most common source of localized pigmentation on the buccal mucosa. They result from traumatic implantation of amalgam into the soft tissue. It clinically presents as a gray to bluish or black macule adjacent to a restored tooth. Diagnosis can be made clinically, or confirmation can be made with biopsy and pathology. No treatment is necessary.

Leukoplakia and Erythroplakia

Leukoplakia is an adherent white plaque on the mucosa that most often is a benign, inflammatory response to triggers such as trauma or tobacco use. It can be premalignant and lead to intraoral squamous cell carcinoma in approximately 20% of patients. Premalignant leukoplakia is more common in certain anatomic sites (floor of the mouth or ventral tongue). The differential diagnosis includes oral candidiasis, which manifests as nonadherent white plaques. Oral hairy leukoplakia is an Epstein-Barr virus infection that occurs almost uniquely in patients with HIV infection. It presents as adherent linear white plaques on the lateral surface of the tongue (**Figure 133**).

Erythroplakia is a red, velvety plaque, which has a higher probability of underlying dysplasia at the time of diagnosis. In both leukoplakia and erythroplakia, biopsy is necessary to evaluate for dysplasia, and erythroplakia should always be biopsied when clinically observed.

Aphthous Ulcers

Aphthous ulcers (canker sores) are common, benign, noninfectious shallow ulcerations of unknown etiology with surrounding erythema that occurs on nonkeratinizing oral and genital surfaces (labial/buccal mucosa, sides of tongue, floor of mouth) (**Figure 134**). Diagnosis is made clinically, although testing to rule out infections can be performed. Aphthous ulcers may be self-limited when the lesions are few or infrequent. When they become recurrent, painful outbreaks that interfere with eating and quality of life, therapy such as topical glucocorticoids or topical lidocaine can be used; oral therapies including colchicine also can be considered when the ulcers are recalcitrant to topical therapies. Severe, recurrent oral

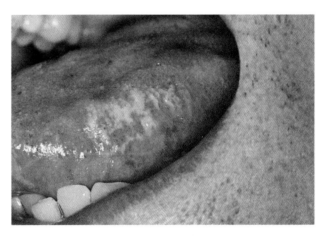

FIGURE 133. Oral hairy leukoplakia in a patient with AIDS. Oral hairy leukoplakia is a precancerous lesion that presents as white patches on the oral mucosa with changes in the surface texture.

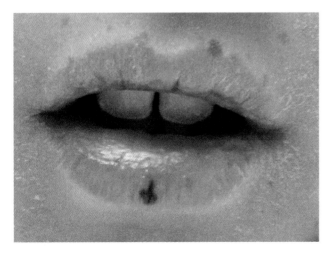

FIGURE 132. Melanotic macule occurring on the vermilion border of the lower lip.

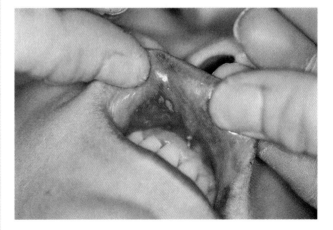

FIGURE 134. Aphthous ulcers are characterized by painful, discrete, shallow, round-to-oval ulcers with a grayish base typically less than 1 cm in diameter.

ulcers may suggest a systemic disease such as Behçet syndrome (associated with eye symptoms and arthralgia), or Crohn disease, HIV infection, or erythema multiforme. The differential diagnosis includes herpes simplex ulcers, which can present as grouped vesicles typically on the keratinizing surfaces, and sexually transmitted infections.

KEY POINT

- Severe, recurrent oral aphthous ulcers may suggest a systemic disease such as Behçet syndrome, Crohn disease, HIV infection, or erythema multiforme.

Lichen Planus

Lichen planus is an inflammatory condition that can affect the skin, nails, or mucosa (see Common Rashes). Clinical presentations include white lines and patches (Wickham striae) or painful erythema and erosions (erosive variant) (**Figure 135**). With mucosal-only disease, evaluation for contact allergens should be considered. Biopsy establishes the diagnosis. Therapies are glucocorticoids (systemic and topical) and immunosuppressive agents in severe disease. Follow-up is important as squamous cell carcinoma can occur in long-standing ulcerative lesions.

Actinic Cheilitis and Squamous Cell Carcinoma

Actinic cheilitis is a premalignant condition that presents with chronic erythema and recurrent scaling of the lower lip. This differs from angular cheilitis, which is inflammation involving one or both corners of the mouth and often related to bacterial or fungal infections. Treatment with topical chemotherapy agents (5-fluorouracil), imiquimod, laser therapy, photodynamic therapy, or cryotherapy is recommended.

Development of a mucosal nodule or ulcer should raise the suspicion of invasive squamous cell carcinoma (SCC). Mucosal SCC also can develop as a result of chronic inflammatory conditions (lichen planus, lichen sclerosus) or in the oral cavity in association with tobacco or alcohol use or human papillomavirus infection. Biopsy is required for diagnosis, and excision often is necessary. SCC of the lip is often underrecognized and leads to delayed diagnosis, more extensive surgery, and a high metastatic rate (see Common Neoplasms).

KEY POINTS

- Actinic cheilitis is a premalignant condition and presents as chronic erythema and recurrent scaling of the lower lip; management is with topical chemotherapy agents, imiquimod, laser therapy, photodynamic therapy, or cryotherapy.
- Development of a nodule or ulcer on the lip area should raise the suspicion of invasive squamous cell carcinoma.

Lichen Sclerosus

Lichen sclerosus is an inflammatory condition that often presents as a white, atrophic patch on the genital and perianal skin, although extragenital lesions can occur (**Figure 136**). It differs from lichen planus in its clinical presentation of white patches that circumferentially involve the vaginal introitus and perianal area ("figure 8" appearance) or the head of the penis. Prepubertal girls and postmenopausal women appear to be at highest risk. The differential diagnosis includes vitiligo, which causes depigmented rather than atrophic plaques. Biopsy establishes the diagnosis and can differentiate it from other inflammatory disorders, as lichen sclerosus has distinct histopathologic features compared with lichen planus. Treatment is with potent topical glucocorticoids (similar to first-line treatment for lichen planus), and frequent clinical follow-up is

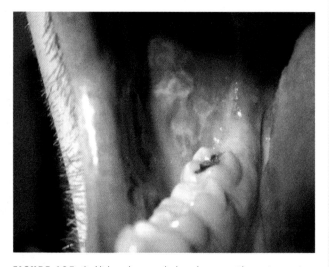

FIGURE 135. Oral lichen planus on the buccal mucosa with prominent reticulated white lines of Wickham striae.

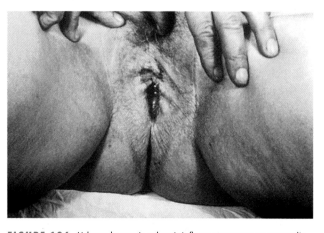

FIGURE 136. Lichen sclerosus is a chronic inflammatory mucocutaneous disease characterized by "parchment-like" or "cigarette paper" skin. Courtesy of CDC Public Health Image Library.

necessary. If left untreated, permanent scarring can occur. SCC may occur in long-standing lesions.

Black Hairy Tongue

Black hairy tongue is a harmless but distinctive presentation of overgrowth of filiform papillae and bacteria or fungi, causing a dark and hairy appearance (**Figure 137**). Poor hygiene, tobacco use, coffee and tea consumption, dry mouth, and medications such as antibiotics can contribute to the appearance. Management includes better oral hygiene, such as tongue scraping, and modifying risk factors, including tobacco and medication use.

Geographic Tongue

Geographic tongue (benign migratory glossitis) is a common, benign inflammatory condition of the dorsal tongue that presents with migratory areas of smooth red surfaces and white patches, creating a map-like appearance (**Figure 138**). Although generally asymptomatic, a burning sensation can occur, and it may be exacerbated by hot or spicy foods. It has been reported in association with psoriasis. Management consists of analgesics and avoidance of triggers.

Oral Candidiasis

Oral candidiasis can present in a variety of ways. The most common presentation is that of white, nonadherent plaques on the tongue, palate, and gingiva with a burning sensation (thrush) (**Figure 139**). It also can present as angular cheilitis, which are painful erythematous patches in one or both corners of the mouth; concomitant bacterial super-infection also can occur. Risk factors are immunosuppression (HIV infection or transplantation), oral glucocorticoid use, antibiotic use, and

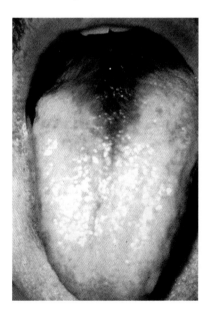

FIGURE 137. Black hairy tongue is most commonly associated with antibiotic use, coffee and tea consumption, poor oral hygiene, and smoking.

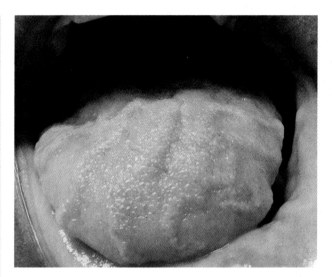

FIGURE 138. Geographic tongue (benign migratory glossitis) showing irregularly shaped, map-like migratory patches on the dorsal tongue.

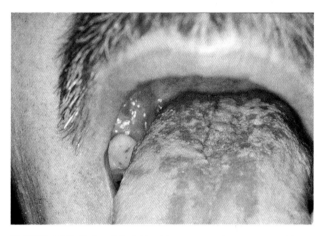

FIGURE 139. Oral candidiasis (thrush) most commonly presents as a white, fluffy, nonadherent film on the tongue, buccal mucosa, or palate.

xerostomia with thrush, and poor-fitting dentures with drooling for angular cheilitis. Diagnosis can be made using potassium hydroxide (KOH) examination, and treatment with oral antifungal preparations such as azole troches or nystatin swish and swallow mouthwash is effective. Oral antifungal agents can be used in patients with severe or recalcitrant candidiasis.

Foot and Leg Ulcers

Lower extremity ulcerations may be divided into several categories, including venous stasis ulcers, arterial insufficiency ulcers, neuropathic ulcers, infectious ulcers, ulcers due to malignancy, drug-induced ulcers, ulcers associated with sickle cell anemia, and ulcers resulting from inflammatory conditions such as pyoderma gangrenosum (see Cutaneous Manifestations of Internal Disease). Discriminating among them is important, as the treatments differ widely depending on the underlying cause.

Venous Stasis Ulcers

Ulcerations are one of the most common complications of long-standing venous stasis disease. Most patients have a history of stasis dermatitis and often have some level of scarring and dyspigmentation on the bilateral lower extremities (see Common Rashes). The same mechanism of impaired venous drainage causing changes in vascular permeability with stretching of the skin may lead to loss of integrity of the dermal barrier and development of ulceration. Venous stasis ulcers usually occur on the distal lower leg, particularly the medial aspect of the ankle, and may result from a minor trauma, a medical procedure, or an acute stasis dermatitis flare. The symptoms vary from negligible discomfort to significant pain. The ulcers tend to have an irregular border and surrounding hyperpigmentation, and the skin and subcutaneous tissues are thickened, resulting in lipodermatosclerosis (fibrosing panniculitis of the subcutaneous tissue) (**Figure 140**). Patients often have varicose veins and peripheral edema.

Treatment is directed toward three main areas: reducing the peripheral edema, creating a wound environment that is conducive to healing, and treating any secondary infection that may be present.

Reduction of peripheral edema is achieved by the use of compression stockings, pneumatic compression boots, and compression dressings (Unna boots). In some patients with evidence of hypervolemia, low salt diets, and diuretics (hydrochlorothiazide or furosemide) may be indicated. Since some patients may have a significant degree of arterial insufficiency as well, determination of their arterial circulation status by measuring the ankle-brachial index may be helpful in patients with significant risk factors for arterial disease to ensure that excessive compression (and resultant arterial ischemia) is not performed. Venous ultrasonography is generally not indicated, however, since the clinical examination is ordinarily sufficient to establish venous insufficiency.

Creating a desirable wound environment is critical to encourage healing. Wounds should be moist but not overly saturated. Wounds that are dry may be covered with hydrogel or hydrocolloid dressings to increase the moisture content. Debridement of necrotic tissue may be necessary. Alginate and foam dressings may be used when excessive exudate is present.

Cultures of many chronic wounds, such as stasis ulcers, will typically reveal a polymicrobial mixture of bacteria; in most patients this represents colonization rather than acute infection. Nevertheless, keeping the bacterial burden low is a desirable goal, since having a significant bacterial burden likely interferes with wound healing. Reduction of the bacterial burden is achieved (when needed) by temporary and judicious use of silver impregnated dressings or similar local antimicrobial preparations. Topical antibiotics should be used with caution, however, because of the potential for the development of contact dermatitis and resistant bacteria and thus should be avoided if possible. Clues to suggest active infection are worsening pain, swelling, and copious exudate; these findings would be an indication for oral antibiotics.

KEY POINTS

- Venous stasis ulcers occur on the distal lower leg and are typically associated with signs of chronic venous insufficiency.
- Treatment consists of compression, creating a wound environment that is conducive to healing, and treating any secondary infection that may be present.

Arterial Insufficiency Ulcers

Arterial insufficiency ulcers develop in patients with a history of significant atherosclerotic disease of the extremities and are caused by a lack of blood flow to these areas. They tend to be painful; discomfort may increase with elevation of the legs, compression, or any other maneuver that further limits circulation. Unlike venous stasis ulcers, which often have somewhat irregular borders and a significant amount of surrounding postinflammatory hyperpigmentation and lipodermatosclerosis, arterial insufficiency ulcers have a "punched out" appearance with surrounding erythema. The extremities as a whole often appear pale, and the skin is thin, taut, and shiny and lacks hair (**Figure 141**). Pedal pulses are often difficult to appreciate, the toes are cold, and capillary refill is poor. If arterial insufficiency is suspected, diagnosis can be confirmed by measuring

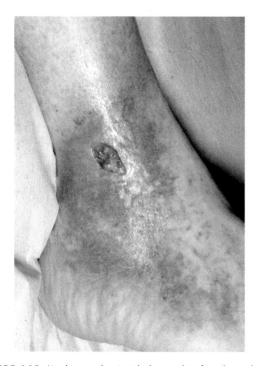

FIGURE 140. Lipodermatosclerosis with ulcer, resulting from chronic thickening of the skin in chronic venous stasis dermatitis.

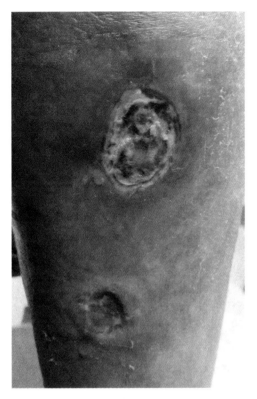

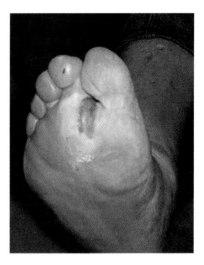

FIGURE 142. Neuropathic ulcers have a hyperkeratotic rim and occur over pressure points such as the metatarsal heads.

from further trauma. Daily examination of the feet in patients with diabetes is encouraged. The ulcers can be quite deep and occasionally extend into the bone; thus, early identification and treatment are crucial to prevent development of osteomyelitis and avoid potential amputation.

KEY POINTS

- Neuropathic ulcers are painless and typically occur in areas prone to trauma, such as the plantar aspects of the feet or friction points.
- Daily examination of the feet in patients with diabetes mellitus is encouraged to check for neuropathic ulcers; early identification and treatment are crucial to avoid potential amputation.

Other Causes of Lower Extremity Ulcers

Pyoderma gangrenosum is an extremely painful ulcerating inflammatory condition seen most commonly in patients with inflammatory bowel disease; it may also be associated with rheumatoid arthritis, hematologic malignancies, and liver disease. It should be suspected in patients with the appropriate history and also when no other obvious cause for ulceration exists. Pyoderma gangrenosum may be confused with various other causes of ulceration such as stasis ulcers, infections, and pressure ulcers. Squamous cell carcinomas may also arise on the lower extremities and present as ulcers that clinically may appear nearly identical to the other types; thus, biopsy should be considered when ulcers fail to improve despite appropriate therapeutic measures. Certain organisms, including fungi and atypical mycobacteria, can cause chronic ulcers and should be suspected in patients who have an appropriate travel history or who are immunocompromised (see Cutaneous Manifestations of Internal Disease).

FIGURE 141. Arterial insufficiency ulcers appear sharply demarcated or "punched out," and the surrounding skin is red, taut, and tender.

the ankle-brachial index. The ulcers are treated with debridement and dressings similar to venous stasis ulcers; the same antibacterial preparations are also used when necessary. One important distinction, however, is that compression will increase pain and worsen arterial insufficiency ulcers, whereas the opposite is true with venous stasis ulcers. Surgical revascularization to improve the lower extremity circulation is often necessary to facilitate wound healing.

KEY POINTS

- Arterial insufficiency ulcers have a "punched out" appearance with surrounding erythema.
- In patients with arterial insufficiency ulcers, surgical revascularization to improve the lower extremity circulation is often necessary to facilitate wound healing.

Neuropathic Ulcers

Neuropathic ulcers arise from recurrent trauma in patients who have lost sensation in a given limb. Diabetes mellitus is the most common underlying predisposing factor, but other causes of nerve damage, or less common disorders such as tertiary syphilis, may be responsible. The ulcers are painless and typically occur in areas prone to trauma, such as the plantar aspects of the feet or friction points created by poorly fitting orthotic devices (**Figure 142**). Treatment consists of debridement, use of appropriate dressings, and protection

Dermatologic Problems of Special Populations

Treatment of Dermatologic Conditions in Pregnancy

Pregnant and nursing women need special consideration because potential medication-related teratogenicity can limit the treatment options for dermatologic diseases. Dermatologic conditions can be chronic and unchanged during pregnancy, and pregnancy itself can induce normal changes (**Table 36**). The FDA assigns categories for every medication to indicate the potential of a drug to cause birth defects if used during pregnancy. These categories and the risk-to-benefit ratio should be considered before prescribing medications to any woman of childbearing potential, including those attempting pregnancy, pregnant women, or nursing mothers. The specific trimester and developmental stage should be considered as medications carry different risks depending on the developmental period.

FDA pregnancy category X medications should never be used in pregnant or nursing women, and those specifically prescribed in dermatology are methotrexate, thalidomide, and retinoids (**Table 37**). Importantly, men who are potential fathers should not take methotrexate. There are regulatory systems that monitor certain medications such as iPledge for isotretinoin and STEPs for thalidomide because of the significant potential detriment to fetuses.

Management with topical agents often is considered before prescribing systemic medications because they are lower risk, with the exception of tazarotene (category X). Glucocorticoids are pregnancy category C, but are generally thought to be safe,

TABLE 37. Selected FDA Pregnancy Category X Drugs to Avoid During Pregnancy and Lactation
Acitretin
Danazol
Estrogens
Finasteride
5-Fluorouracil
Flutamide
Isotretinoin
Methotrexate
Stanozolol
Tazarotene (topical)
Thalidomide

especially topical formulations. The lowest required amount for therapeutic efficacy is used. Antihistamines also are considered safe in pregnancy (except hydroxyzine in the first trimester), but they should be avoided in breastfeeding mothers because of risks of sedation in infants.

Tetracyclines are frequently used in dermatology; however, they should be avoided because of the risk of staining the teeth and bone during fetal development (category D). Trimethoprim-sulfamethoxazole should also be avoided because it can interfere with folic acid metabolism (category C). Other antibiotic classes such as the penicillins (category B) and cephalosporins (category B) are safer choices during pregnancy. Spironolactone may be used to treat acne but should not be used for acne in pregnant women because of risks of feminization in a fetus.

TABLE 36.	Normal Dermatologic Changes Observed During Pregnancy	
	Finding	**Characteristics**
Hyperpigmentation	Melasma	"Mask of pregnancy," brown patches on face and neck, occasionally extremities
	Linea nigra	Line of pigmentation on the abdomen that may extent centrally from the pubis to xiphoid
	Nipples, areolae, axillae, genitals	Skin may darken in pregnancy; moles also may darken
Striae gravidarum	Stretch marks	May start pink to red and then become paler over time
Hair and Nails	Hair	May thicken during pregnancy, and then loss of hair about 3 months postpartum is common (telogen effluvium)
	Nails	May grow faster during pregnancy
Vascular changes	Spider angiomas	Common on face, neck, extremities
	Hemorrhoids and varicose veins	Occur in about 40% of women
	Palmar erythema	Increased redness on palms seen in two thirds of women
	Edema	Diffuse swelling can occur; lower leg edema is common
	Vaginal erythema (Chadwick sign) and blue discoloration of cervix (Goodell sign)	Due to increased blood flow and congestion
	Gingival hyperemia and edema	Occurs in some extent to all women; pyogenic granulomas also can occur

If dermatologic surgical procedures during pregnancy are indicated, low doses of local anesthetics, including lidocaine and epinephrine are safe to use; however, sedatives and opioids should be avoided in pregnant and breastfeeding women.

KEY POINTS

- FDA pregnancy category X medications should never be used in pregnant or breastfeeding women, and those specifically prescribed in dermatology are methotrexate, thalidomide, and retinoids.
- Management with topical agents often is considered before prescribing systemic medications to pregnant women because they are lower risk than systemic medications, with exception of topical tazarotene (FDA pregnancy category X).

Aging

Several common and uncommon skin conditions become more prevalent during aging, and the skin structure and function change with age. Autoimmune blistering diseases are rare, but bullous pemphigoid is more common after the age of 60 years, and the risk increases each year thereafter. The most common skin conditions to affect older patients are pruritus, inflammatory dermatoses, fungal infections, and bacterial and viral infections.

Changes Due to Chronologic Aging and Photoaging

A myriad of changes occur in the skin over time; these can be due to chronologic aging alone or influenced by the cumulative effects of ultraviolet light exposure (**Table 38**).

Xerosis (dry skin) is more common in older patients and is often associated with pruritus (see Pruritus). Actinic purpura is caused by age-related capillary fragility and bleeding under atrophic skin. It is common on the forearms and dorsal hands, but may be seen anywhere on the body (**Figure 143**). It is not a sign of vasculitis, a bleeding disorder, or nutritional deficiency, and does not require additional evaluation or therapy. Stellate

TABLE 38. Common Skin Findings of Intrinsic Aged Versus Photoaged Skin

Intrinsic Aging	Photoaging
Thinned epidermis	Coarse furrows
Loss of subcutaneous fat	Fine wrinkles
Fine wrinkles	Diffuse pigmentation; "bronzing"
Dry, flaky skin	Lentigines
Loss of elasticity	Pebbly texture of skin (elastosis)
Skin pallor	Solar purpura
Decreased skin temperature	Telangiectasia

pseudoscars are jagged or linear atrophic scars that primarily occur on the forearms of patients with chronic actinic damage. Patients may or may not recall antecedent trauma. Stellate pseudoscars are often seen in conjunction with actinic purpura.

Inflammatory Skin Conditions

Xerotic eczema occurs in areas of excessively dry skin. The lower legs are common areas. Patients with severe xerotic eczema can develop poorly demarcated, scaly patches interspersed with superficial red fissures in a netlike distribution (**Figure 144**). The appearance has been likened to cracked porcelain or a dry lake bed (see Common Rashes).

Seborrheic dermatitis is more common as age increases. Greasy scaling of the scalp, brows, nose, and cheeks may develop. Areas such as the axillae and central chest may be affected (see Common Rashes).

Infection

Herpes zoster and postherpetic neuralgia are more frequent in older persons, and the risk of these conditions can be reduced with immunization (see MKSAP 17 General Internal Medicine). Infestations by scabies, lice, or bedbugs can occur in group

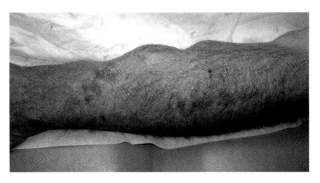

FIGURE 143. Actinic purpura on the forearm of a patient with an iatrogenic fistula.

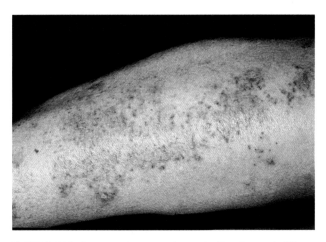

FIGURE 144. Severe xerotic eczema is characterized by redness and a "tile-like" pattern on dry skin (xerosis) with evidence of trauma from scratching. This typically occurs during midwinter in northern climates.

living arrangements. Fungal infections of the feet and toenails are very common in older populations; however, not all nail changes are caused by fungus. The nail changes in color, texture, and thickness with age. These changes can be mistaken for onychomycosis (see Nail Disorders).

Skin of Color

Melanocytes are responsible for the wide variety of skin colors observed. The variation in skin color among individuals is due to variability in the size, distribution, and melanin concentration of the melanosomes. Melanin absorbs and scatters energy from ultraviolet (UV) light, so persons with darker skin have a lower risk of sun damage, but are more likely to develop pigmentation alteration, both hyper- and hypopigmentation. Persons with skin of color can be affected by novel and common skin conditions. Inflammatory dermatoses can have a more subtle appearance since the pink-red color that is a sign of inflammation can be difficult to see on darker skin (**Figure 145**). The most common skin problems in people with skin of color are acne, dyschromia or any alteration in skin color (darker or lighter), seborrheic dermatitis, atopic dermatitis, or other causes of dermatitis.

Differences in Pigmentation

Persons with skin of color often have normal variations in skin color with areas of hyperpigmentation along the gingiva and lines of demarcation on the trunk and extremities. Traumatic or inflammatory skin damage can also cause pigment altera-

tion. Scrapes, bug bites, or acne often heal with hyperpigmentation. Areas of active inflammation from seborrhea, eczema, or psoriasis may develop hypopigmentation. Topical or intralesional glucocorticoids can also cause hypopigmentation, which can be difficult to distinguish from the effects of a rash; upon cessation of the medication the dyschromia will improve. Partial or complete depigmentation is also seen in idiopathic guttate hypomelanosis, which manifests as 2- to 6-mm hypopigmented macules on the trunk and extremities.

Vitiligo affects about 1% to 2% of the general population but is more difficult to treat for patients with darker skin color because of the dramatic difference in the depigmented (white) skin and preserved areas of natural pigmented skin (**Figure 146**). The peak onset is between 10 and 30 years of age, and the most common form is a generalized form that has a predilection for the eyes, nostrils, and mouth and is often bilaterally symmetric. Topical glucocorticoids are the most frequent therapies for vitiligo and can be used for patients with limited or generalized disease. Ultraviolet light therapy is frequently used for generalized disease since it can be difficult to apply medications diffusely. When depigmentation affects nearly the entire body and is unresponsive to treatment, depigmentation of the remaining normal skin is considered.

Treatment of hyperpigmentation is challenging. Depigmenting agents such as hydroquinone, azelaic acid, and kojic acid target different steps in the production of melanin. Topical retinoids can be used in combination with depigmenting agents for additional effect. Procedures including chemical peeling and laser therapy, can be effective but can be expensive, and adverse effects can be severe. Cosmetic camouflage is an affordable option for most patients. Sunscreen can reduce the recurrence of pigment.

Acne Keloidalis Nuchae and Pseudofolliculitis Barbae

Both acne keloidalis nuchae (AKN) and pseudofolliculitis barbae (PFB) are characterized by firm, skin-colored, pink, or hyperpigmented papules that are often centered on hair

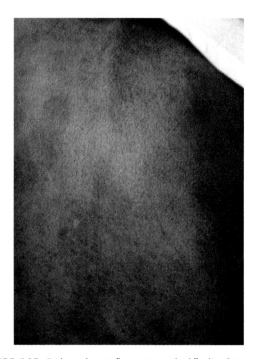

FIGURE 145. Erythema due to inflammation can be difficult to distinguish in people with more skin color. This patient has secondary syphilis manifesting as dark brown patches without erythema.

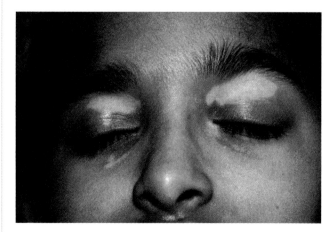

FIGURE 146. Symmetric patches of generalized vitiligo on the eyelids.

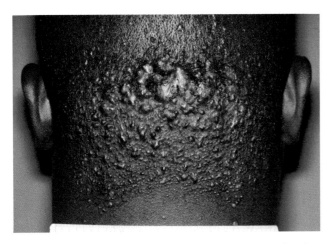

FIGURE 147. Skin-colored papules and plaques on the posterior scalp and nape of the neck from acne keloidalis nuchae.

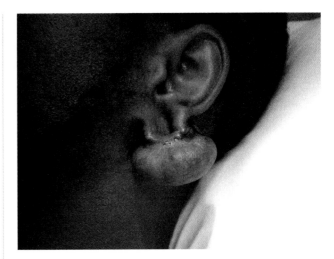

FIGURE 148. Large keloid on the earlobe as a result of an ear piercing.

follicles. AKN often occurs on the posterior scalp and neck (**Figure 147**), whereas PFB occurs on the face and anterior neck. These conditions are most likely caused by the trauma of an ingrown hair. The hair follicle in people with skin of color is often curved, and the hair grows out of the skin in a spiral. Rather than spiral outward smoothly, occasionally the hair punctures the side of the follicle and can incite an inflammatory response and subsequent skin lesions that range from small papules to large keloids (see Hair Disorders). The differential diagnosis includes acne and bacterial folliculitis. Acne will often occur at any site on the face rather than being limited to areas of terminal hairs. Infectious folliculitis presents with red papules and pustules; however, it is often distributed across an area such as the scalp or trunk rather than preferentially in the beard or posterior scalp. Acne and folliculitis do not usually heal with fibrotic papules. Therapy aims to minimize inflammation and secondary infection, flatten scars, and alter damage done by hairs. Topical and oral antibiotics, glucocorticoids (topical or intralesional), changes in shaving habits, and laser hair removal can be used, often in combination.

Keloids

Black persons are at least twice as likely as white persons to develop keloids. Keloids are an overgrowth of dermal collagen often in response to skin injury such as piercing, tattoo, surgery, or acne (**Figure 148**). The upper trunk, neck, and ears are frequent sites. Keloids can be asymptomatic, painful, or pruritic. In contrast to hypertrophic scars and typical scars, keloids extend beyond the border of the original injury. There is no single preferred treatment. Options include topical and intralesional glucocorticoids, laser therapy, intralesional chemotherapy, and radiation therapy. Intralesional glucocorticoids are often the first-line therapy but must be repeated about every 8 weeks and three to four injections are needed to demonstrate significant improvement. Topical glucocorti-

coids are generally ineffective for keloids but can be effective for hypertrophic scars. Surgical excision alone is avoided as recurrence is frequent, and surgery is often paired with intralesional glucocorticoids. Similar to surgery, laser therapy, for example with a pulsed dye laser, is often paired with intralesional glucocorticoids.

Skin Cancers

Although less common, both nonmelanoma and melanoma skin cancers occur in skin of color populations. Although skin cancer rates are lower, cancers are often found later than in white populations. Both patients and physicians need to be suspicious of growing, bleeding, or ulcerating lesions.

The frequency of basal cell carcinoma (BCC) is inversely correlated with the degree of pigmentation in the skin; those most commonly affected are fair-skinned white persons, followed by Hispanics, and the least frequently affected are black persons. Pigmented BCC is more common in those with darker skin. Otherwise the behavior and treatment are the same, and metastasis is rare.

Darkly pigmented persons can develop squamous cell carcinoma (SCC); however, in contrast to the UV-induced type seen in the white population, SCC often develops in areas of chronic inflammation or scarring and is found more often on the legs. SCC developing in these settings has a metastasis rate of 20% to 40%, compared with a rate of 1% to 4% in white persons with UV-induced SCC.

Acral lentiginous melanoma (ALM) constitutes 5% to 10% of all melanomas yet is the most common type in those with skin of color. The most common sites are the palms, soles, and nails (**Figure 149**). Melanoma rates are lower in persons of color than in the white population; however, the average time to diagnosis is 2 years. Even after adjusting for age, stage, site, and socioeconomic status, the 5-year survival rates of blacks and Hispanics are lower than those of white persons.

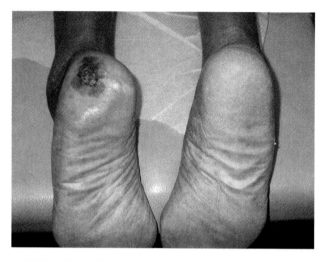

FIGURE 149. Acral lentiginous melanoma presents on an acral site such as the foot or hand and may involve the nail. It often has an irregular shape, color variation, and in later stages may ulcerate.

Melanonychia

Melanonychia refers to brown or black coloration of the nails. Longitudinal melanonychia is a common form in which brown lines traverse the nail proximally to distally. This is a normal variant that is found in 50% of black persons. The thumb and forefinger are most commonly affected (**Figure 150**). The condition is often bilateral. The prevalence and number of nails affected increases with age. The differential diagnosis includes other pigmented lesions of the nail such as a nevus, acral lentiginous melanoma, postinflammatory hyperpigmentation, pigmented squamous cell carcinoma, blood extravasation from trauma, and drug pigmentation. A biopsy of a pigmented band in the nail should be considered only if a single digit is affected, if it developed during the fourth decade or later, if there is associated nail dystrophy, if the diameter is 4 mm or greater, if the characteristics of the band changes, or if there is a personal or family history of melanoma.

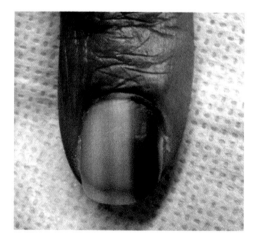

FIGURE 150. Longitudinal melanonychia showing hyperpigmentation at the proximal nail fold, a clinical sign suggesting the presence of subungual melanoma.

The Homeless

Skin problems, most commonly infections and infestations, are the main reasons the homeless seek medical attention. The foot is the most frequent site of disorders such as ulcers, cellulitis, erysipelas, and gas gangrene. Poor foot hygiene, inadequate footwear, and excessive moisture are frequent and result in high rates of tinea pedis (30% to 40%) and pitted keratolysis (20%). Infestations with scabies, lice, and bedbugs are frequent and affect 25% of those in a shelter. The body louse can transmit *Bartonella quintana*, which has caused trench fever, bacillary angiomatosis, endocarditis, and chronic afebrile bacteremia in the homeless. Epidemic typhus caused by *Rickettsia prowazekii* and relapsing fever caused by *Borrelia recurrentis* are also louse borne.

Pruritus is a common problem of the homeless and may be attributed to a primary skin dermatosis, medications or illicit drug use, or occult or uncontrolled internal disease. Pruritus is often accompanied by bacterial infection from poor hygiene and secondary infection of excoriations. Common skin dermatoses, such as psoriasis, seborrheic dermatitis, and atopic eczema, occur in the homeless. It isn't known if inflammatory dermatoses are more frequent in this population; however, it is possible that common dermatoses are more severe because of poor hygiene, exposure to cold, moisture, and difficult medical access.

Dermatologic Diseases of Overweight Patients

Intertrigo

Intertrigo is an inflammatory process found in skin fold areas such as the inframammary region, abdominal pannus, and crural folds. It is particularly problematic in hot, moist conditions, and thus annual exacerbations during the summer are commonly seen. The rash consists of confluent, well-demarcated erythema, generally symmetrically distributed. Secondary infection by yeast can often occur and is generally characterized by multiple small red macules that surround the main rash (satellitosis). Treatment consists of keeping the area dry and well-ventilated. Antifungal powders may be useful in controlling moisture and are frequently used to reduce the likelihood of flares. Low- or mid-potency topical glucocorticoid creams may be used for a short period of time, but prolonged use should be avoided to prevent skin thinning and stretch mark formation. If secondary infection with yeast is present, concomitant treatment with topical antifungal agents may be added.

Stasis Dermatitis

Obese persons and those with poor venous circulation are particularly prone to stasis dermatitis. Treatment consists of compression stockings and topical glucocorticoids (see Common Rashes). Long-standing untreated peripheral edema can also lead to massive localized lymphedema and elephantiasis nostras verrucosa, a debilitating condition characterized by substantial swelling of the lower extremities with skin thickening and the development of multiple warty-appearing nodules in the affected area.

Acrochordons

Acrochordons (skin tags) are commonly found in obese persons in areas of recurrent friction, such as the axillae and groin. They may also be seen on the eyelids and around the neck. Although harmless, they are often of cosmetic concern. The combination of acanthosis nigricans and skin tags around the neck and in the axillae is often seen in obese patients with diabetes mellitus.

Bibliography

Approach to the Patient with Dermatologic Disease

Ashton RE. Teaching non-dermatologists to examine the skin: a review of the literature and some recommendations. Br J Dermatol. 1995 Feb;132(2):221-5. [PMID: 7888358]

Choudhury K, Volkmer B, Greinert R. Christophers E, Breitbart EW. Effectiveness of skin cancer screening programmes. Br J Dermatol. 2012 Aug;167 Suppl 2:94-8. [PMID: 22881593]

Wolff T, Taie E, Miller T. Screening for skin cancer: an update of the evidence for the US Preventive Services Task Force. Ann Intern Med. 2009 Feb 3;150(3):194-8. [PMID: 19189909]

Therapeutic Principles in Dermatology

Cook D. FDA experience: topical corticosteroids and HPA axis suppression. www.fda.gov/ohrms/dockets/ac/03/slides/3999s1_03_cook.ppt. Accessed January 6, 2014.

Tan X, Feldman SR, Chang J, Balkrishnan R. Topical drug delivery systems in dermatology: a review of patient adherence issues. Expert Opin Drug Deliv. 2012 Oct;9(10):1263-71. [PMID: 22861153]

Weiss SC. Conventional topical delivery systems. Dermatol Ther. 2011 Sep-Oct;24(5):471-6. [PMID: 22353153]

Common Rashes

Chamlin SL, Kao J, Frieden IJ, et al. Ceramide-dominant barrier repair lipids alleviate childhood atopic dermatitis: Changes in barrier function provide a sensitive indicator of disease activity. J Am Acad Dermatol. 2002 Aug;47(2):198-208. [PMID: 12140465]

DeAngelis YM, Gemmer CM, Kaczvinsky JR, Kenneally DC, Schwartz JR, Dawson TL Jr. Three etiologic facets of dandruff and seborrheic dermatitis: Malassezia fungi, sebaceous lipids, and individual sensitivity. J Investig Dermatol Symp Proc. 2005 Dec;10(3):295-7. [PMID: 16382685]

Gelfand, JM Neimann, AL. et al. Risk of myocardial infarction in patients with psoriasis. JAMA. 2006 Oct 11;296(14):1735-41. [PMID: 17032986]

Huerta C, Rivero E, Rodríguez LA. Incidence and risk factors for psoriasis in the general population. Arch Dermatol. 2007 Dec;143(12):1559-65. [PMID: 18087008]

Jensen P, Zachariae C, Christensen R, et al. Effect of weight loss on the severity of psoriasis: a randomized clinical study. JAMA Dermatol. 2013 Jul;149(7):795-801. [PMID: 23752669]

Kagami S, Rizzo HL, Lee JJ, Koguchi Y, Blauvelt A. Circulating Th17, Th22, and Th1 cells are increased in psoriasis. J Invest Dermatol. 2010 May;130(5):1373-83. [PMID: 20032993]

Lodi G, Pellicano R, Carrozzo M. Hepatitis C virus infection and lichen planus: a systematic review with meta-analysis. Oral Dis. 2010 Oct;16(7):601-12. [PMID: 20412447]

Martignoni E, Godi L, Pacchetti C, et al. Is seborrhea a sign of autonomic impairment in Parkinson's disease? J Neural Transm. 1997;104(11-12):1295-304. [PMID: 9503275]

Sánchez-Pérez J, De Castro M, Buezo GF, Fernandez-Herrera J, Borque MJ, García-Díez A. Lichen planus and hepatitis C virus: prevalence and clinical presentation of patients with lichen planus and hepatitis C virus infection. Br J Dermatol. 1996 Apr;134(4):715-9. [PMID: 23752669]

Wollenberg A, Räwer HC, Schauber J. Innate immunity in atopic dermatitis. Clin Rev Allergy Immunol. 2011 Dec;41(3):272-81. [PMID: 21181301]

Acneiform Eruptions

Alikhan A, Lynch PJ, Eisen DB. Hidradenitis suppurativa: a comprehensive review. J Am Acad Dermatol. 2009 Apr;60(4):539-61. [PMID: 19293006]

Kennedy Carney C, Cantrell W, Elewski BE. Rosacea: a review of current topical, systemic and light-based therapies. G Ital Dermatol Venereol. 2009 Dec;144(6):673-88. [PMID: 19907406]

Rambhatla PV, Lim HW, Hamzavi I. A systematic review of treatments for hidradenitis suppurativa. Arch Dermatol. 2012 Apr;148(4):439-46. [PMID: 22184715]

Stone DU, Chodosh J. Ocular rosacea: an update on pathogenesis and therapy. Curr Opin Ophthalmol. 2004 Dec;15(6):499-502. [PMID: 15523195]

Strauss JS, Krowchuk DP, Leyden JJ, et al; American Academy of Dermatology/American Academy of Dermatology Association. Guidelines of care for acne vulgaris management. J Am Acad Dermatol. 2007 Apr;56(4):651-63. [PMID: 17276540]

Thiboutot D, Gollnick H, Bettoli V, et al. New insights into the management of acne: an update from the Global Alliance to Improve Outcomes in Acne group. J Am Acad Dermatol. 2009 May;60(5 suppl):S1-50. [PMID: 19376456]

van Zuuren EJ, Kramer SF, Carter BR, Graber MA, Fedorowicz Z. Effective and evidence-based management strategies for rosacea: summary of a Cochrane systematic review. Br J Dermatol. 2011 Oct;165(4):760-81. [PMID: 21692773]

Common Skin Infections

Avci O, Tanyildizi T, Kusku E. A comparison between the effectiveness of erythromycin, single-dose clarithromycin and topical fusidic acid in the treatment of erythrasma. J Dermatol Treat. 2013 Feb;24(1):70-4. [PMID: 21923567]

Cohen JI. Clinical practice: herpes zoster. N Engl J Med. 2013 Jul 18;369(3):255-63. [PMID: 23863052]

Daum RS. Clinical practice: skin and soft-tissue infections caused by methicillin-resistant Staphylococcus aureus. N Engl J Med. 2007 Jul 26;357(4):380-90. [PMID: 17652653]

Gormley RH, Kovarik CL. Human papillomavirus-related genital disease in the immunocompromised host: part I, II. J Am Acad Dermatol. 2007 Jul 26;357(4):380-90. [PMID: 22583721]

Gupta AK, Batra R, Bluhm R, Boekhout T, Dawson TL Jr. Skin diseases associated with Malassezia species. J Am Acad Dermatol. 2004 Nov;51(5):785-98. [PMID: 15523360]

Huang SS, Septimus E, Kleinman K, et al. Targeted versus universal decolonization to prevent ICU infection. N Engl J Med. 2013 Jun 13;368(24):2255-65. [PMID: 23718152]

Liu C, Bayer A, Cosgrove SE, et al. Clinical practice guidelines by the Infectious Diseases Society of America for the treatment of methicillin-resistant Staphylococcus aureus infections in adults and children. Clin Infect Dis. 2011 Feb 1;52(3):285-92. [PMID: 21217178]

Moriarty B, Hay R, Morris-Jones R. The diagnosis and management of tinea. BMJ. 2012 Jul 10;345:e4380. [PMID: 22782730]

Oon S-F, Winter DC. Perianal condylomas, anal squamous intraepithelial neoplasms and screening: a review of the literature. J Med Screen. 2010;17(1):44-9. [PMID: 20356945]

Rigopoulos D, Larios G, Gregoriou S, Alevizos A. Acute and chronic paronychia. Am Fam Physician. 2008 Feb 1;77(3):339-46. [PMID: 18297959]

Thomas KS, Crook AM, Nunn AJ, et al. Penicillin to prevent recurrent leg cellulitis. N Engl J Med. 2013 May 2;368(18):1695-703. [PMID: 23635049]

Bibliography

Infestations

Currie BJ, McCarthy JS. Permethrin and ivermectin for scabies. N Engl J Med. 2010 Feb 25;362(8):717-25. [PMID: 20181973]

Kolb A, Needham GR, Neyman KM, High WA. Bedbugs. Dermatol Ther. 2009 Jul-Aug;22(4):347-52. [PMID: 19580578]

Pariser DM, Meinking TL, Bell M, Ryan WG. Topical 0.5% ivermectin lotion for treatment of head lice. N Engl J Med. 2012 Nov;367(18):1687-93. [PMID: 23113480]

Shimose L, Munoz-Price LS. Diagnosis, prevention, and treatment of scabies. Curr Infect Dis Rep. 2013 Aug 1 [epub ahead of print]

Wolf R, Davidovici B. Treatment of scabies and pediculosis: facts and controversies. Clin Dermatol. 2010 Sep-Oct;28(5):511-8. [PMID: 20797511]

Bites and Stings

Haddad V Jr, Cardoso JL, Lupi O, Tyring SK. Tropical dermatology: venomous arthropods and human skin: part I. Insecta. J Am Acad Dermatol. 2012 Sep;67(3):331.e1-14. [PMID: 22890734]

Haddad V Jr, Cardoso JL, Lupi O, Tyring SK. Tropical dermatology: venomous arthropods and human skin: part II. Diplopoda, Chilopoda, and Arachnida. J Am Acad Dermatol. 2012 Sep;67(3):347.e1-9. [PMID: 22890735]

Miller MJ, Gomez HF, Snider RG. Stephens EL, Czop RM, Warren JS. Detection of Loxosceles venom in lesional hair shafts and skin: application of a specific immunoassay to identify dermonecrotic arachnidism. Am J Emerg Med. 2000 Sep;18(5):626-8. [PMID: 10999583]

Cuts, Scrapes, and Burns

Alsbjörn B, Gilbert P, Hartmann B, Kaźmierski M, Monstrey S, Palao R, Roberto MA, Van Trier A, Voinchet V. Guidelines for the management of partial-thickness burns in a general hospital or community setting–recommendations of a European working party. Burns. 2007 Mar;33(2):155-60. [PMID: 17280913]

Hettiaratchy S Initial management of a major burn: II–assessment and resuscitation. BMJ. 2004 July 10; 329(7457):101-3. [PMID: 15242917]

Alharbi Z, Piatkowski A, Dembinski R, et al. Treatment of burns in the first 24 hours: simple and practical guide by answering 10 questions in a step-by-step form. World J Emerg Surg. 2012 May 14;7(1):13. [PMID: 22583548]

Common Neoplasms

Alam M, Ratner D. Cutaneous squamous-cell carcinoma. N Engl J Med. 2001 Mar 29;344(13):975-83. [PMID: 11274625]

Balch CM, Gershenwald JE, et al. Final version of 2009 AJCC melanoma staging and classification. J Clin Oncol. 2009 Dec 20;27(36):6199-206. [PMID: 19917835]

Duffy K, Grossman D. The dysplastic nevus: from historical perspective to management in the modern era: Part I. Historical, histologic, and clinical aspects. J Am Acad Dermatol. 2012 Jul;67(1):19.e1-12. [PMID: 22703916]

Luba MC, Bangs SA, Mohler AM, Stulberg DL. Common benign skin tumors. Am Fam Physician. 2003 Feb 15;67(4):729-38. [PMID: 12613727]

Rigel DS, Gold LF. The importance of early diagnosis and treatment of actinic keratosis. J Am Acad Dermatol. 2013 Jan;68(1 Suppl 1):S20-7. [PMID: 23228303]

Rubin AI, Chen EH, Ratner D. Basal cell carcinoma. N Engl J Med. 2005 Nov 24;353(21):2262-9. [PMID: 16306523]

Tsao H, Atkins MB, Sober AJ. Management of cutaneous melanoma. N Engl J Med. 2004 Sep 2;351(10):998-1012. [PMID: 15342808]

Pruritus

Cassano N, Tessari G, Vena GA, Girolomoni G. Chronic pruritus in the absence of specific skin disease: an update on pathophysiology, diagnosis, and therapy. Am J Clin Dermatol. 2010 Dec 1;11(6):399-411. [PMID: 20866115]

Reamy BV, Bunt CW, Fletcher S. A diagnostic approach to pruritus. Am Fam Physician. 2011 Jul 15;84(2):195-202. [PMID: 21766769]

Ständer S, Weisshaar E, Mettang T, et al. Clinical classification of itch: a position paper of the International Forum for the Study of Itch. Acta Derm Venereol. 2007;87(4):291-4. [PMID: 17598029]

Yosipovitch G, Bernhard JD. Clinical practice: chronic pruritus. N Engl J Med. 2013 Apr 25;368(17):1625-34. [PMID: 23614588]

Urticaria

Spector, SL, Tan, SL. Effect of omalizumab on patients with chronic urticaria. Annals of Allergy, Asthma & Immunology. 2007 Aug;99(2):190-3. [PMID: 17718108]

Autoimmune Blistering Diseases

Di Zenzo G. Marazza G, Borradori L. Bullous pemphigoid; physiopathology, clinical features and management. Adv Dermatol. 2007;23:257-88. [PMID: 18159905]

Egan CA, Lazarova Z, Darling TN, Yee C, Coté T, Yancey KB. Anti-epiligrin cicatricial pemphigoid and relative risk for cancer. Lancet. 2001 Jun 9;357(9271):1850-1. [PMID: 11410196]

Hervonen K, Vornanen M, Kautiainen H, Collin P, Reunala T. Lymphoma in patients with dermatitis herpetiformis and their first-degree relatives. Br J Dermatol. 2005 Jan;152(1):82-6. [PMID: 15656805]

Reddy H, Shipman AR, Wojnarowska F. Epidermolysis bullosa acquisita and inflammatory bowel disease: a review of the literature. Clin Exp Dermatol. 2013 Apr;38(3):225-30. [PMID: 23517353]

Ruocco E, Wolf R, Caccavale S, Brancaccio G, Ruocco V, Lo Schiavo A. Bullous pemphigoid: Associations and management guidelines: Facts and controversies. Clin Dermatol. 2013 Jul-Aug;31(4):400-12. [PMID: 23806157]

Saw VP, Dart JK. Ocular mucous membrane pemphigoid; diagnosis and management strategies. Ocul Surf. 2008 Jul;6(3):128-42. [PMID: 18781259]

Schmidt E, Bröcker EB, Goebeler M. Rituximab in treatment-resistant autoimmune blistering skin disorders. Clin Rev Allergy Immunol. 2008 Feb;34(1):56-64. [PMID: 18270859]

Schmidt E, Zillikens D. Modern diagnosis of autoimmune blistering skin diseases. Autoimmun Rev. 2010 Dec;10(2):84-9. [PMID: 20713186]

Zone JJ. Skin manifesations of celiac disease. Gastroenterology. 2005 Apr;128 (4 suppl 1):S87-91. [PMID: 15825132]

Cutaneous Manifestations of Internal Disease

Dabade TS, Davis MS. Diagnosis and treatment of the neutrophilic dermatoses (pyoderma gangrenosum, Sweet's syndrome). Dermatol Ther. 2011 Mar-Apr;24(2):273-84. [PMID: 21410617]

Haimovic A, Sanchez M, Judson MA, Prystowsky S. Sarcoidosis: a comprehensive review and update for the dermatologist: part I. Cutaneous disease. J Am Acad Dermatol. 2012 May;66(5):699.e1-18 [PMID: 22507585]

Haimovic A, Sanchez M, Judson MA, Prystowsky S. Sarcoidosis: a comprehensive review and update for the dermatologist: part II. Extracutaneous disease. J Am Acad Dermatol. 2012 May;66(5):719.e1-10. [PMID: 22507586]

Lowe G, Henderson CL, Grau RH, Hansen CB, Sontheimer RD. A systematic review of drug-induced subacute cutaneous lupus erythematosus. Br J Dermatol. 2011 Mar;164(3):465-72. [PMID: 21039412]

Micheletti R, Rosenbach M. An approach to the hospitalized patient with urticaria and fever. Dermatol Ther. 2011 Mar-Apr;24(2):187-95. [PMID: 21410608]

Miller J, Yentzer BA, Clark A, Jorizzo JL, Feldman SR. Pyoderma gangrenosum: a review and update on new therapies. J Am Acad Dermatol. 2010 Apr;62(4):646-54. [PMID: 20227580]

Morganroth PA, Kreider ME, Okawa J, Taylor L, Werth VP. Interstitial lung disease in classic and clinically amyopathic dermatomyositis: a retrospective study with screening recommendations. Arch Dermatol. 2010 Jul;146(7):729-38. [PMID: 20644033]

Okon LG, Werth VP. Cutaneous lupus erythematosus: diagnosis and treatment. Best Pract Res Clin Rheumatol. 2013 Jun;27(3):391-404. [PMID: 24238695]

Ramos-Casals M, Stone JH, Cid MC, Bosch X. The cryoglobulinaemias. The Lancet. 2012 Jan 28;379(9813):348-60. [PMID: 21868085]

Ross EA. Evolution of treatment strategies for calciphylaxis. Am J Nephrol. 2011;34(5):460-7. [PMID: 21986387]

Thornsberry LA, LoSicco KI, English JC 3rd. The skin and hypercoaguable states. J Am Acad Dermatol. 2013 Sep;69(3):450-62. [PMID: 23582572]

Yagub A, Chung L, Rieger KE, Fiorentino DF. Localized cutaneous fibrosing disorders. Rheum Dis Clin North Am. 2013 May;39(2):347-64. [PMID: 23597968]

Zaba LC, Fiorentino DF. Skin disease in dermatomyositis. Curr Opin Rheumatol. 2012 Nov;24(6):597-601. [PMID: 22907594]

Dermatologic Urgencies and Emergencies

Bastuji-Garin S, Fouchard N, Bertocchi M, et al. SCORTEN: a severity-of-illness score for toxic epidermal necrolysis. J Invest Dermatol. 2000 Aug;115(2):149-53. [PMID: 10951229]

Bruno TF, Grewal P. Erythroderma: a dermatologic emergency. Clin J Endocrinol Metab. 2009 May;11(3):244-6. [PMID: 19523275]

Khaled A, Sellami A, Fazaa B, et al. Acquired erythroderma in adults: a clinical and prognostic study. J Eur Acad Dermatol Venereol. 2010 Jul;24(7):781-8. [PMID: 20028449]

Okoduwa C, Lambert WC, Schwartz RA, et al. Erythroderma: review of a potentially life-threatening dermatosis. Indian J Dermatol. 2009;54(1):1-6. [PMID: 20049259]

Poon SH, Baliog CR Jr, Sams RN, Robinson-Bostom L, Telang GH, Reginato AM. Syndrome of cocaine-levamisole-induced cutaneous vasculitis and immune-mediated leukopenia. Semin Arthritis Rheum. 2011 Dec;41(3):434-44. [PMID: 21868067]

Scully C, Bagan J. Oral mucosal diseases: erythema multiforme. Br J Oral Maxillofac Surg. 2008 Mar;46(2):90-5. [PMID: 17767983]

Wetter DA, Camilleri MJ. Clinical, etiologic, and histopathologic features of Stevens-Johnson syndrome during an 8-year period at Mayo Clinic. Mayo Clin Proc. 2010 Feb;85(2):131-8. [PMID: 20118388]

Wysong A, Venkatesan P. An approach to the patient with retiform purpura. Dermatol Ther. 2011 Mar-Apr;24(2):151-72. [PMID: 21410606]

Hair Disorders

Curran DR, Moore C, Huber T. Clinical inquiries: what is the best approach to the evaluation of hirsutism? J Fam Pract. 2005 May;54(5):465-7. [PMID: 15865908]

González U, Seaton T, Bergus G, Jacobson J, Martínez-Monzón C. Systemic antifungal therapy for tinea capitis in children. Cochrane Database Syst Rev. 2007 Oct 17;(4):CD004685. [PMID: 17943825]

Hordinsky M. Cicatricial alopecia: discoid lupus erythematosus. Dermatol Ther. 2008 Jul-Aug;21(4):245-8. [PMID: 18715293]

Moriarty B, Hay R, Morris-Jones R. The diagnosis and management of tinea. BMJ. 2012 Jul 10;345:e4380. [PMID: 22782730]

Mounsey AL, Reed SW. Diagnosing and treating hair loss. Am Fam Physician. 2009 Aug 15;80(4):356-62. [PMID: 19678603]

Rácz E, Gho C, Moorman PW, Noordhoek Hegt V, Neumann HA. Treatment of frontal fibrosing alopecia and lichen planopilaris: a systematic review. J Eur Acad Dermatol Venereol. 2013 Mar 26. [PMID: 23531029]

Nail Disorders

Cohen PR, Scher RK. Geriatric nail disorders: diagnosis and treatment. J Am Acad Dermatol. 1992 Apr;26(4):521-31. [PMID: 1597537]

Holzberg M. Common nail disorders. Dermatol Clin. 2006 Jul;24(3):349-54. [PMID: 16798432]

Rigopoulos D, Larios G, Gregoriou S, Alevizos A. Acute and chronic paronychia. Am Fam Physician. 2008 Feb 1;77(3):339-46. [PMID: 18297959]

Singh G, Haneef NS, Uday A. Nail changes and disorders among the elderly. Indian J Dermatol Venereol Leprol. 2005 Nov-Dec;71(6):386-92. [PMID: 16394478]

Disorders of Mucous Membranes

Ebrahimi M, Lundqvist L, Wahlin YB, Nylander E. Mucosal lichen planus, a systemic disease requiring multidisciplinary care: a cross-sectional clinical review from a multidisciplinary perspective. J Low Genit Tract Dis. 2012 Oct;16(4):377-80. [PMID: 22622344]

Gonsalves WC, Chi AC, Neville BW. Common oral lesions: Part I. Superficial mucosal lesions. Am Fam Physician. 2007 Feb 15;75(4):501-7. [PMID: 17323710]

McPherson T, Cooper S. Vulval lichen sclerosus and lichen planus. Dermatol Ther. 2010 Sep-Oct;23(5):523-32. [PMID: 20868406]

Mirowski GW, Schlosser BJ. The diagnosis and treatment of oral mucosal lesions. Dermatol Ther. 2010 May-Jun;23(3):207-8. [PMID: 20597939]

Reamy BV, Derby R, Bunt CW. Common tongue conditions in primary care. Am Fam Physician. 2010 Mar 1;81(5):627-34. [PMID: 20187599]

Silverman S Jr. Mucosal lesions in older adults. J Am Dent Assoc. 2007;138 (Suppl):41S-46S. [PMID: 17761845]

van der Waal I. Potentially malignant disorders of the oral and oropharyngeal mucosa; terminology, classification and present concepts of management. Oral Oncol. 2009 Apr-May;45(4-5):317-23. [PMID: 18674954]

Foot and Leg Ulcers

Alavi A, Sibbald RG, Mayer D, et al. Diabetic foot ulcers: Part I. Pathophysiology and prevention. J Am Acad Dermatol. Jan;70(1):1.e1-1.e18. [PMID: 24355275]

Grey JE, Enoch S, Harding KG. Venous and arterial leg ulcers. BMJ. 2006 Feb 11;332(7537):347-50. [PMID: 16470058]

Richmond NA, Maderal AD, Vivas AC. Evidence-based management of common lower extremity ulcers. Dermatol Ther. 2013 May-Jun;26(3):187-96. [PMID: 23742279]

Dermatologic Problems of Special Populations

Brouqui P, Raoult D. Arthropod-borne diseases in homeless. Ann N Y Acad Sci. 2006 Oct;1078:223-35. [PMID: 17114713]

Callender VD, St Surin-Lord S, Davis EC, Maclin M. Postinflammatory hyperpigmentation: etiologic and therapeutic considerations. Am J Clin Dermatol. 2011 Apr 1;12(2):87-99. [PMID: 21348540]

Gloster HM Jr, Neal K. Skin cancer in skin of color. J Am Acad Dermatol. 2006 Nov;55(5):741-64. [PMID: 17052479]

Huggins RH, Schwartz RA, Janniger CK. Vitiligo. Acta Dermatolovenereol Alp Panonica Adriat. 2005;14(4):137-42. [PMID: 16435042]

Jefferson J, Rich P. Melanonychia. Dermatol Res Pract. 2012;2012:952186. [PMID: 22792094]

Leachman SA, Reed BR. The use of dermatologic drugs in pregnancy and lactation. Dermatol Clin. 2006 Apr;24(2):167-97. [PMID: 16677965]

Manuskiatti W, Fitzpatrick RE. Treatment response of keloidal and hypertrophic sternotomy scars: comparison among intralesional corticosteroid, 5-fluorouracil, and 585-nm flashlamp-pumped pulsed-dye laser treatments. Arch Dermatol. 2002 Sep;138(9):1149-55. [PMID: 12224975]

Moy JA, Sanchez MR. The cutaneous manifestations of violence and poverty. Arch Dermatol. 1992 Jun;128(6):829-39. [PMID: 1599274]

Patel T, Yosipovitch G. The management of chronic pruritus in the elderly. Skin Therapy Lett. 2010 Sep;15(8):5-9. [PMID: 20844849]

Raoult D, Foucault C, Brouqui P. Infections in the homeless. Lancet Infect Dis. 2001 Sep;1(2):77-84. [PMID: 11871479]

Richards KA, Stasko T. Dermatologic surgery and the pregnant patient. Dermatol Surg. 2002 Mar;28(3):248-56. [PMID: 11896778]

Schmidt E, della Torre R, Borradori L. Clinical features and practical diagnosis of bullous pemphigoid. Immunol Allergy Clin North Am. 2012 May;32(2): 217-32. [PMID: 22560135]

Stratigos AJ, Stern R, Gonzalez E, et al. Prevalence of skin disease in a cohort of shelter-based homeless men. J Am Acad Dermatol. 1999 Aug;41(2 Pt 1): 197-202. [PMID: 10426888]

Tyler KH, Zirwas MJ. Pregnancy and dermatologic therapy. J Am Acad Dermatol. 2013 Apr;68(4):663-71. [PMID: 23182064]

Venugopal SS, Murrell DF. Diagnosis and clinical features of pemphigus vulgaris. Immunol Allergy Clin North Am. 2012 May;32(2):233-43. [PMID: 22560136]

Yalçin B, Tamer E, Toy GG, Oztaş P, Hayran M, Alli N. The prevalence of skin diseases in the elderly: analysis of 4099 geriatric patients. Int J Dermatol. 2006 Jun;45(6):672-6. [PMID: 16796625]

Yosipovitch G, DeVore A, Dawn A. Obesity and the skin: Skin physiology and skin manifestations of obesity. J Am Acad Dermatol. 2007 Jun;56(6):901-16. [PMID: 17504714]

Dermatology Self-Assessment Test

This self-assessment test contains one-best-answer multiple-choice questions. Please read these directions carefully before answering the questions. Answers, critiques, and bibliographies immediately follow these multiple-choice questions. The American College of Physicians is accredited by the Accreditation Council for Continuing Medical Education (ACCME) to provide continuing medical education for physicians.

The American College of Physicians designates MKSAP 17 **Dermatology** for a maximum of **12** *AMA PRA Category 1 Credits*™. Physicians should claim only the credit commensurate with the extent of their participation in the activity.

Earn "Instantaneous" CME Credits Online

Print subscribers can enter their answers online to earn Continuing Medical Education (CME) credits instantaneously. You can submit your answers using online answer sheets that are provided at mksap.acponline.org, where a record of your MKSAP 17 credits will be available. To earn CME credits, you need to answer all of the questions in a test and earn a score of at least 50% correct (number of correct answers divided by the total number of questions). Take any of the following approaches:

➢ Use the printed answer sheet at the back of this book to record your answers. Go to mksap.acponline.org, access the appropriate online answer sheet, transcribe your answers, and submit your test for instantaneous CME credits. There is no additional fee for this service.

➢ Go to mksap.acponline.org, access the appropriate online answer sheet, directly enter your answers, and submit your test for instantaneous CME credits. There is no additional fee for this service.

➢ Pay a $15 processing fee per answer sheet and submit the printed answer sheet at the back of this book by mail or fax, as instructed on the answer sheet. Make sure you calculate your score and fax the answer sheet to 215-351-2799 or mail the answer sheet to Member and Customer Service, American College of Physicians, 190 N. Independence Mall West, Philadelphia, PA 19106-1572, using the courtesy envelope provided in your MKSAP 17 slipcase. You will need your 10-digit order number and 8-digit ACP ID number, which are printed on your packing slip. Please allow 4 to 6 weeks for your score report to be emailed back to you. Be sure to include your email address for a response.

If you do not have a 10-digit order number and 8-digit ACP ID number or if you need help creating a user name and password to access the MKSAP 17 online answer sheets, go to mksap.acponline.org or email custserv@acponline.org.

CME credit is available from the publication date of July 31, 2015, until July 31, 2018. You may submit your answer sheets at any time during this period.

Item 1

A 62-year-old woman is evaluated for multiple areas of scaling and rough skin on her forehead and cheeks, the backs of her hands, and forearms. These areas are painless but persist despite application of moisturizer. She is in good overall health and takes no medications. She has a history of multiple sunburns.

On physical examination, vital signs are normal. Skin findings are shown.

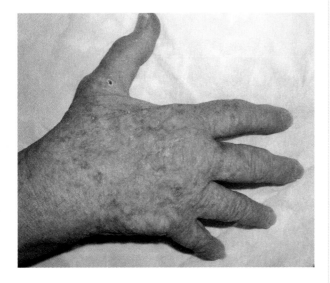

The remainder of the physical examination is unremarkable.

Which of the following is the most likely diagnosis?

(A) Actinic keratosis
(B) Seborrheic keratosis
(C) Squamous cell carcinoma
(D) Superficial basal cell carcinoma

Item 2

A 19-year-old man is evaluated for a 3-year history of firm bumps in his hairline at the back of his neck. He is concerned because they are increasing in number and occasionally are itchy. Skin findings are shown.

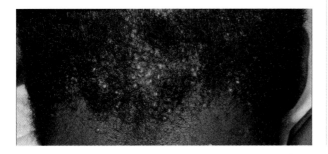

The rest of his skin examination is normal.

Which of the following is the most likely diagnosis?

(A) Acne keloidalis nuchae
(B) Acne vulgaris
(C) Bacterial folliculitis
(D) Keloids

Item 3

A 41-year-old man is evaluated because of his "red face." He notices that his face gets redder when he goes out in the sun, gets out of the shower, or drinks hot coffee. He is most bothered by the pimples he gets on his cheeks and chin. His skin is not itchy or painful. He takes no medications, drinks three or four beers on the weekend, and otherwise feels well. General physical examination findings are unremarkable. Skin findings are shown.

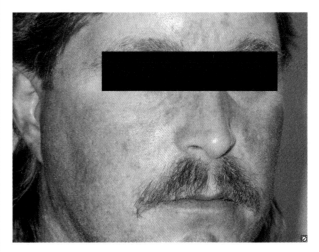

Which of the following is the most likely diagnosis?

(A) Acute cutaneous lupus erythematosus
(B) Periorificial dermatitis
(C) Rosacea
(D) Seborrheic dermatitis

Item 4

A 75-year-old woman is evaluated for a 7-month history of an ulcer on the inner portion of her right ankle. In addition to the ulcer, she notes that an oozing, weeping rash periodically develops in the surrounding area, and that a similar rash sometimes occurs on her other leg. She also experiences intermittent lower extremity edema on the legs bilaterally. Medical history is significant for long-standing type 1 diabetes mellitus and hypertension. Medications are insulin glargine, metformin, and lisinopril.

On physical examination, vital signs are normal. BMI is 32. Pedal pulses are palpable, and the patient has good capillary refill in the toes. The ulcer is not tender. She has multiple venous varicosities. Skin findings are shown.

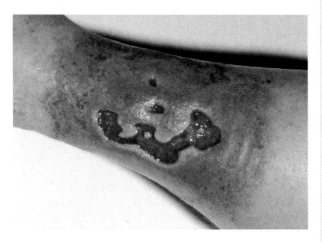

Which of the following is the most likely diagnosis?

(A) Arterial ulcer
(B) Neuropathic ulcer
(C) Pyoderma gangrenosum
(D) Venous stasis ulcer

Item 5

A 72-year-old man is evaluated for discoloration of the tongue and bad breath. He notes the gradual onset of the tongue changes, with development of significant halitosis in recent weeks. He otherwise feels well and has no other symptoms. Medical history is unremarkable. He smokes a half-pack of cigarettes per day and drinks two to three glasses of wine or beer each night. He takes no medications.

On physical examination, the patient is afebrile and vital signs are normal. The appearance of the tongue is shown.

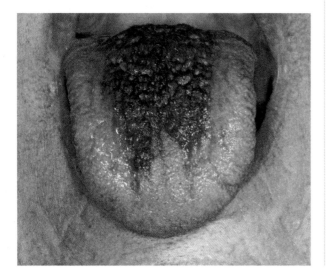

Dentition is poor, but there are no other lesions in the oral cavity. There is no lymphadenopathy in the head or neck. The remainder of the examination is unremarkable.

Which of the following is the most appropriate management?

(A) Amoxicillin-clavulanate
(B) Biopsy of the discolored area
(C) Brushing of the tongue
(D) Fluconazole

Item 6

A 30-year-old man presents to the clinic with a concern about the appearance of his fingernails. His fingernails on both hands have been pitting, yellowing, and lifting off the nail bed for the past 6 months. He has not tried to treat his nail changes.

On physical examination, there are no changes in his toenails or the skin of his feet. There are well-demarcated pink, scaling plaques on his elbows and knees. Fingernail findings are shown.

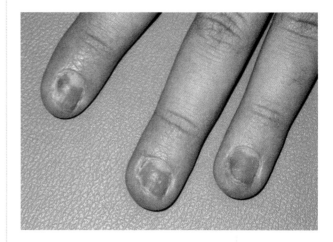

Which of the following is the most likely cause of this patient's fingernail changes?

(A) Candidal infection
(B) Eczema
(C) Psoriasis
(D) Tinea manuum

Item 7

A 20-year-old male farmer is evaluated for a several-month history of increasing odor and wetness involving both of his feet during the summer months. He otherwise feels well and has no pain or other foot-related symptoms. Medical history is unremarkable, and he takes no medications.

Oh physical examination, vital signs are normal. Examination of the feet is notable for a significant malodor. Skin findings are shown (see top of next page).

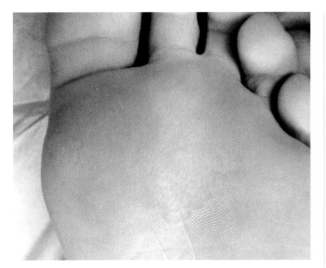

The remainder of his examination is noncontributory.

Which of the following is the most appropriate topical treatment?

(A) Clotrimazole cream
(B) Clotrimazole-betamethasone cream
(C) Erythromycin lotion
(D) Hydrocortisone cream

Item 8

A 27-year-old woman is evaluated for a 1-week history of an intensely pruritic rash on her eyelids. She applied a new brand of eye makeup just prior to the onset of the rash. She immediately discontinued its use and has been applying a moisturizing lotion to both eyelids since then without improvement in her symptoms. She notes no other areas of rash and generally feels well. The patient has no significant medical history and takes no medications.

On physical examination, vital signs are normal. There is erythema, mild edema, and some serous crusting over the upper eyelids bilaterally. No erythema is present on the scalp, face, neck, upper back, shoulders, arms, or fingers. The remainder of the examination is normal.

A 2-week course of which of the following is the most appropriate treatment for this patient?

(A) Betamethasone dipropionate
(B) Clobetasol propionate
(C) Halobetasol propionate
(D) Hydrocortisone valerate

Item 9

A 72-year-old man sustains a laceration on his left index finger while preparing chicken. He immediately washes the area and applies neomycin and an occlusive bandage. He changes the bandage and reapplies the medication twice daily. Two days later, he develops itching and redness at the wound site. He has had no fever or other systemic

symptoms. Medical history is significant for well-controlled type 2 diabetes mellitus. His only medication is metformin.

On physical examination, vital signs are normal. The left index finger shows a 1.0-cm superficial wound with well-approximated margins without purulence or drainage, and no pain on palpation. There are pinpoint papules and vesicles in an area extending 0.5 cm around the laceration site in a rectangular pattern approximating the bandage. There is no lymphangitic streaking. The remainder of the physical examination is unremarkable.

Which of the following is the most likely diagnosis?

(A) Allergic contact dermatitis
(B) Group A streptococcal infection
(C) Herpes simplex virus infection
(D) *Staphylococcus aureus* infection

Item 10

A 44-year-old woman is evaluated for a 2-year history of hair loss. She has noticed hair loss on the top of her scalp, but not from the sides or back of her scalp. Her father and brother have "bald spots," but she states that her mother and grandmother are "normal."

On physical examination, vital signs are normal. Her scalp findings are shown.

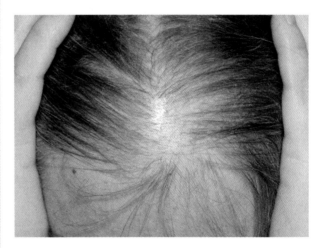

Which of the following is the most likely cause of the patient's alopecia?

(A) Alopecia areata
(B) Androgenetic alopecia
(C) Frontal fibrosing alopecia
(D) Telogen effluvium

Item 11

A 34-year-old man is evaluated for several slow-growing lesions on his penis. He first noticed the wart-like growths 3 years ago, and they have progressively enlarged. He was treated with topical cryotherapy six times and topical imiquimod over the past year without improvement; the lesions have continued to enlarge. Medical history is significant for HIV infection. Medications are tenofovir, emtricitabine, and efavirenz.

On physical examination, vital signs are normal. Multiple red to brown verrucous papules with underlying induration and focal erosions are present on the penile shaft.

There is no lymphadenopathy. There are no other skin findings, and the remainder of the physical examination is normal.

Laboratory studies are significant for a CD4 cell count of 875/μL (0.875 × 10⁹/L) and an undetectable viral load.

Which of the following is the most appropriate management?

(A) Biopsy
(B) Cryotherapy
(C) Human papillomavirus (HPV) vaccination
(D) Topical triamcinolone cream

Item 12

A 53-year-old woman is evaluated for an ulcer on the bottom of her foot. Medical history is significant for type 2 diabetes mellitus and hypertension. Medications are metformin and lisinopril.

On physical examination, blood pressure is 128/78 mm Hg; other vital signs are also normal. A painless ulcer is present on the plantar aspect of the right foot. Skin findings are shown.

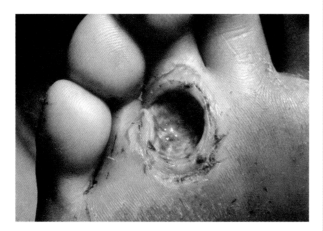

Pedal pulses are intact.

Which of the following is the most likely diagnosis?

(A) Arterial ulcer
(B) Neuropathic ulcer
(C) Squamous cell carcinoma
(D) Venous stasis ulcer

Item 13

A 20-year-old woman is evaluated for growth of dark brown hairs on her cheeks and neck. The growth began 5 years ago, and she finds it bothersome. She has tried to manage the growth by using depilatory creams. She otherwise feels

well, her medical history is unremarkable, and she takes no medications. She notes irregular menstrual cycles, having fewer than six periods in a calender year. There is no history of similar hair growth affecting the women in her family.

On physical examination, vital signs are normal. BMI is 30. Skin findings on the face are shown.

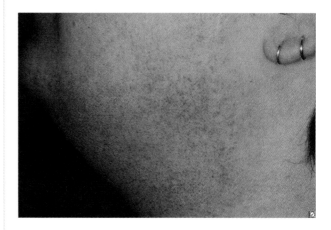

Breast development and external gynecologic examination are normal. The remainder of the physical examination is normal.

Which of the following is the most likely cause of this patient's facial hair?

(A) Familial hair growth pattern
(B) Hyperthyroidism
(C) Polycystic ovary syndrome
(D) Porphyria

Item 14

A 35-year-old woman is evaluated for a rash on her hands and arms. The previous day she was clearing vines in her backyard. The skin eruption is red and intensely itchy, and she has scratched multiple areas. She experiences a burning sensation when she applies moisturizer. The patient has a history of depression for which she takes sertraline.

On physical examination, vital signs are normal. Skin findings are shown.

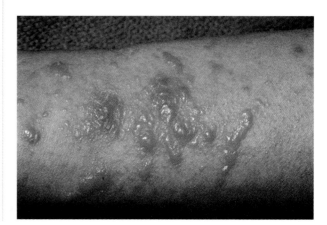

The remainder of the examination is unremarkable.

Which of the following is the most appropriate topical therapy for this patient's skin eruption?

(A) Bacitracin
(B) Diphenhydramine
(C) High-potency glucocorticoid ointment
(D) Low-potency glucocorticoid cream

Item 15

A 61-year-old woman with long-standing pedal edema is evaluated for redness on the bilateral lower legs. She notes that the edema worsens over the course of the day but is improved with elevation of her legs. She reports no pain or pruritus, no calf tenderness, no shortness of breath, no palpitations, and otherwise feels well. Medical history is significant for obesity but is otherwise unremarkable. She takes no medications.

On physical examination, vital signs are normal. BMI is 36. There is no jugular venous distention. The lungs are clear, and an S_3 is not present. Pedal pulses are normal, and there is no calf tenderness. Skin findings are shown.

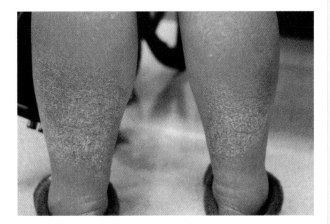

The remainder of the physical examination is non-contributory.

Which of the following is the most appropriate treatment?

(A) Compression stockings
(B) Oral cephalexin
(C) Oral furosemide
(D) Topical mupirocin

Item 16

A 49-year-old woman has a 20-year history of painful papules and nodules of the perineum and perianal skin. Her underarms are not involved. She develops several concurrent nodules every other month, and these prevent her from working for a week or more. Occasionally some of the nodules will spontaneously drain foul-smelling fluid. The nodules have been unresponsive to antibacte-rial soaps and lotions and topical and systemic antibiotic therapy, and recur following incision and drainage. The patient has no other medical problems other than obesity and cigarette smoking.

On physical examination, vital signs are normal. BMI is 30. Skin findings are shown.

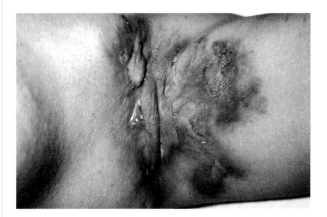

Which of the following is the most likely diagnosis?

(A) Bacterial abscesses
(B) Bacterial folliculitis
(C) Hidradenitis suppurativa
(D) Ruptured epidermal cysts

Item 17

A 68-year-old man is evaluated for a 6-month history of a rapidly growing nodule on the lower lip. He notes mild tenderness surrounding this area. Medical history is significant for a 40-pack-year history of smoking, moderate alcohol consumption, and significant sun exposure. He is otherwise in good health and takes no medications.

On physical examination, vital signs are normal. The nodule is shown.

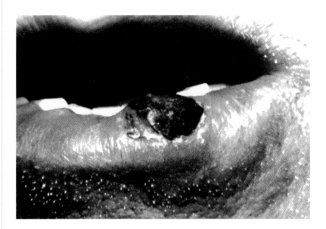

The remainder of the physical examination is unre-markable.

Which of the following is the most appropriate next step in management?

(A) Bacterial culture

(B) Cryotherapy

(C) Electrodesiccation and curettage

(D) Lesional biopsy

(E) Topical 5-fluorouracil

Item 18

A 62-year-old woman is evaluated for a 4-month history of decreased exercise tolerance, joint stiffness, mild weakness, and a rash on her hands. She has noted increasing difficulty carrying heavy objects and feels exhausted after climbing stairs. Although her joints are stiff, she has not had any joint swelling. Her rash developed around the time of her other symptoms and has not responded to over-the-counter topical agents. She has no other symptoms, including cough or dyspnea. Medical history is unremarkable, and she takes no medications.

On physical examination, temperature is 37.2 °C (99.0 °F), blood pressure is 109/72 mm Hg, pulse rate is 82/min, and respiration rate is 20/min. Oxygen saturation is 98% on ambient air. Cardiopulmonary examination is unremarkable. Joint examination is normal. Skin findings are shown.

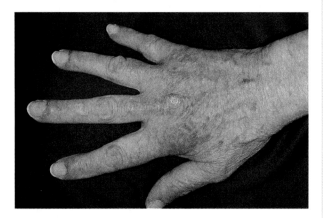

Laboratory studies:

Creatine kinase	320 U/L
Antinuclear antibodies	Positive (titer of 1:640)
Anti-dsDNA antibodies	Negative
Anti-Ro/SSA antibodies	Negative
Anti-La/SSB antibody	Negative
Complete blood count	Normal
Metabolic profile	Normal

A plain chest radiograph is normal.

Which of the following pulmonary conditions is associated with this patient's clinical presentation?

(A) Bronchiectasis

(B) Diffuse alveolar hemorrhage

(C) Hilar lymphadenopathy

(D) Interstitial lung disease

(E) Pleuritis

Item 19

A 53-year-old woman is evaluated for a slowly enlarging, telangiectatic, pearly, ulcerated 1-cm plaque on the left temple. It bleeds periodically when traumatized. Medical history is significant for atrial fibrillation. She takes warfarin daily. She is otherwise in good health.

On physical examination, vital signs are normal. Cardiac examination shows an irregular heart rate but is otherwise normal. The remainder of the examination is unremarkable.

Biopsy of the lesion reveals a basal cell carcinoma with micronodular and infiltrative features.

Which of the following is the most appropriate treatment for this lesion?

(A) Cryotherapy

(B) Electrodesiccation and curettage

(C) Mohs micrographic surgery

(D) Radiation therapy

(E) Topical imiquimod

Item 20

A 32-year-old woman is evaluated at a well-patient visit. Both her parents have a history of nonmelanoma skin cancer within the past year, and she is seeking counseling regarding skin cancer prevention. She has a history of remote sunburns and had previously tanned as a teenager. She requests advice on how to approach sun protection to limit both future skin cancer risk as well as to prevent wrinkles and cosmetic photodamage.

The patient has no other significant medical history and takes no medications.

On physical examination, vital signs are normal. She has mild scattered wrinkling, scattered solar lentigines, and an average number of benign-appearing nevi.

Which of the following is the most appropriate advice for this patient?

(A) Maintain a baseline tan

(B) Sunscreen with sun protection factor (SPF) 2 to 14

(C) Sunscreen with SPF 15 or greater

(D) Sunscreen with SPF 15 or greater plus UVA protection

Item 21

A 67-year-old woman is evaluated for a chronic rash under her breasts and arms, and in the groin and upper thigh region. She notes that the rash is intermittent and tends to be worse in the summer months. Medical history is significant for type 2 diabetes mellitus, hypertension, and hyperlipidemia. Medications are metformin, lisinopril, and simvastatin.

On physical examination, vital signs are normal. BMI is 39. Skin findings are shown (see top of next page).

The remainder of the examination is normal.

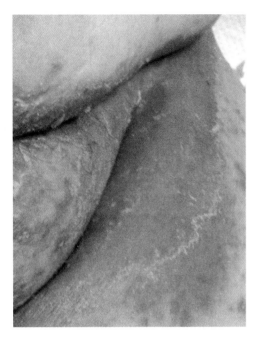

Which of the following is the most likely diagnosis?

(A) Allergic contact dermatitis

(B) Atopic dermatitis

(C) Cellulitis

(D) Intertrigo

Item 22

A 53-year-old man is evaluated for itching lasting 5 months. He reports that his whole body is itchy and that a short course of emollients and antihistamine medication did not improve his symptoms. He feels well otherwise. Review of systems is negative including findings for fever, fatigue, and unintentional weight loss. He does not take any medications.

On physical examination, vital signs are normal. Examination of the skin reveals no signs of xerosis or inflammation. Excoriations are noted on his legs, shoulders, and back. The remainder of the physical examination, including thyroid and lymph node examinations, is normal.

A complete blood count, metabolic profile, serum thyroid-stimulating hormone level, liver chemistry tests, and HIV antibody assay are normal.

Which of the following is the most appropriate next step in management?

(A) Chest radiograph

(B) CT scan of the chest, abdomen, and pelvis

(C) Skin biopsy

(D) No further testing

Item 23

A 19-year-old man is evaluated for a month-long history of rash. He states that the rash is extremely itchy; he has areas of involvement under his arms, around his waist, on his

wrists, between his fingers, and on his palms. Medical history is unremarkable, and he takes no medications. He has not attempted to treat the rash. He is temporarily homeless and has been staying with different friends or in the local shelter. Two months ago, he left the apartment of a friend who had a similar rash.

The general physical examination is unremarkable. Skin examination shows scattered, excoriated lesions that spare the feet. Skin lesions on the hand are shown.

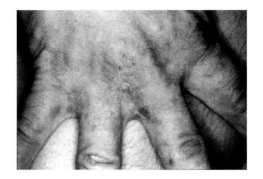

Which of the following is the most likely diagnosis?

(A) Allergic contact dermatitis

(B) Bedbug bites

(C) Scabies infestation

(D) Tinea manuum

Item 24

A 72-year-old woman is evaluated for a pruritic rash on the abdomen. She reports previous episodes of similar symptoms in the past. Medical history is significant for type 2 diabetes mellitus and hypertension. Medications are metformin, valsartan, hydrochlorothiazide, and a clonidine patch.

On physical examination, vital signs are normal. Skin findings are shown.

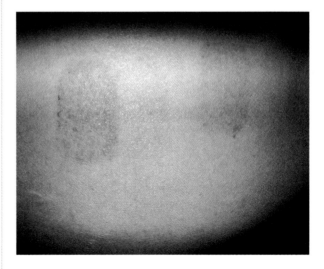

The remainder of the physical examination is unremarkable.

Which of the following is the most likely cause of this patient's skin findings?

(A) Allergic contact dermatitis

(B) Fixed drug eruption

(C) Irritant dermatitis

(D) Tinea corporis

Item 25

A 25-year-old man is evaluated in the emergency department for fever of 48 hours' duration and a rash for 24 hours. His illness began with fever followed by fine, red, itchy papules on the trunk, arms, and legs. The rash soon became painful. This morning, he awoke with the rash on his face and sores in his mouth, and when he touched his skin it peeled off. Two weeks ago, he began minocycline and tretinoin cream for acne. He has no other medical problems.

On physical examination, he is toxic appearing and in pain. Temperature is 39.4 °C (102.9 °F), blood pressure is 110/60 mm Hg, pulse rate is 116/min, and respiration rate is 18/min. His eyes are red, and his mouth and lips are covered with a bloody film. Representative skin findings are shown.

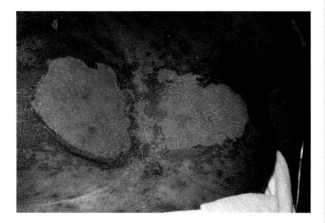

Which of the following management options is most likely to benefit this patient?

(A) Infliximab

(B) Intravenous methylprednisone

(C) Intravenous vancomycin and ceftriaxone

(D) Supportive care and discontinuation of minocycline

Item 26

A 52-year-old woman is evaluated for a 1-month history of a spreading rash on her back, chest, and arms. She has been using over-the-counter topical glucocorticoids without relief. She does not have any other associated symptoms and otherwise feels well. Medical history is significant for hypertension. Medications are hydrochlorothiazide and metoprolol.

On physical examination, temperature is 37.1 °C (98.7 °F), blood pressure is 141/83 mm Hg, pulse rate is 72/min, and respiration rate is 18/min. Skin findings are shown (see top of next column).

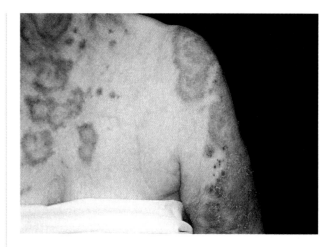

There are no lesions in the scalp or ears, no finger or nail changes, no joint inflammation, and no oral ulcers. The remainder of the physical examination is unremarkable.

Laboratory studies:

Antinuclear antibodies	Positive (titer of 1:320)
Anti-Ro/SSA antibodies	Positive
Anti-La/SSB antibodies	Negative
Antihistone antibodies	Negative
Creatine kinase	Normal

Which of the following is the most likely diagnosis?

(A) Dermatomyositis

(B) Pemphigus foliaceus

(C) Psoriasis

(D) Subacute cutaneous lupus erythematosus

Item 27

A 78-year-old woman is hospitalized for management of acute worsening of chronic kidney disease. On the third hospital day, she develops a painful nodule under the tape adjacent to the site of a peripheral intravenous catheter on her left forearm. Medical history is also significant for hypertension and type 2 diabetes mellitus. She currently takes amlodipine, insulin, and furosemide.

On physical examination, temperature is 38.3 °C (100.9 °F), blood pressure is 125/85 mm Hg, pulse rate is 70/min, and the respiration rate is 12/min. A tender, fluctuant, erythematous nodule with 2 cm of surrounding erythema is present on the left forearm. There is no lymphadenopathy. The remainder of the physical examination is noncontributory.

The leukocyte count is 13,000/µL (13×10^9/L). The nodule is incised and drained. Microscopic examination shows numerous leukocytes and small gram-positive cocci; culture results are pending.

Which of the following is the most appropriate antibiotic therapy for this patient?

(A) Amoxicillin-clavulanate

(B) Cephalexin

(C) Meropenem

(D) Vancomycin

Item 28

A 20-year-old man is evaluated for a 6-week history of a patch of alopecia on his scalp. The hair loss was asymptomatic. He has not tried to treat it, and he has noticed some hairs re-growing in the patch. He has no history of hair loss. There is no family history of hair loss, but his mother has hypothyroidism. He takes no medications.

The general physical examination is unremarkable. Scalp findings are shown.

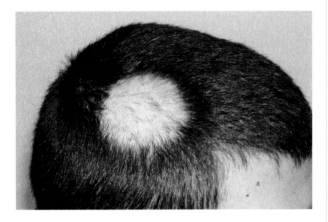

Which of the following is the most likely diagnosis?

(A) Alopecia areata

(B) Androgenetic alopecia

(C) Discoid lupus erythematosus

(D) Telogen effluvium

(E) Tinea capitis

Item 29

A 74-year-old woman is evaluated in the hospital for management of a painful skin lesion on her left lower leg that has been present for 3 weeks. The initial lesion began as a small darkened area that progressively increased in size with worsening pain. Her pain is now so severe that she is unable to walk. Medical history is significant for end-stage kidney disease requiring hemodialysis, type 2 diabetes mellitus, and hypertension. Medications are insulin, calcitriol, calcium carbonate, erythropoietin, aspirin, and lisinopril, although the patient has significant difficulty with medication adherence.

On physical examination, temperature is 37.3 °C (99.1 °F), blood pressure is 143/80 mm Hg, pulse rate is 102/min, and respiration rate is 15/min. The left lower extremity lesion is shown (see top of next column).

Which of the following is the most likely diagnosis?

(A) Calciphylaxis

(B) Cutaneous vasculitis

(C) Pyoderma gangrenosum

(D) Spider bite

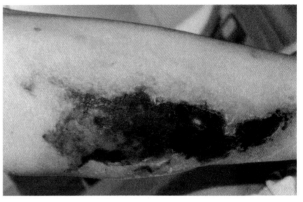

ITEM 29

Item 30

A 21-year-old woman is evaluated for mosquito bites on her arms and legs that she received 1 week ago that she has been scratching regularly. One of the bites on her left thigh is now is painful with a small amount of drainage. She otherwise feels well, has no significant medical history, and takes no medications.

On physical examination, vital signs are normal. A weeping red papule with overlying honey-colored crust is present on the anterior left thigh. There is no surrounding or extension of the redness, no lymphadenopathy, and no systemic symptoms. The remainder of the examination is unremarkable.

Which of the following is the most appropriate treatment?

(A) Cephalexin

(B) Doxycycline

(C) Mupirocin ointment

(D) Triamcinolone ointment

Item 31

A 20-year-old man is evaluated for a new scaling rash on the trunk. He had been well until 3 weeks ago when he developed subjective fever for 2 days with cough and rhinitis that resolved without treatment. One week later, he developed a spot on the right shoulder, and now the rash has spread to his entire trunk and proximal extremities. He has not noted any lesions in the genital area. Medical history is unremarkable, and he takes no medications. He is sexually active.

On physical examination, vital signs are normal. Skin findings are shown (see top of next page).

He has no oral or genital lesions. The remainder of the examination is unremarkable.

Which of the following is the most appropriate management?

(A) Hepatitis C virus antibody testing

(B) Polymerase chain reaction testing

(C) Rapid plasma reagin testing

(D) No further evaluation

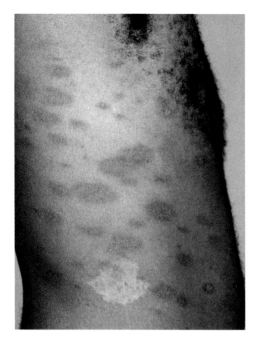

ITEM 31

Item 32

A 27-year-old man is evaluated for numerous moles scattered over his chest, back, abdomen, and extremities. He is concerned about the possibility of developing melanoma, although he does not believe that any of the moles have recently changed in size or appearance. His mother and two of his brothers also have similar lesions. Family history is significant for two early melanomas in his mother. Medical history is unremarkable, and he takes no medications.

On physical examination, vital signs are normal. Skin findings are shown.

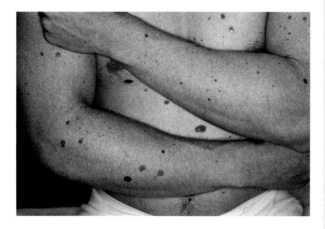

The remainder of the physical examination is normal.

Which of the following is the most appropriate next step in management?

(A) Monthly self-examinations and referral to a dermatologist

(B) Partial biopsy of multiple pigmented lesions

(C) Removal of the largest pigmented lesions

(D) Removal of as many pigmented lesions as feasible

Item 33

A 40-year-old man is evaluated for several ulcers located near his ostomy site. He has a 15-year history of ulcerative colitis and underwent elective proctocolectomy with ostomy placement 3 months ago to decrease his risk of colorectal cancer. His ostomy has functioned well without previous problems. The ulcers, which are moderately painful, developed 1 month ago and have failed to respond to topical care, including barrier methods and changing adhesives. He is otherwise healthy and takes no medications.

On physical examination, vital signs are normal. BMI is 19. Skin findings are shown.

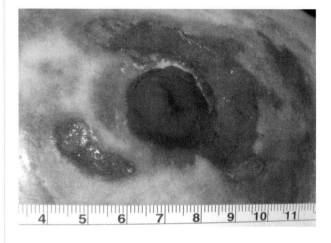

Which of the following is the most appropriate treatment?

(A) Replace ostomy to the opposite side

(B) Rituximab

(C) Surgical debridement

(D) Topical clobetasol

Item 34

A 35-year-old woman is evaluated for a 6-month history of skin changes on her legs. She initially noted scaling and thickening of the skin on her anterior shins that has persisted despite application of a topical moisturizer and an over-the-counter glucocorticoid. She was evaluated at a walk-in clinic approximately 3 months ago. Antifungal agents and topical glucocorticoids were prescribed, which she applied without relief. She reports that the involved areas have continued to thicken. Medical history is significant for type 1 diabetes mellitus, hyperthyroidism, and vitiligo. Medications are insulin glargine and methimazole.

On physical examination, temperature is 37.3 °C (99.1 °F), blood pressure is 132/90 mm Hg, pulse rate is 90/min, and respiration rate is 20/min. BMI is 19. The thyroid is diffusely enlarged without nodularity. The remainder of the general physical examination is normal. Skin findings are shown (see top of next page).

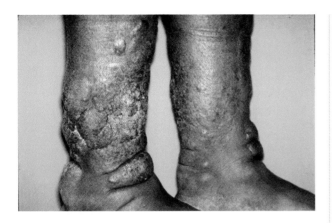

Which of the following is the most likely diagnosis?

(A) Lipodermatosclerosis
(B) Necrobiosis lipoidica
(C) Pretibial myxedema
(D) Stasis dermatitis

Item 35

A 52-year-old man is evaluated for multiple extremely itchy spots on his arms, legs, chest, and neck. His symptoms started approximately 1 month ago. He continues to develop new groups of lesions daily along with healing of previous areas. His wife also recently began to experience similar findings. Medical history is unremarkable, and he takes no medications.

On physical examination, vital signs are normal. Examination of the skin shows multiple lesions scattered primarily across the lower neck, the proximal arms, and the lower legs. Representative lesions are shown.

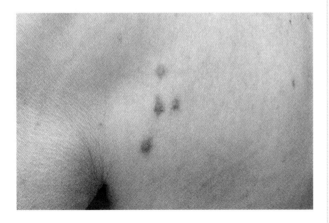

The remainder of the physical examination is normal.

Which of the following is the most likely cause of these lesions?

(A) Bedbugs
(B) Body lice

(C) Fleas
(D) Scabies
(E) Spider bites

Item 36

A 66-year-old man is evaluated for a 6-week history of a red, very itchy rash "all over" his body. It began as patches and plaques but over the past 2 weeks has progressed to a generalized red skin rash. The pruritus keeps him awake at night. His only other medical problem is hypertension for which he has taken hydrochlorothiazide for the past 12 years.

On physical examination, vital signs are normal. Generalized lymphadenopathy is present, and there is 1+ edema involving the feet and legs to the knees. Skin findings are shown.

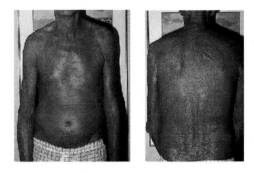

Which of the following is the most likely diagnosis?

(A) Angioedema
(B) Drug-induced subacute cutaneous lupus erythematosus
(C) Erythroderma
(D) Pityriasis rosea

Item 37

A 52-year-old woman had a burning sensation involving the right side of her forehead and the tip of her nose for 2 days, followed by increased redness and the development of lesions involving the tip of her nose. Medical history is significant for hypertension, and her only medication is ramipril.

On physical examination, vital signs are normal. Skin examination shows an erythematous patch on the right side of the forehead with scattered overlying grouped vesicles and a vesicle on the tip of the nose with background erythema. Mild conjunctival erythema is noted. The remainder of the physical examination is unremarkable.

In addition to starting antiviral medications, which of the following is the most appropriate next step in management?

(A) Administer herpes zoster vaccine
(B) Start mupirocin
(C) Urgent ophthalmologic evaluation
(D) Urgent otolaryngology evaluation

Item 38

A 38-year-old woman is hospitalized for a rash that developed during antibiotic treatment for pyelonephritis. She was diagnosed 1 week ago and was started on a 10-day course of trimethoprim-sulfamethoxazole based on urine culture results. Although her urinary tract symptoms have resolved, yesterday she noted the onset of a widespread, itchy rash. She also notes some facial swelling but has no difficulty breathing. Medical history is otherwise unremarkable, and she is taking no other medications.

On physical examination, temperature is 38.5 °C (101.3 °F). Her mucous membranes are normal. She has 3-cm lymph nodes in the anterior cervical and axillary regions and a liver edge palpable 4 cm below the costal margin. Skin findings are shown.

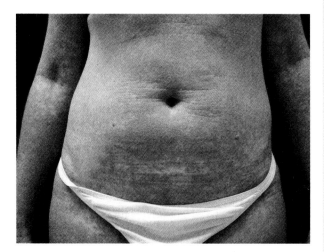

In addition to discontinuing the antibiotic, which of the following is the most appropriate next step in the management of this patient?

(A) Complete blood count and liver chemistry tests
(B) Lymph node biopsy
(C) Skin biopsy
(D) No further testing

Item 39

A 62-year-old woman is evaluated for pain with sexual intercourse and genital itching. Her symptoms began several years ago and have been progressively worsening. She has used lubricants and topical moisturizers without improvement. She notes no vaginal discharge or odor. She has no significant medical history and takes no medications.

On physical examination, vital signs are normal. The general physical examination is unremarkable. Skin findings are shown (see top of next column).

There is no vaginal discharge or odor.

Which of the following ointments is the most appropriate treatment?

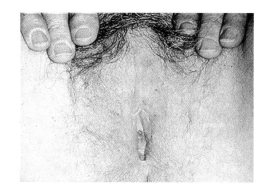

(A) Clobetasol, 0.05%
(B) Hydrocortisone, 1%
(C) Mupirocin
(D) Nystatin

Item 40

A 32-year-old man is evaluated for a painful purple area on the penis and the thigh that appeared 2 days ago. He describes a burning and stinging sensation associated with the lesion. He recalls having a similar episode several months ago that resolved spontaneously. He otherwise feels well. Medical history is unremarkable, and his only medication is as-needed ibuprofen for occasional musculoskeletal pain. He has had no sexual partners in the past 6 months.

On physical examination, vital signs are normal. Skin lesions are shown.

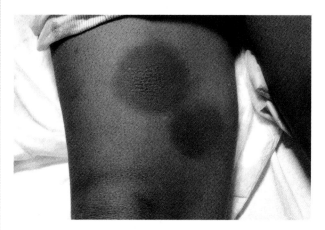

There is no inguinal lymphadenopathy. The remainder of the physical examination is unremarkable.

Which of the following is the most likely diagnosis?

(A) Contact dermatitis
(B) Fixed drug eruption
(C) Herpes simplex virus infection
(D) Primary syphilis

Item 41

A 52-year-old man is evaluated in the hospital for several skin lesions on his back, chest, and arms. The patient has acute myeloid leukemia and was hospitalized after developing neutropenic fever 10 days following his initial course of chemotherapy. The skin lesions first appeared the day his fever started. Medications are vancomycin and cefepime.

On physical examination, temperature is 38.4 °C (101.2 °F), blood pressure is 110/70 mm Hg, pulse rate is 95/min, and respiration rate is 18/min. A representative skin lesion is shown.

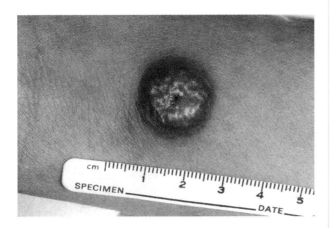

Laboratory studies:

Hemoglobin	8.2 g/dL (82 g/L)
Leukocyte count	400/µL (0.4 × 10⁹/L) with 95% neutrophils
Platelet count	10,000/µL (10 × 10⁹/L)
Metabolic profile	Normal
Urinalysis	Normal

Chest radiograph is normal. Blood cultures show no growth to date.

Which of the following is the most likely diagnosis?

(A) Candidiasis
(B) Keratoacanthoma
(C) Pyogenic granuloma
(D) Sweet syndrome

Item 42

A 32-year-old man is evaluated for a 2-week history of a rash on his face and midchest. He describes the rash as consisting of small, reddish "lumps" that are intensely itchy; they develop and begin to resolve with development of new lesions. He otherwise feels well. Medical history is significant for a recent diagnosis of HIV infection. Medications are tenofovir, emtricitabine, efavirenz, and trimethoprim-sulfamethoxazole. On physical examination, vital signs are normal. The patient has 1- to 3-mm papules and pustules on the face and central chest. There is no crusting or scaling in the web spaces, and no lesions on the umbilicus or penis. There is no lymphadenopathy or facial swelling. The remainder of the physical examination is unremarkable.

Laboratory studies:

Hemoglobin	Normal
Leukocyte count	3200/µL (3.2 × 10⁹/L) with 9% eosinophils
Platelet count	Normal
CD4 cell count	170/µL
HIV viral load	8000 copies/mL
Creatinine	Normal
Liver chemistry tests	Normal

Which of the following is the most likely diagnosis?

(A) Drug-induced acne
(B) Drug reaction with eosinophilia and systemic symptoms (DRESS)
(C) Eosinophilic pustular folliculitis
(D) Scabies infestation

Item 43

A 20-year-old male college student on the wrestling team is evaluated for a superficial skin infection. He has a history of several episodes of folliculitis and furunculosis over the past year that has required systemic treatment. His recurrent infections were treated with various oral antibiotics, including cephalexin, clindamycin, and trimethoprim-sulfamethoxazole. He currently takes no medications, has no drug allergies, and is otherwise in good health.

On physical examination, vital signs are normal. There are multiple, scattered erythematous papulopustules and nodules on the buttocks and upper thighs, some with a collarette of scale. He has no background erythema or lymphadenopathy. The remainder of the physical examination is unremarkable.

Which of the following is the most appropriate next step in management?

(A) Culture a pustule
(B) Perform a Tzanck smear
(C) Start linezolid
(D) Start vancomycin

Item 44

A 31-year-old woman is evaluated during a routine physical examination. She feels well but notes skin changes on her legs that have been present for several years. The skin changes persist regardless of position or temperature. Medical history is unremarkable except for three episodes of first trimester spontaneous pregnancy loss. She takes no medications.

On physical examination, vital signs are normal. The general medical examination is normal. Skin findings are shown (see top of next page).

The skin changes are more prominent when she is sitting or standing, but persist while supine. They don't go away when she is warmed. There is no lower extremity edema.

Which of the following is the most likely diagnosis?

(A) Amyloidosis
(B) Antiphospholipid antibody syndrome

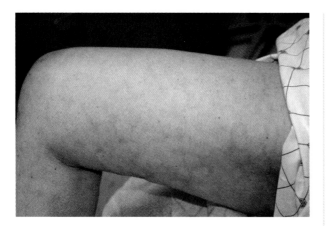

(C) Autoimmune thyroid disease

(D) Systemic sclerosis

Item 45

A 76-year-old woman is evaluated for a new lesion on her trunk. The lesion appeared a few months ago and has grown steadily. It may be itchy and becomes irritated when traumatized and sometimes bleeds. The patient is otherwise in good health. She takes no medications.

On physical examination, vital signs are normal. Skin findings are shown.

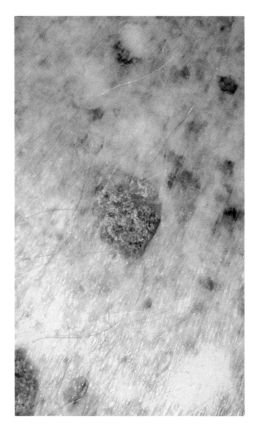

The remainder of her physical examination is normal.

Which of the following is the most likely diagnosis?

(A) Dermatofibroma

(B) Malignant melanoma

(C) Pigmented basal cell carcinoma

(D) Seborrheic keratosis

(E) Solar lentigo

Item 46

A 35-year-old man is evaluated for a 1-day history of a rash on the trunk and extremities. A few days earlier, he had a nonpurulent cough and rhinitis that resolved without treatment. Each individual skin lesion is very pruritic and lasts only a few hours before disappearing. He has no difficulty with swallowing or breathing. Medical history is unremarkable, and he takes no medications.

On physical examination, vital signs are normal. There is no evidence of lip or tongue swelling. The lungs are clear without wheezing. Skin findings are shown.

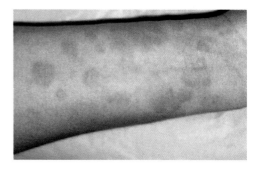

The remainder of the physical examination is unremarkable.

Which of the following is the most appropriate management?

(A) Amoxicillin

(B) Cetirizine

(C) Prednisone

(D) Ranitidine

Item 47

An 80-year-old man is evaluated for a facial skin rash. He reports dry skin, scaling, and redness most notably around his eyebrows and nose. He has regularly applied moisturizer without improvement. He washes his face with gentle soap and moisturizes with petrolatum jelly. The skin in the affected areas is not pruritic or painful. The patient has a history of hypertension and hypothyroidism. Medications are hydrochlorothiazide and levothyroxine.

On physical examination, vital signs are normal. Skin findings are shown (see top of next page).

The remainder of the physical examination is unremarkable.

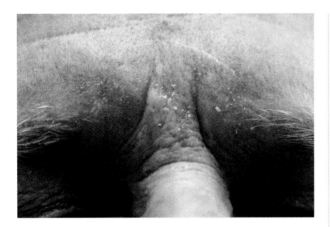

Which of the following is the most appropriate treatment for this patient?

(A) Benzoyl peroxide gel
(B) Ketoconazole cream
(C) Metronidazole gel
(D) Mupirocin ointment
(E) Triamcinolone ointment

Item 48

A 68-year-old man is evaluated for a slowly growing nodule on his nose. The lesion has been present for 6 months and is asymptomatic. Medical history is unremarkable, and he takes no medications. He does not smoke or drink.

On physical examination, vital signs are normal. The remainder of his examination is normal. Skin findings are shown.

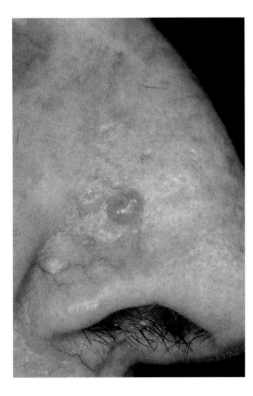

Which of the following is the most likely diagnosis?

(A) Angiofibroma
(B) Basal cell carcinoma
(C) Sebaceous hyperplasia
(D) Squamous cell carcinoma

Item 49

A 28-year-old woman is evaluated for an acne flare on her face. She is approximately 8 weeks pregnant. She has had acne for several years, which was well-controlled when she was using a combination benzoyl peroxide-clindamycin gel, salicylic acid wash, and tazarotene cream. She stopped all of these after her preconception counseling. Skin findings are shown.

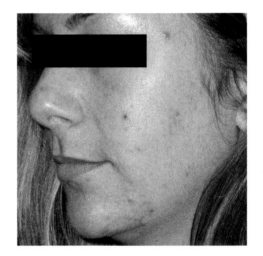

Which of the following is the most appropriate therapy for this patient?

(A) Azelaic acid cream
(B) Oral doxycycline
(C) Tazarotene cream
(D) Tretinoin cream

Item 50

A 24-year-old man is evaluated in the office for blisters that have developed on his lips and tongue. He has not had any similar episodes previously. He developed a tingling and burning sensation of the lip that was followed by redness and development of blisters. The patient has a recent diagnosis of HIV infection but has not started any medications.

On physical examination, vital signs are normal. Skin lesions are shown (see top of next page).

The remainder of the examination is normal.

Which of the following is the most appropriate diagnostic test to perform next?

(A) Bacterial culture
(B) Direct-fluorescent antibody testing
(C) Herpes simplex virus serologic testing
(D) Viral culture

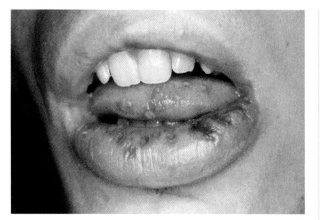

ITEM 50

Item 51

A 62-year-old man was admitted to the ICU for high fevers associated with sepsis following hip replacement surgery. Since the procedure he has been relatively immobile except when receiving physical therapy. Two days after surgery, he developed fine superficial vesicles on the back. Except for pain following the procedure, he has felt well. Medical history is otherwise unremarkable, and his only medication is as-needed acetaminophen-oxycodone.

On physical examination, temperature is 37.9 °C (100.2 °F). The rest of his vital signs are normal. Skin findings are shown.

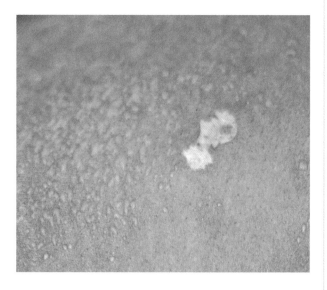

The surgical site is clean and dry. The remainder of the examination is unremarkable.

Which of the following is the most likely cause of this acute eruption?

(A) Allergic contact dermatitis
(B) *Candida albicans* infection
(C) Miliaria crystallina
(D) *Staphylococcus aureus* folliculitis

Item 52

A 67-year-old man is evaluated for an ulcer on his right ankle. The ulcer developed several weeks ago and does not appear to be healing despite application of a topical dressing. He reports that the ulcer is painful and is worse with leg elevation and improved with the leg in a dependent position. Medical history is significant for hypertension and a 40-pack-year smoking history. His only medication is amlodipine.

On physical examination, vital signs are normal. Skin findings are shown.

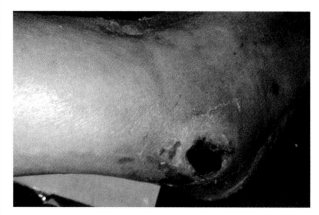

The remainder of the examination is unremarkable.

Which of the following is the most appropriate next step in management?

(A) Biopsy of ulcer edge
(B) External compression
(C) Measurement of the ankle-brachial index
(D) Oral antibiotics

Item 53

A 32-year-old woman is evaluated for a 1-week history of a rash affecting both feet. She recently traveled to Jamaica for vacation and was well during that trip, but noted the onset of symptoms after returning home. The rash is mildly painful but intensely itchy and is keeping her awake at night. She has no other symptoms and otherwise feels well. Medical history is unremarkable, and she takes no medications.

On physical examination, vital signs are normal. Skin findings are shown (see top of next page).

The remainder of the physical examination is normal.

Laboratory studies are significant for a leukocyte count of 9000/µL (9.0×10^9/L) with 9% eosinophils.

Which of the following is the most appropriate treatment?

(A) Cephalexin
(B) Ivermectin
(C) Prednisone
(D) Terbinafine

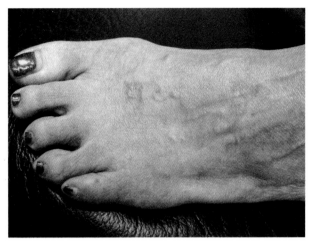

ITEM 53

Item 54

A 50-year-old man is evaluated for a firm, darkly pigmented papule on his back that has been growing steadily over a period of several months. His medical history is unremarkable, and he takes no medications.

On physical examination, vital signs are normal. The skin lesion is a 0.5-cm darkly pigmented, raised plaque with irregular borders and inconsistent coloration. The remainder of his physical examination, including the rest of his skin examination, is unremarkable.

A skin biopsy is performed and shows malignant melanoma on pathologic examination.

Which of the following is the primary feature used to determine prognosis?

(A) Lesion depth
(B) Mitotic rate
(C) Presence of ulceration
(D) Radial diameter of the lesion

Item 55

A 22-year-old woman is evaluated for a red, itchy rash on her chest, back, abdomen, arms, and legs for 1 week. She notes that an area of redness and swelling arises and lasts less than 24 hours, followed by development of a new area in a new location. She has no lip, tongue, or throat swelling. She is unable to recall any new medication, food, or other exposures prior to onset of the rash. Medical history is unremarkable, and she takes no medications.

On physical examination, vital signs are normal. There is no lip or tongue swelling. The lungs are clear without wheezes. Skin findings are shown (see top of next column).

The remainder of the examination is normal.

Which of the following is the most appropriate next diagnostic step?

(A) Chest radiograph
(B) Complete blood count with differential
(C) Food allergy testing

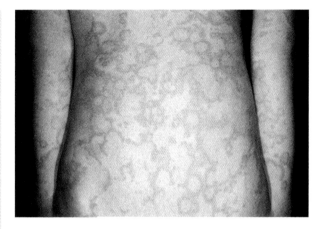

(D) Thyroid function tests
(E) No further evaluation

Item 56

A 45-year-old woman is evaluated for a "dark spot under her nail." She is healthy, feels well, and takes no medications. She thought the streak started after she "banged" her finger, but it has not gone away after 6 months.

On physical examination, she has a hyperpigmented longitudinal band on her index finger that is 4 mm wide. Vital signs are normal. Nail findings are shown.

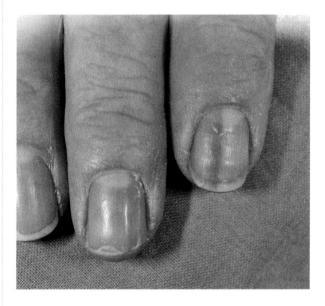

Which of the following is the most appropriate next step in the management of this dark nail streak?

(A) Culture of nail clipping
(B) Histologic examination of nail clipping
(C) Nail matrix biopsy
(D) Observation

Item 57

An 80-year-old woman is evaluated in the emergency department for a red, blistering rash. Her symptoms began 1 week ago with significant itching with the subsequent development of blisters that do not break easily. The blisters have occurred on her chest, abdomen, and extremities; she has not noted any blisters involving her lips or mouth. The patient has no other significant medical history.

On physical examination, vital signs are normal. Representative skin findings are shown.

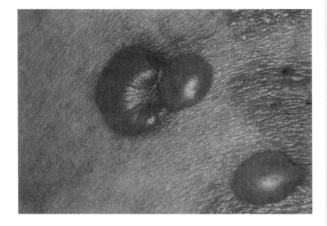

There are no oral or mucosal lesions. The remainder of the physical examination is normal.

Which of the following is the most likely diagnosis?

(A) Bullous pemphigoid
(B) Pemphigus foliaceus
(C) Pemphigus vulgaris
(D) Toxic epidermal necrolysis

Item 58

A 34-year-old man is evaluated for asymptomatic skin changes in his groin that have been present for weeks to months. He has a long-standing history of plaque psoriasis without psoriatic arthritis, for which he uses a combination of topical medications. A few months ago, he developed redness and pruritus in his groin and tried using some of his psoriasis medications to treat the itching. For the plaque psoriasis, he uses clobetasol ointment twice daily on weekends and calcipotriene cream twice daily on weekdays.

On physical examination, vital signs are normal. There are large red plaques with silvery scale over the elbows, knees, and around the umbilicus. Skin findings are shown (see top of next column).

There is no nail pitting, joint swelling, redness, or tenderness. The remainder of the examination is unremarkable.

Which of the following is the most likely diagnosis?

(A) Contact dermatitis
(B) Inverse psoriasis
(C) Striae distensae
(D) Tinea cruris

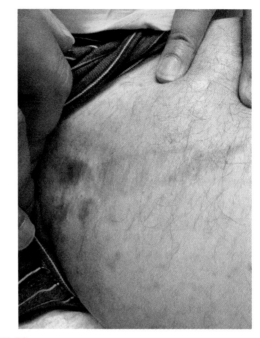

ITEM 58

Item 59

A 24-year-old man is evaluated for persistent acne. He has been treated for approximately 1 year with multiple therapies but has noticed minimal improvement. Medical history is unremarkable. His medications for the past 6 months are oral doxycycline, tretinoin cream, clindamycin lotion, and benzoyl peroxide wash.

On physical examination, vital signs are normal. His general medical examination is unremarkable. Skin findings are shown.

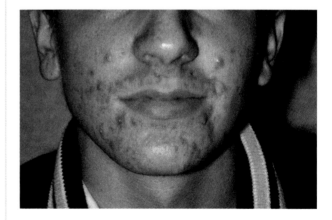

Which of the following is the most appropriate next step in management?

(A) Add metronidazole cream
(B) Change to tazarotene cream
(C) Switch doxycycline to oral minocycline
(D) Discontinue current medications and start oral isotretinoin

Item 60

A 55-year-old man is evaluated for a 6-week history of blisters on his hands. The blisters are tender, break easily after they develop, and occur in different regions on the backs of his hands. Medical history is notable for alcoholic liver disease. The patient does not use tobacco but drinks 6 beers daily. He takes no medications.

On physical examination, temperature is 36.4 °C (97.5 °F), blood pressure is 98/70 mm Hg, pulse rate is 85/min, and respiration rate is normal. BMI is 22. Cardiopulmonary examination is normal. The abdominal examination is significant for mild splenomegaly; there is no evidence of ascites. The patient has slight darkening of his skin and scattered spider telangiectasias. Mild hypertrichosis is evident on the face. The hand findings are shown.

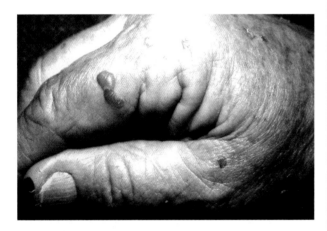

There are no oral erosions or ocular inflammation.

Which of the following is the most likely diagnosis?

(A) Allergic contact dermatitis
(B) Bullous lupus erythematosus
(C) Bullous pemphigoid
(D) Porphyria cutanea tarda

Item 61

A 32-year-old man is evaluated for a 2-month history of a persistent skin rash. He describes the rash as lesions that develop rapidly, are very itchy with burning and tingling, last for 2 to 3 days, and then leave bruises once they resolve. He has felt feverish at times since the rash started and had also had some stiffness and pain in his hands and fingers. Medical history is unremarkable, and his only medications are cetirizine daily and diphenhydramine as needed, which have not helped the condition.

On physical examination, temperature is 37.9 °C (100.2 °F), blood pressure is 138/83 mm Hg, pulse rate is 85/min, and respiration rate is 18/min. Skin findings are shown (see top of next column).

There are also numerous ecchymoses and hyperpigmented patches at sites where he reports lesions to have resolved. The skin of the face is uninvolved, and there are

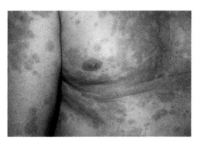

no oral ulcers. Joint examination reveals mild tenderness of the wrists bilaterally but no synovitis. Range of motion is full and intact. The remainder of the examination is unremarkable.

Which of the following is the most appropriate management?

(A) Gluten-free diet
(B) Radioallergosorbent test (RAST)
(C) Skin biopsy
(D) Thyroid function tests

Item 62

A 53-year-old woman is evaluated in the emergency department for a 1-week history of increased swelling, redness, and pain in her lower legs. She has not had trauma to her legs and has not noted any drainage. She has not had fevers and has otherwise felt well. Medical history is significant for heart failure. Medications are ramipril, metoprolol, and furosemide, which she has not been taking recently as she has not had her prescriptions refilled.

On physical examination, vital signs are normal. The neck veins are prominent. Mild bibasilar crackles are present. There is no inguinal lymphadenopathy, and the remainder of the general examination is unremarkable. Skin findings are shown.

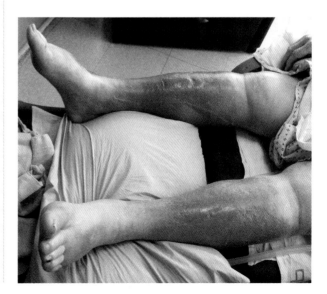

Which of the following is the most likely diagnosis?

(A) Cellulitis
(B) Contact dermatitis
(C) Deep venous thrombosis
(D) Stasis dermatitis

Item 63

A 24-year-old woman with longstanding atopic dermatitis is evaluated for an acute worsening of her disease in the past week. She has had increased pruritus and now has multiple painful areas within the involved skin. She has been applying petrolatum jelly and triamcinolone ointment and washing with gentle cleansers without improvement. She is otherwise well and takes no medications.

On physical examination, vital signs are normal. She has eczematous plaques with scattered pustules in the involved areas. The remainder of the physical examination is unremarkable.

Which of the following is the most likely cause of this patient's acute flare?

(A) Herpes simplex virus infection
(B) Soap allergy
(C) *Staphylococcus aureus* infection
(D) Topical glucocorticoids

Item 64

A 20-year-old woman is evaluated for a 3-year history of pink papules and pustules on her face and neck. Her menstrual periods are regular, and she feels well. She says she gets a few "pimples" at a time, but they leave dark marks that take months to fade. She has not had any prior treatment, and she is not using any over-the-counter products. Skin findings are shown.

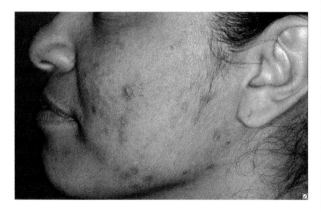

Which of the following is the most appropriate treatment?

(A) Bleaching cream
(B) Topical antimicrobial agent
(C) Topical glucocorticoid
(D) Topical retinoid

Item 65

A 47-year-old man is evaluated for a several-month history of itching and scaling on his feet that has not been improving with moisturizing lotion. He has no significant medical history and takes no medications.

On physical examination, vital signs are normal. Skin findings are shown.

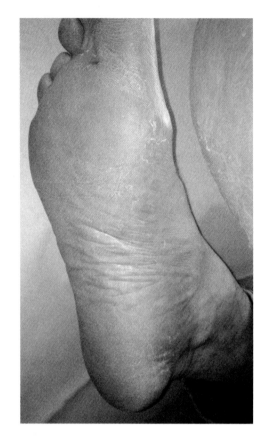

There is scaling and fissuring between the toes as well.

Which of the following is the most appropriate topical treatment?

(A) Betamethasone
(B) Clotrimazole
(C) Clotrimazole-betamethasone
(D) Nystatin

Item 66

H

A 57-year-old man is evaluated in the emergency department for a rash on his legs, arthralgia, myalgia, and fever of 4 days' duration. Over the past week, he has developed pain and numbness in the left foot, and he has tripped several times when walking.

On physical examination, temperature is 37.7 °C (99.8 °F), blood pressure is 150/100 mm Hg, pulse rate is 88/min, and respiration rate is 18/min. Cardiopulmonary examination is normal. The liver is palpable. Skin findings are shown (see top of next page).

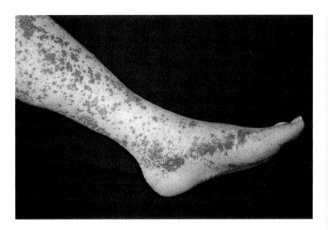

H
CONT. **Which of the following is the most likely dermatologic diagnosis?**

(A) Erythema multiforme

(B) Lichen planus

(C) Traumatic ecchymosis

(D) Vasculitis

Item 67

A 34-year-old woman is evaluated for very dry, painful hands. She works in a daycare center and washes her hands 15 to 20 times daily, often for 2 to 3 minutes at a time. She has been applying lotion multiple times daily with no relief of the pain. She has a history of obsessive-compulsive disorder and takes no medications.

On physical examination, vital signs are normal. She has xerosis on the dorsal aspect of her hands with lichenification, erythema, and fissuring.

The remainder of the physical examination is unremarkable.

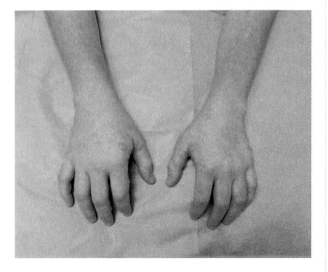

In addition to decreasing the frequency of hand washing, which of the following is the most appropriate therapy?

(A) Petrolatum moisturizer

(B) Topical diphenhydramine

(C) Topical lidocaine gel

(D) Topical neomycin

Item 68

A 44-year-old man was admitted to the hospital 2 weeks ago with fever and a new heart murmur and was diagnosed with native valve endocarditis. He was treated initially with broad-spectrum antibiotics with narrowing of his antimicrobial therapy to intravenous nafcillin based on culture and sensitivity results. He was discharged on the third hospital day to complete a 6-week course of intravenous antibiotic therapy. Although he had done well since discharge, he presents 11 days later with new fever and a rash.

On physical examination, temperature is 38.3 °C (100.9 °F), blood pressure is 115/78 mm Hg, pulse rate is 110/min, and respiration rate is 12/min. There is mild facial edema and lymphadenopathy of his cervical and axillary lymph nodes. The lungs are clear. Cardiac examination shows mild tachycardia and a grade 2/6 systolic murmur, unchanged from his last examination. Skin examination reveals diffuse erythema on his trunk, proximal extremities, and face. The remainder of his examination is unremarkable.

Laboratory studies:

Leukocyte count	12,100/µL (12.1 × 10^9/L) with 54% neutrophils, 31% lymphocytes, and 15% eosinophils
Albumin	Normal
Alanine aminotransferase	147 U/L
Aspartate aminotransferase	156 U/L
Bilirubin	Normal

Repeat blood culture results are pending.

Which of the following is the most likely diagnosis?

(A) Drug reaction with eosinophilia and systemic symptoms

(B) Morbilliform drug exanthem

(C) Stevens-Johnson syndrome

(D) Vasculitis

Item 69

A 44-year-old woman is evaluated for pruritus that has been present for about 3 months. She reports that she feels the itch on her upper back only, and the only thing that gives her relief is to scratch hard enough to "make it bleed." She says there were no preceding papules, pustules, or rash. Antihistamines, emollients, topical glucocorticoid ointment, and application of ice provided no relief. Her symptoms developed shortly after she lost her job. She has a history of depression and anxiety for which she sometimes takes fluoxetine.

On physical examination, vital signs are normal. The general physical examination is normal. Skin findings are shown (see top of next page).

Which of the following is the most likely diagnosis?

(A) Fluoxetine-induced morbilliform drug eruption

(B) Neuropathic itch

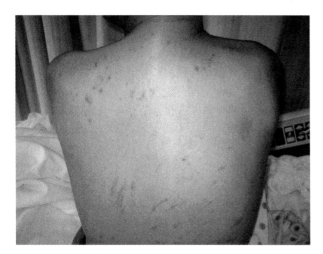

(C) Occult colorectal adenocarcinoma

(D) Psychogenic itch

Item 70

A 32-year-old woman is evaluated for a 6-month history of a new rash on her elbows, knees, and scalp. The rash is intensely pruritic, and she is concerned that it has resulted from insect bites. She has not noticed any other skin lesions but does relate a 4.5-kg (10-lb) unintentional weight loss over the past 6 months. Medical history is significant for irritable bowel syndrome for which she takes loperamide as needed.

On physical examination, the patient is afebrile and vital signs are normal. Skin findings are shown.

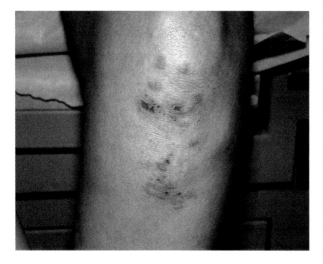

There is no mucosal involvement, and the remainder of the skin examination is normal. The general physical examination is otherwise unremarkable.

Which of the following associated conditions is most likely in this patient?

(A) Celiac disease

(B) Hepatitis C

(C) Non-Hodgkin lymphoma

(D) Ulcerative colitis

Item 71

A 32-year-old woman is evaluated for a rash on her face and arms of 2 months' duration. The rash developed progressively and has not responded to topical moisturizers and an over-the-counter glucocorticoid. The patient also has a moderate nonproductive cough, but otherwise feels well. Medical history is significant only for a 15-pack-year smoking history, although she quit smoking 4 months ago. She takes no medications.

On physical examination, vital signs are normal. BMI is 23. The lungs are clear. Skin findings are shown.

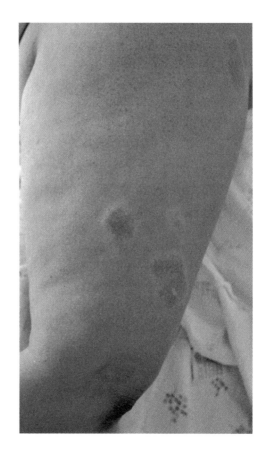

Her hair is normal, and she has no scarring or lesions in the ears or on the cheeks.

A chest radiograph is shown (see top of next page).

Which of the following is the most likely diagnosis?

(A) Dermatomyositis

(B) Hodgkin lymphoma

(C) Limited systemic sclerosis

(D) Sarcoidosis

(E) Systemic lupus erythematosus

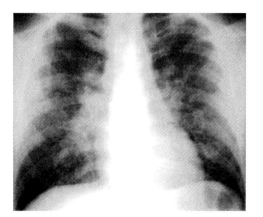

ITEM 71

Item 72

A 30-year-old woman is evaluated for a 3-year history of chronic lesions on her scalp, cheeks, and ears. She has lost hair and is concerned she may become bald. She has been treated with a number of topical medications, including topical hydrocortisone and tacrolimus. The patient does not have any antecedent triggers or associated systemic symptoms. Medical history is unremarkable. Her sister has systemic lupus erythematosus. She takes no medications and is not currently using any topical therapy for her rash.

On physical examination, vital signs are normal. Skin findings are shown (see top of next column).

She has no oral ulcers and no lesions below the head and neck. The remainder of the examination is unremarkable.

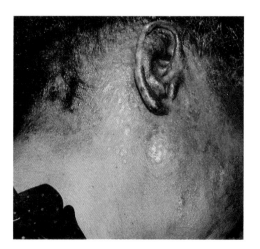

Laboratory studies:

Antinuclear antibodies	Positive (titer of 1:160)
Anti-Ro/SSA antibodies	Negative
Anti-La/SSB antibodies	Negative
Anti-dsDNA antibodies	Negative
Anti-Smith antibodies	Negative
Complete blood count	Normal
Urinalysis	Normal

Which of the following is the most appropriate treatment?

(A) Dapsone

(B) Hydroxychloroquine

(C) Prednisone

(D) Vitamin D supplementation

Answers and Critiques

Item 1   Answer: A

Educational Objective: Diagnose actinic keratosis.

This patient has actinic keratoses (AKs). AKs are precancerous lesions that generally occur in fair-skinned persons on sun-exposed areas such as the face, dorsal arms, hands, legs, and upper back. They are strongly correlated with cumulative sun exposure; the more sun exposure an individual has had, the more numerous they are. A small percentage of lesions (1% to 5%) may evolve into invasive squamous cell carcinomas. However, they never develop into other types of skin cancer such as basal cell carcinoma or melanoma, although many of the factors that predispose one to develop AKs are also risk factors for these other malignancies. The diagnosis of AKs is generally based on the clinical history and the typical tactile and visual appearance of the lesions; biopsy is not routinely needed. Liquid nitrogen is most commonly used to treat AKs, although other destructive methods (shave removal or curettage) are options, and topical therapies (5-fluorouracil, imiquimod) are often used for extensive disease. Efforts to decrease risk for developing AKs include sun avoidance and diligent use of sunscreen.

Seborrheic keratoses are a benign proliferation of keratinocytes that typically appear as hyperpigmented, well-circumscribed, "stuck on" lesions that most commonly develop on the trunk, upper extremities, and face. This patient's skin lesions are not consistent with this appearance, and their location on the dorsal surface of the hands would be uncommon.

Squamous cell carcinomas (SCCs) are typically larger and present as papules or nodules rather than macules. Also, in immunocompetent persons, it is rare to find multiple SCCs occurring simultaneously. Distinguishing between advanced AKs (also referred to as hypertrophic AKs) and early SCCs can sometimes be challenging. Therefore presumptive AKs that fail to respond to treatment should be biopsied to rule out early SCC.

Superficial basal cell carcinomas (SBCCs) often present as scaly macules and sometimes can resemble AKs. SBCCs tend to be more reddish-violet in color, and in contrast to AKs which are often seen in large numbers, patients typically have only a few of these at any given time.

KEY POINT

- Actinic keratoses are premalignant, erythematous, scaly macules that occur on sun-exposed areas of older persons with fair skin.

Bibliography

Rigel DS, Gold LF. The importance of early diagnosis and treatment of actinic keratosis. J Am Acad Dermatol. 2013 Jan;68(1 Suppl 1):S20-7. [PMID: 23228303]

Item 2   Answer: A

Educational Objective: Diagnose acne keloidalis nuchae.

This patient has acne keloidalis nuchae (AKN), which is characterized by firm, skin-colored, pink, or hyperpigmented papules that are often centered on hair follicles. AKN often occurs on the back of the neck and is similar in appearance to pseudofollicular barbae, which occurs on the hair-bearing face and anterior neck. These conditions are most likely due to ingrown hair and are more frequent in persons of color with curly hair owing to the shape of the hair and hair follicle. AKN can cause keloid formation associated with chronic folliculitis at the back of the neck. Therapy aims to minimize inflammation and secondary infection, flatten scars, and alter damage done by hairs. Topical and oral antibiotics, glucocorticoids (topical or intralesional), changes in shaving habits, and laser hair removal can be utilized, often in combination. Changes to shaving habits that are recommended include liberal use of shaving cream, avoidance of stretching the skin when shaving, and use of a single-blade razor rather than a multi-blade razor.

The differential diagnosis includes acne vulgaris and bacterial folliculitis. Inflammatory acne consists of erythematous pustules, nodules, or cysts (deeper and often painful) and are the result of inflammation in and around the hair follicles. This patient has only inflammatory papules and lacks comedones, which would be expected if this was acne. Bacterial folliculitis presents with red papules and pustules centered on hair follicles. The beard, pubic areas, axillae, and thighs are most often affected. Acne and folliculitis do not usually heal with fibrotic papules.

Keloids are areas of exuberant scar formation. A keloid is a tuberous growth of scar tissue that extends beyond the limits of the original injury. Any type of injury to the skin, including internal (acne) or external (trauma or surgery), can trigger keloids. Keloids most frequently occur on the earlobe and upper torso. People of African or Asian descent have a higher risk of keloid formation.

KEY POINT

- Acne keloidalis nuchae is characterized by firm, skin-colored, pink, or hyperpigmented papules that are often centered on hair follicles and appear most frequently on the back of the neck in people of color.

Bibliography

Mounsey AL, Reed SW. Diagnosing and treating hair loss. Am Fam Physician. 2009 Aug 15;80(4):356-62. [PMID: 19678603]

Item 3   Answer: C

Educational Objective: Diagnose rosacea.

This patient has rosacea, which presents as central facial erythema with transient papules or pustules. Burning and stinging may be present. The pathogenesis of rosacea is unknown. There are two types, erythematotelangiectatic (vascular) and papulopustular (inflammatory) rosacea. Vascular rosacea presents as persistent flushing, especially of the central face, with prominent telangiectasias. Pustules and papules are seen in the inflammatory variant, but in contrast to acne, rosacea pustules are not follicular based. Bulbous thickening of the nose (rhinophyma) can also occur. Eye involvement, with dry, gritty-feeling eyes and conjunctival injection, is common. Multiple studies have demonstrated that rosacea is associated with cutaneous inflammation; however, the trigger is highly debated. Alcohol, sun exposure, and other triggers can cause a transient increase in facial erythema but do not cause rosacea. Flushing is a common characteristic of rosacea; the differential diagnosis of this includes carcinoid syndrome, mastocytosis, and pheochromocytoma. The differential diagnosis for rosacea also includes entities that cause central facial erythema and/or inflammatory papules, namely acne, periorificial dermatitis, cutaneous lupus erythematosus, sarcoidosis, contact dermatitis (eczema), seborrheic dermatitis, actinic damage, and folliculitis due to *Pityrosporum* or *Demodex* spp.

The malar rash of acute cutaneous lupus erythematosus, typically seen in patients with systemic lupus erythematosus, is a transient erythematous patch over the cheeks that often spares the nasolabial fold. Certain forms of rosacea may resemble the rash of malar erythema, but patients with rosacea will often have a prominent telangiectatic component, as well as inflammatory papules, pustules, and occasionally rhinophymatous changes of the nose.

Periorificial dermatitis shares some clinical characteristics with rosacea. It occurs in both young children, commonly around the mouth and eyes, and adults, who are usually affected around the mouth. Monomorphous pink papules (1 to 2 mm) that sting or burn rather than itch are grouped around the mouth or eyes. Periorificial dermatitis is sometimes caused by the use of topical glucocorticoids on the face.

Seborrheic dermatitis causes white, scaling macules and papules that are sharply demarcated on yellowish-red skin and may be greasy or dry. Sticky crusts and fissures often develop behind the ears, and significant dandruff or scaling of the scalp frequently occurs. Seborrheic dermatitis may develop in a "butterfly"-shaped pattern but also may involve the nasolabial folds, eyebrows, and forehead. This condition usually improves during the summer and worsens in the fall and winter.

KEY POINT

- Papulopustular rosacea is a chronic inflammatory condition characterized by central facial erythema with transient papules or pustules.

Bibliography

Powell FC. Clinical practice. Rosacea. N Engl J Med. 2005 Feb 24;352(8):793-803. [PMID: 15728812]

Item 4   Answer: D

Educational Objective: Diagnose venous stasis ulcers.

The patient's skin findings are most consistent with a venous stasis ulcer. Venous stasis ulcers are commonly found on the lower extremities, particularly on or near the medial malleoli. They often occur in patients with recurrent bouts of stasis dermatitis, which is an eczematous rash on the lower legs associated with impaired venous drainage of the lower extremities caused by venous insufficiency, or by chronic peripheral edema of any cause. Venous stasis leads to changes in vascular permeability with stretching of the skin and loss of integrity of the dermal barrier. Initial changes involve development of dermatitis, seen as dark discoloration (postinflammatory hyperpigmentation) and "woody" induration known as lipodermatosclerosis. Impaired skin function in areas of venous stasis may also lead to breakdown of the dermal barrier with development of ulceration. Venous stasis ulcers tend to be shallow rather than deep. They may be asymptomatic or quite tender.

Arterial ulcers also occur on the lower extremities, but in contrast to venous stasis ulcers, they are not surrounded by stasis dermatitis changes or lipodermatosclerosis. They tend to be more demarcated than venous stasis ulcers and are often painful. The surrounding skin tends to be white or erythematous, and there is a loss of leg hair. These ulcers typically occur in the setting of peripheral atherosclerotic disease, with diminished pedal pulses and impaired capillary refill.

Neuropathic ulcers arise from repetitive trauma in patients with a history of sensory loss in the lower extremities. The ulcers are well-demarcated, often quite deep, and lack surrounding inflammation; they develop on pressure points or other areas where recurrent trauma may occur. They are most commonly seen in patients with peripheral neuropathy associated with diabetes mellitus.

Pyoderma gangrenosum is an uncommon inflammatory process that often occurs on the pretibial aspects of the lower legs and is often associated with an underlying systemic disease, such as inflammatory bowel disease or monoclonal gammopathy. The ulcers are well-demarcated, often very deep and painful, and show progression of the ulcer under the overlying skin (undermined borders). The ulcers tend to lack surrounding evidence of stasis, as is present in this patient.

KEY POINT

- Venous stasis ulcers appear on the distal lower leg, particularly the medial aspect of the ankle, and often occur in patients with recurrent bouts of stasis dermatitis.

Bibliography

Richmond NA, Maderal AD, Vivas AC. Evidence-based management of common lower extremity ulcers. Dermatol Ther. 2013 May-Jun;26(3):187-96. [PMID: 23742279]

Item 5   Answer: C
Educational Objective: Manage black hairy tongue.

This patient has black hairy tongue, and the correct management is tongue brushing as part of aggressive oral hygiene. Black hairy tongue is a benign and self-limited disorder related to several predisposing factors such as alcohol and tobacco use, poor oral hygiene, and medications (including bismuth, tetracycline, and linezolid). The clinical appearance of black discoloration and a thickened tongue without other symptoms is characteristic. Treatment includes aggressive oral hygiene with tongue brushing and scraping and modification of any risk factors (smoking cessation, avoidance of alcohol or medications inducing the change).

Amoxicillin-clavulanate is an antibiotic that is often used to treat oral infections. Black hairy tongue is not an infection that requires antibiotic treatment. The clinical appearance and the absence of oral or systemic symptoms make an oral infection as a cause of his findings unlikely.

A biopsy of the lesion is not indicated as this is a benign and self-limited condition. If the lesion is recalcitrant to therapy or if there are concerning manifestations such as leukoplakia or erythroplakia, a biopsy may be considered. Management with aggressive oral hygiene before biopsy is recommended.

Oral fluconazole is used for candidiasis oral infections, whereas black hairy tongue is a keratin build-up related to risk factors and poor oral hygiene.

KEY POINT
- Management of black hairy tongue consists of tongue brushing as part of aggressive oral hygiene.

Bibliography
Nisa L, Giger R. Black hairy tongue. Am J Med. 2011 Sep;124(9):816-7. [PMID: 21854889]

Item 6   Answer: C
Educational Objective: Diagnose psoriatic nail disease.

This patient has the classic features of psoriatic nail dystrophy with onycholysis (lifting of nail off the nail bed) that appears as areas of white nail at the lateral edges of the nail plate. This patient also has pitting of the nails, which manifests as small indentations on the surface of the nail plate. Lastly this patient also has "oil spots," which are the areas of yellow-tan discoloration at the distal end of the nail plate. Psoriasis most commonly presents as long-standing, discrete, erythematous plaques with silvery-white scale. Other patterns include inverse (intertriginous), guttate, pustular, and erythrodermic types. Nail changes occur in about 75% of patients with psoriasis. The most common psoriatic nail abnormality is subungual hyperkeratosis. Pitting and ridging are more common on fingernails as compared with toenails. The "oil drop" sign, which is yellow-tan discoloration, is another typical manifestation. Multiple nails are generally affected, both on the hands and feet. Over time, a significant amount of nail dystrophy can

occur, and the changes may be indistinguishable from onychomycosis. Patients with psoriatic nail dystrophy are more often affected by psoriatic arthritis, but nail findings do not necessarily correlate with the severity of disease.

Candidal infection can cause intertrigo, recognized as pink-red patches with satellite lesions in skin folds but is an uncommon cause of nail dystrophy.

The eczematous dermatoses are a diverse group of skin disorders that share clinical features of itching and a red, scaly, vesicular-to-crusted rash. Eczema can cause changes in the nail plate (nail dystrophy), but it is secondary to inflammation of the nearby skin of the proximal and lateral nail folds, which is not present in this patient.

Tinea manuum is a dermatophyte infection involving the hand. Dermatophytes are the most common fungi that infect skin. Tinea manuum characteristically involves only one hand (and two feet). The findings are characterized by a dry scale, and if chronic, the nails can be involved. The diagnosis of tinea manuum is unlikely if the feet are not involved.

KEY POINT
- Pitting, onycholysis, and the "oil drop" sign are typical manifestations of psoriatic nail dystrophy.

Bibliography
Holzberg M. Common nail disorders. Dermatol Clin. 2006 Jul;24(3):349-54. [PMID: 16798432]

Item 7   Answer: C
Educational Objective: Treat pitted keratolysis.

This patient has pitted keratolysis and should be treated with erythromycin lotion. Pitted keratolysis presents with small indented pits on a background of hyperkeratosis and results from increased sweating or perspiration (hyperhidrosis) of the feet. It is a superficial bacterial infection secondary to *Kytococcus sedentarius*, *Corynebacterium*, or *Actinomyces* spp. First-line treatment includes clindamycin lotion or erythromycin lotion in conjunction with keeping the feet dry. Oral therapy with clarithromycin or erythromycin also can be used.

Topical clotrimazole and other antifungal agents are effective for tinea pedis or candidal infections of the feet, which often have macerated web spaces with superficial scale and erythema. The patient's web spaces were not affected, and the clinical picture is consistent with pitted keratolysis, not tinea pedis.

Clotrimazole-betamethasone cream also is ineffective for pitted keratolysis. The combination of a topical antifungal and a topical glucocorticoid will not improve a superficial bacterial infection and will allow it to worsen. In addition, combination treatment can decrease diagnostic accuracy, as combined agents can treat an underlying entity (fungus), but the topical glucocorticoid may also cause the infection to worsen. Combination treatment may be associated with more side effects at an increased cost.

Another topical glucocorticoid, hydrocortisone, may cause the superficial bacterial infection to worsen and will not treat the underlying infection. Topical glucocorticoids may be used for eczematous dermatitis, but not for pitted keratolysis.

KEY POINT

- Pitted keratolysis is a superficial bacterial infection, and first-line treatment is clindamycin lotion or erythromycin lotion in conjunction with keeping the feet dry.

Bibliography

Pranteda G, Carlesimo M, Pranteda G, et al. Pitted keratolysis, erythromycin, and hyperhidrosis. Dermatol Ther. 2014 Mar-Apr;27(2):101-4. [PMID: 24703267]

Item 8   Answer: D

Educational Objective: Treat inflammatory skin disease on an area of thin skin.

This patient has allergic contact dermatitis of her eyelids, and a low-potency hydrocortisone ointment such as hydrocortisone valerate is the most appropriate treatment. Treatment courses should be of limited duration (2 weeks or less), which can be controlled by dispensing a small size tube (15 g) when treating areas of thin, sensitive skin such as the face or skin folds. There are multiple formulations of hydrocortisone that range in potency (hydrocortisone valerate, fumarate, and more); not all are low potency, and it is important when selecting a topical hydrocortisone to consider the anatomic site to be treated. The eyelids are very thin skin and are exposed to multiple irritants and allergens. Cosmetics, including nail products, shampoo, and fragrances, frequently result in an allergy on the eyelids, even when not directly applied to that location, because of the thin eyelid skin. This patient has mild allergic contact dermatitis; she should avoid the trigger, and topical glucocorticoids will relieve her symptoms.

The other three medications are all very potent topical glucocorticoids. The potencies of topical glucocorticoids in the United States are designated by classification into one of seven groups, with group 7 (1% and 2.5% hydrocortisone) being the least potent and group 1 being the most potent (up to 600 times more potent than the group 7 agents). Higher-potency glucocorticoids can rapidly lead to adverse effects, including lightening of the skin, atrophy, and telangiectasias, when used on areas of thin skin such as the eyelids. In addition, patients are at risk of ocular exposure and eventual cataract formation if chronically exposed. Therefore, treatment of facial lesions is usually limited to low-potency (groups 6 and 7) glucocorticoids.

KEY POINT

- Hydrocortisone valerate is a very-low-potency topical glucocorticoid that is safe to use on the eyelids.

Bibliography

Wolf R, Orion E, Tüzün Y. Periorbital (eyelid) dermatides. Clin Dermatol. 2014 Jan-Feb;32(1):131-40. [PMID: 24314387]

Item 9   Answer: A

Educational Objective: Diagnose allergic contact dermatitis.

This patient most likely has allergic contact dermatitis from the neomycin. Neomycin is a commonly used over-the-counter topical aminoglycoside antibiotic (often used either alone or as part of combination topical antibiotic preparations). With repeated use, especially on abraded or lacerated skin, neomycin can lead to contact sensitization, which is a T-cell mediated hypersensitivity reaction. Patients and clinicians often mistake this for a wound infection, but if the area is pruritic and there is a geometric, well-defined pattern generally corresponding with the contact area, a contact allergy should be suspected. Discontinuation of the medication and future avoidance are generally recommended.

Group A streptococcal infections would cause skin infections such as impetigo, cellulitis, or erysipelas. None of these infections tend to present with a well-demarcated pattern of involvement, as seen in this patient. This patient has no pain, wound drainage, or discharge that could be associated with bacterial impetigo. There is no pain or lymphangitic streaking typical of cellulitis. Erysipelas would appear as violaceous-red, edematous, well-demarcated plaques on the face or lower extremities, unlike this patient's presentation.

The classic presentation of herpes simplex virus infection is a group of painful, small vesicles on an erythematous base, transitioning to pustules and subsequent crusting of the lesions over time. Herpetic infection would be painful with no pruritus.

Staphylococcus aureus infection would present with eczematous plaques and open erosions on the flexural folds with pustules in those areas, not in a geometric pattern on a compromised skin barrier typical of allergic contact dermatitis.

KEY POINT

- Use of neomycin on abraded or lacerated skin can lead to contact sensitization, which is often mistaken for a wound infection; a contact allergy should be suspected if the area is pruritic and there is a geometric, sharply bordered pattern.

Bibliography

Sasseville D. Neomycin. Dermatitis. 2010 Jan-Feb;21(1):3-7. [PMID: 20137735]

Item 10   Answer: B

Educational Objective: Diagnose androgenetic alopecia in a woman.

This woman has androgenetic alopecia, which can affect both men and women. Hair loss (alopecia) is generally divided into two categories: scarring and nonscarring. Distinguishing between the two types is important because hair loss that occurs with scarring alopecia is permanent, whereas the hair loss that occurs with nonscarring alopecia is usually reversible, although the hair does not always completely regrow.

Androgenetic alopecia is categorized as a nonscarring alopecia. The prevalence of androgenetic alopecia in white men is 50% at age 50 years and over 70% at age 70 years. The prevalence is lower for women. In men, the temples and vertex are often affected. In contrast, in women the top of the head is affected, and balding is not complete. Androgenetic alopecia results in hair follicles that are thinner in caliber or "miniaturized" and, ultimately, the loss of hair follicles; however, androgenetic alopecia causes a decreased density of hair but not areas of complete loss of hair as seen in alopecia areata. A classic examination finding is "widening" of central part compared with the occipital part as a result of the decreased density of hairs. On examination, there is generalized rather than localized hair loss and decreased density of hair rather than complete smooth patch of hair.

Alopecia areata is an autoimmune disease characterized by well-demarcated areas of nonscarring total alopecia. The involved areas are often circular or oval but may coalesce to form more extensive areas of involvement. The affected areas are devoid of erythema or scale and are asymptomatic. Tapered "exclamation point" hairs may be seen at the periphery; these hairs have shafts that are thicker at the distal portion and narrower near the scalp. This patient's diffuse hair loss is not consistent with alopecia areata.

Frontal fibrosing alopecia is a scarring alopecia and is considered a variant of lichen planopilaris. The frontal scalp shows a band pattern of hair loss associated with follicular hyperkeratosis and perifollicular erythema. This patient's distribution of hair loss is not consistent with frontal fibrosing alopecia.

Telogen effluvium is a form of diffuse, nonscarring alopecia that is usually triggered by a systemically stressful event such as a serious illness, surgery, or childbirth. It is most commonly seen in women in the postpartum period. It is caused by the realignment of a higher-than-average number of hair follicles into the telogen, or final, phase of hair development. Approximately 3 to 5 months after the inciting event, numerous hairs are shed, leading to noticeably thinned hair. A small hair bulb may be visible at the scalp end of the shed hair. The hair loss tends to be patchy and diffuse; foci of total alopecia are not seen, and inflammation is absent. In most patients, the follicular maturation cycling returns to normal after a few months. This patient's history of gradual hair loss over 2 years is not consistent with telogen effluvium.

KEY POINT

- Female pattern androgenetic alopecia results in a decreased density of hair on top of the head but not complete loss of hair as seen in alopecia areata.

Bibliography
Mounsey AL, Reed SW. Diagnosing and treating hair loss. Am Fam Physician. 2009 Aug 15;80(4):356–62. [PMID: 19678603]

Item 11   Answer: A

Educational Objective: Manage recalcitrant condylomata acuminata.

This patient has condylomata acuminata, and his lesions should be biopsied. This is especially important in a patient with underlying HIV infection. These lesions have been refractory to therapy, and the incidence is continuing to grow. Condyloma acuminatum is a form of human papillomavirus (HPV) infection in the genital area, most often secondary to HPV 6 and HPV 11. Therapy for condylomata acuminata includes destructive techniques such as cryotherapy, cantharidin, podophyllin, laser therapy, and topical application of salicylic acid. Immune modulators such as imiquimod also can be used. When these lesions are recalcitrant to therapy or large and atypical in appearance, biopsy is essential to establish the diagnosis and rule out verrucous carcinoma or squamous cell carcinoma.

Although use of cryotherapy for condylomata acuminata and other verruca vulgaris is standard care, repeat cryotherapy is not appropriate in this setting since the lesion has been previously treated multiple times without improvement and with worsening.

HPV vaccination is currently recommended for routine vaccination in males and females at 11 to 12 years of age, with catch-up vaccination up to age 21 years in men and up to age 26 years in women and men who have sex with men or are immunocompromised or have HIV infection. However, its use outside of these risk groups, and particularly in those who already have the infection, is unknown at this time. This vaccine is used to help prevent cervical and anal cancer, and whether the vaccine prevents development of condylomata is not known yet. The quadrivalent vaccine against four types of HPV is currently recommended for men and provides additional protection; a bivalent vaccine also is available.

Topical triamcinolone can be effective in the treatment of dermatitis and multiple inflammatory disorders but does not have a role in the treatment of condylomata or potential cancers.

KEY POINT

- Condylomata acuminata that is recalcitrant to therapy should be biopsied to rule out premalignant or malignant transformation of lesions.

Bibliography
Gormley RH, Kovarik CL. Human papillomavirus-related genital disease in the immunocompromised host: part II. J Am Acad Dermatol. 2012 Jun;66(6):883.e1–17. [PMID: 22583721]

Item 12   Answer: B

Educational Objective: Diagnose neuropathic ulcers.

This patient has a neuropathic ulcer. Neuropathic ulcers often occur on the lower extremities in patients with peripheral neuropathy and other disorders of sensation. They result from repetitive trauma; patients are often unaware of the injury because of the lack of pain or other discomfort. The asymptomatic nature of most neuropathic ulcers highlights the need for clinical testing for neuropathy (by monofilament testing) and routine surveillance for ulcers in patients at high risk, such as this woman with long-standing diabetes mellitus. Neuropathic ulcers are usually noninflamed, have well-demarcated borders, and are often surrounded by signs of recurrent friction such as callus. The ulcers may be quite deep and occasionally extend to bone, increasing the risk for osteomyelitis. They typically occur over pressure points on the feet. Treatment consists of debridement of devitalized tissue, removal of friction, protection of the area, and treatment of any co-existing infection.

Arterial ulcers may also occur over bony prominences in patients with diabetes (since many patients with diabetes mellitus have peripheral vascular disease), but they are usually quite tender and have significant surrounding erythema. They may also occur on the pretibial aspects of the lower legs.

Squamous cell carcinomas may occur on the lower extremities and appear as nonhealing ulcers. They typically occur in sun-exposed areas such as the pretibial lower legs rather than the plantar feet. They are usually inflamed and are not surrounded by callus or other signs of chronic friction.

Venous stasis ulcers generally occur on the medial aspects of the lower legs and are surrounded by dyspigmentation and induration consistent with lipodermatosclerosis. Intermittent stasis dermatitis flares are also commonly seen.

KEY POINT

- Neuropathic ulcers occur on the lower extremities in patients with peripheral neuropathy and other disorders of sensation and often result from repetitive trauma.

Bibliography

Alavi A, Sibbald RG, Mayer D, et al. Diabetic foot ulcers: Part I. Pathophysiology and prevention. J Am Acad Dermatol. 2014 Jan;70(1):1. e1-18. [PMID: 24355275]

Item 13   Answer: C

Educational Objective: Recognize hirsutism associated with polycystic ovary syndrome.

This woman has hirsutism, and polycystic ovary syndrome (PCOS) is the most likely cause. PCOS is the cause of hirsutism in 50% to 70% of premenopausal women with excess hair growth. Hirsutism is defined as the excessive growth of thick, pigmented hair (terminal hairs) in androgen-responsive areas (a "male pattern") and affects about 8% of women. In androgen-dependent sites such as the jawline, the fine vellus hairs can be converted to thicker, courser terminal hairs like those on the underarms. The most to least common sites are the lower abdomen and areola, the chin and upper lip, between the breasts, and on the lower back.

The most important goal of the evaluation of a patient with hirsutism is to exclude the most serious causes, including androgen-secreting tumors (ovarian or adrenal). The patient must first be assessed for virilization, which is commonly due to an ovarian or adrenal tumor. Signs and symptoms of virilization include a deepening of the voice, severe acne, clitoromegaly, a decrease in breast size, and male-pattern balding. Other concerning features are rapid onset and progressive hirsutism over a short period of time (such as 1 year) or hirsutism that develops after 30 years of age. The diagnosis of PCOS is confirmed if two of the three following criteria are met: (1) oligo-ovulation or anovulation, (2) clinical or biochemical evidence of hyperandrogenism, and (3) polycystic ovarian morphology on an ultrasound when other endocrine disorders are excluded. In this patient, a transvaginal ultrasound will not be necessary to establish the diagnosis of PCOS.

Women in some family groups are predisposed to having more terminal hair growth in androgen-responsive areas. These women often develop the hairs slowly around the time of puberty and have normal menses. There is often a history of similar findings in other women in the family; however, this patient does not have a history of similar hair growth affecting the women in her family.

Hyperthyroidism may be associated with hypertrichosis, which is an excessive growth of hair but, as opposed to hirsutism, is not limited to androgen-responsive areas. The hairs often do not get as dark or thick as the terminal hairs that develop in hirsutism. Patients with hyperthyroidism may develop longer and more prominent hair growth all over their bodies, rather than in androgen-responsive sites. The hair growth is usually associated with other symptoms such as weight loss, anxiety, tachycardia, or hyperhidrosis.

Similarly, patients with porphyria can develop longer, thicker hairs in areas of sun exposure. Patients with porphyria are likely to have some skin blistering, fragility, or scarring in areas of sun exposure.

KEY POINT

- Polycystic ovary syndrome is the cause of hirsutism in 50% to 70% of premenopausal women with excess hair growth, and the evaluation begins with a medical and family history as well as examination for breast discharge and findings associated with androgen excess.

Bibliography

Curran DR, Moore C, Huber T. Clinical inquiries. What is the best approach to the evaluation of hirsutism? J Fam Pract. 2005 May;54(5):465-7. [PMID: 15865908]

Item 14   Answer: C

Educational Objective: Treat rhus dermatitis.

This patient should be treated with high-potency glucocorticoid ointment. She has pruritic linear red papules and plaques concentrated on exposed areas 1 day after exposure to a vine, which is typical of rhus dermatitis. Rhus dermatitis is caused by urushiol resin in poison ivy, oak, or sumac.

A topical antibiotic such as bacitracin would be indicated for impetigo, a highly contagious bacterial skin infection, but not for rhus dermatitis.

Diphenyhydramine is an antihistamine. Contact dermatitis is a type IV hypersensitivity reaction that is mediated by lymphocytes and not a primary histamine process. Therefore, an antihistamine would be ineffective.

Because this is an intensely pruritic eruption with localization on the hands and arms, a low-potency topical glucocorticoid cream would be unlikely to control her symptoms. In addition, ointments, which are preparations made up of approximately 80% oil and 20% water, would be less likely to cause a burning sensation in a patient with open skin compared with a cream, which is a preparation consisting of approximately half oil and half water.

KEY POINT

- Topical high-potency glucocorticoid ointment will reduce the redness and pruritus of rhus dermatitis.

Bibliography

Craig K, Meadows SE. What is the best duration of steroid therapy for contact dermatitis (rhus)? Fam Pract. 2006 Feb;55(2):166-7. [PMID: 16451787]

Item 15   Answer: A

Educational Objective: Treat stasis dermatitis.

This patient has stasis dermatitis, and compression stockings should be used. Stasis dermatitis is characterized by red, inflamed, pitted skin on the lower legs. It occurs in patients with venous stasis disease or other causes of chronic lower extremity edema. Decreased venous drainage causes an increase in extravascular tissue fluid that results in stretching of the skin and a subsequent propensity for loss of barrier integrity. Also, because the shins are often one of the driest parts of the body and are easily excoriated, dermatitis in this area is common. Compression stockings help to increase the venous return, decrease the stretching of the skin, and reduce the risk of ulceration.

Stasis dermatitis is frequently confused with cellulitis. The four cardinal signs of cellulitis are erythema, pain, warmth, and swelling; associated lymphadenopathy can occur. Systemic symptoms, including fever, chills, and malaise, also may be present. This patient does not have fever, pain, or clinical findings consistent with cellulitis, and it is unlikely for cellulitis to present on both legs simultaneously. Compared with cellulitis, the redness on the anterior shins in patients with stasis dermatitis is often bilateral and warm to the touch but typically is not tender. Therefore oral cephalexin is not indicated.

This patient has edema related to the venous stasis but has no jugular venous distension, no crackles, and no S_3. Given the absence of volume overload, furosemide would not be indicated.

Topical mupirocin would be indicated for impetigo, but this patient has no bullae, crusts, or erosions that would be seen in impetigo.

KEY POINT

- Stasis dermatitis is typically characterized by red, inflamed, pitted skin on the lower legs and occurs in patients with venous stasis disease or other causes of chronic lower extremity edema.

Bibliography

Keller EC. Tomecki KJ. Alraies MC. Distinguishing cellulitis from its mimics. Cleve Clin J Med. 2012 Aug; 79(8):547-52. [PMID: 22854433]

Item 16   Answer: C

Educational Objective: Diagnose hidradenitis suppurativa.

This patient has hidradenitis suppurativa (HS) or "acne inversa," a chronic inflammatory disease that predominantly affects the apocrine gland-bearing areas of the skin. HS is a disease of follicular occlusion. The common sites are the axillae, breasts and inframammary creases, inguinal folds, and gluteal cleft. HS is marked by comedones, inflammatory papules, nodules, cysts, and scarring. The lesions are painful, and the drainage is often foul smelling. The distribution and severity of disease can range from minor to debilitating.

HS is estimated to affect 1% to 4% of the general population and frequently begins in the second to third decade. It is more common in women. Almost 40% of patients with HS report a family history of the disease. About half of patients with HS have breast and armpit involvement and hypertrophic scars.

Smoking is strongly associated with worsening of the disease. Antibacterial soaps and topical antibiotics provide minimal benefit. Oral tetracyclines are used long term for their anti-inflammatory properties, and bacterial cultures may be helpful. Intralesional injections of triamcinolone may hasten resolution of particularly tender areas. Counseling regarding weight loss and smoking cessation should be provided if applicable.

An abscess is a soft-tissue infection with a collection of pus that is walled off from adjacent tissue. Abscesses are warm, tender, fluctuant red-to-purple nodules, which may have an overlying collarette of scale. Bacterial abscesses tend to occur singly and do not typically recur repeatedly in the same general area.

Folliculitis results from infection of the hair follicle. Bacteria, fungi, and even herpes simplex virus can cause folliculitis; however, *Staphylococcus aureus* is the most common cause. Folliculitis appears as erythematous papules and pustules around a follicle on the face, chest, back, and buttocks. The lesions do not cause large painful nodules about the genitals, axillae, or breasts.

Ruptured epidermal cysts appear as red subcutaneous nodules, much like an abscess. These also tend to be solitary and also do not chronically recur.

KEY POINT

- Hidradenitis suppurativa is a chronic inflammatory disease characterized by comedones, inflammatory papules, nodules, cysts, draining sinuses, and scarring of the axillae, breasts and inframammary creases, inguinal folds, and gluteal cleft.

Bibliography

Jemec GB. Clinical practice. Hidradenitis suppurativa. N Engl J Med. 2012 Jan 12;366(2):158–64. [PMID: 22236226]

Item 17   Answer: D

Educational Objective: Diagnose squamous cell carcinoma.

The patient likely has a squamous cell carcinoma (SCC), which is the second most common type of skin cancer, and skin biopsy is the appropriate next step in management. Risk factors for SCC are smoking and sun exposure, as in this patient; other risk factors include human papillomavirus infection, immunosuppression, and arsenic exposure. Prompt recognition of SCCs is crucial for optimizing patient outcomes since these lesions can grow rapidly and occasionally metastasize. Lesions on the lip are particularly aggressive and are associated with worse outcomes. The relatively large size of this patient's lesion and tenderness both suggest a malignancy rather than a precancerous lesion. SCCs can sometimes resemble infectious processes such as furuncles, mycobacterial infections, or fungal infections; however, the patient's clinical presentation is most consistent with an SCC, and thus a skin biopsy would be crucial for diagnosis.

Tissue culture for bacteria would not yield useful diagnostic information and may confuse the diagnosis since SCCs are often colonized by bacteria.

Cryotherapy and topical 5-fluorouracil are used for the treatment of precancerous lesions (actinic keratoses) and occasionally SCC in situ, but would not be an appropriate choice for this patient since the lesion appears to be an invasive SCC in a high-risk site.

Similarly, electrodesiccation and curettage may be used for SCC in situ and in certain settings for low-risk well-differentiated SCCs, but would not be an appropriate choice for this location, particularly prior to obtaining a tissue diagnosis.

KEY POINT

- The diagnosis of squamous cell carcinoma of the lip is best established by skin biopsy since these lesions are particularly aggressive and are likely to metastasize.

Bibliography

Alam M, Ratner D. Cutaneous squamous-cell carcinoma. N Engl J Med. 2001 Mar 29;344(13):975–83. [PMID: 11274625]

Item 18   Answer: D

Educational Objective: Diagnose interstitial lung disease associated with dermatomyositis.

This patient has a clinical picture consistent with dermatomyositis, and she is at increased risk for developing interstitial lung disease. Polymyositis and dermatomyositis are idiopathic inflammatory myopathies. Dermatomyositis also has various characteristic cutaneous manifestations. There are two forms of dermatomyositis: the classic form with both skin and muscle inflammation and either hypomyopathic or amyopathic dermatomyositis with skin findings but minimal or absent muscle inflammation. Patients with polymyositis and those with any form of dermatomyositis (classic, hypomyopathic, or amyopathic) are at increased risk for malignancy, with patients with dermatomyositis at higher risk than those with polymyositis. Similarly, patients with polymyositis or dermatomyositis (regardless of subtype) are at risk for developing interstitial lung disease. Several histopathologic patterns of interstitial lung disease are associated with polymyositis and dermatomyositis. Patients with certain serologic abnormalities may be at higher risks for interstitial lung disease, such as those with anti–Jo-1 antibody positivity. Current screening recommendations include performing pulmonary function tests with measurement of D$_{LCO}$. Patients often require additional testing, including high-resolution chest CT scans. In patients with mild disease, observation may be appropriate. Increasing levels of immunosuppression may be required for patients with more severe interstitial lung disease.

Bronchiectasis is an acquired disorder characterized by permanent abnormal dilatation and destruction of the bronchial walls and requires an infectious insult plus impaired bronchial drainage to develop. Bronchiectasis is an uncommon finding in patients with dermatomyositis, and this patient has no clinical findings consistent with this diagnosis, including existing pulmonary disease, cough, or sputum production.

Diffuse alveolar hemorrhage may occur in a variety of settings, including in patients with active pulmonary vasculitis. Diffuse alveolar hemorrhage is a rare complication in patients with dermatomyositis and is inconsistent with this patient's clinical features.

Hilar lymphadenopathy is often seen in patients with sarcoidosis; the skin manifestations of sarcoidosis, if present, include violaceous infiltrated papules around the nasal ala and periorbitally or periorally or within scars or tattoos. This patient's skin findings are not consistent with a diagnosis of sarcoidosis.

Pleuritis is an uncommon pulmonary complication of systemic lupus erythematosus (SLE). Generally this will occur in patients with true SLE, as opposed to the cutaneous forms of lupus such as chronic cutaneous lupus erythematosus (discoid lupus). Patients with SLE will generally have a bright red patch symmetrically over their cheeks, the so-called butterfly or malar rash.

KEY POINT

- Dermatomyositis is associated with an increased risk of interstitial lung disease.

Bibliography

Morganroth PA, Kreider ME, Okawa J, Taylor L, Werth VP. Interstitial lung disease in classic and clinically amyopathic dermatomyositis: a retrospective study with screening recommendations. Arch Dermatol. 2010 Jul;146(7):729–38. [PMID: 20644033]

Item 19   Answer: C

Educational Objective: Treat basal cell carcinoma.

Mohs micrographic surgery is the most appropriate treatment for this patient's basal cell carcinoma (BCC). Many modalities are available for the treatment of BCCs. Selection of the most appropriate technique depends on a number of factors, including the size of the lesion, the location, the patient's age and comorbidities, the histologic subtype of the tumor, and the cost of the procedure. Although standard surgical therapy is appropriate treatment with high cure rates (>95%) for tumors and a low risk of recurrence, micrographic surgery (Mohs) is preferred for tumors with high-risk pathology (micronodular, infiltrative, or sclerosing) or lesions in sites where a cosmetic outcome is important. For this patient, the size of the lesion and location on the temple indicate that a tissue-sparing procedure would be desirable because of cosmetic considerations. The histologic subtype indicates that this lesion has a relatively high risk of recurrence, and given the patient's age, she will presumably live long enough for recurrence to be likely. Mohs micrographic surgery offers a very high cure rate (>98%) coupled with the likelihood of a good cosmetic result. It is also a cost-effective choice in this setting. The fact that the patient is on anticoagulation therapy is not a contraindication to surgery.

Cryotherapy may be used to treat superficial BCCs and some nodular BCCs, but it is not generally used for other histologic subtypes because of an unacceptably high risk of recurrence. It also has an unpredictable cosmetic result and is not generally used for tumors on the head and neck.

Electrodesiccation and curettage is a reasonable treatment for nodular and superficial BCCs that occur on the trunk and extremities. It is not appropriate for more infiltrative subtypes since the recurrence rate is quite high. It is rarely used for tumors on the face because of a relatively high recurrence rate and an unpredictable cosmetic result.

Radiation therapy is a reasonable choice for BCCs in patients who are either not surgical candidates or who refuse surgery. It carries the risk of chronic radiation skin changes in subsequent years, and given the patient's age, this makes it a less desirable option. Radiation therapy is also less cost-effective and less convenient for the patient, since it requires multiple treatments over the course of several weeks.

Topical imiquimod treatment is often used for superficial BCCs and sometimes used off-label for nodular BCCs, but it is generally not used for other subtypes of BCC because

of an unacceptably high risk of recurrence. This is particularly true for lesions on the head and neck.

KEY POINT

- For basal cell carcinoma, Mohs micrographic surgery offers a very high cure rate coupled with good cosmetic results.

Bibliography

American Academy of Dermatology; American College of Mohs Surgery; American Society for Dermatologic Surgery Association; American Society for Mohs Surgery; Ad Hoc Task Force, Connolly SM, Baker DR, Coldiron BM, et al. AAD/ACMS/ASDSA/ASMS 2012 appropriate use criteria for Mohs micrographic surgery: a report of the American Academy of Dermatology, American College of Mohs Surgery, American Society for Dermatologic Surgery Association, and the American Society for Mohs Surgery. J Am Acad Dermatol. 2012 Oct;67(4):531–50. [PMID: 22958088]

Item 20   Answer: D

Educational Objective: Recommend appropriate sun protection.

This patient should use sunscreen with SPF 15 or greater plus UVA protection. Ultraviolet light is divided into categories based on wavelength: UVA (long wavelength) is the most deeply penetrating and can cause photoaging, tanning, and skin cancer, and UVB (shorter wavelength) penetrates less deeply but can cause both sunburns and skin cancer. The sun protection factor (SPF) measures the ability of a sunscreen to block UVB radiation and produce skin erythema determined under laboratory conditions. The SPF refers to the ratio of the dose of solar radiation needed to cause erythema on sunscreen-protected skin to the dose needed to cause erythema on unprotected skin, indicating the degree of protection. However, the relationship between SPF and degree of protection is not linear, such that an SPF of 30 is not twice as protective as an SPF of 15. SPF of 15 or more is required for adequate UVB protection; sunscreens with values lower than this can only be labeled to help decrease the risk of sunburn. To be considered "broad spectrum" sunscreens, the FDA mandates that products also provide protection against UVA. Only sunscreens that have SPF 15 or higher and broad spectrum protection are known to reduce the risk of both skin cancer and signs of photoaging. Additionally, sunscreens may not be labeled as "waterproof" or "sweatproof" because they have not been proved to be effective for more than 2 hours, at which point they should be reapplied.

Although tanning is a natural defense mechanism in response to chronic sun exposure, it requires exposure to ultraviolet light, which increases the risk of photoaging and both melanoma and nonmelanoma skin cancers. Additionally, some patients are unable to tan and may simply burn with ultraviolet light exposure. Therefore, tanning should be discouraged.

Although randomized controlled data are lacking and there is no consensus U.S. Preventive Services Task Force guideline, mathematical modeling and small-scale studies note benefits in populations in which patients perform skin self-examinations. All patients at risk for skin cancer may benefit from performing monthly skin self-examinations, as many suspicious lesions, including melanomas, are detected initially by attentive patients. Although the sensitivity of skin self-examination is low, it has fair specificity, and patients who engage in skin self-examinations often detect skin cancers at an earlier stage when they are easier to treat and cure.

KEY POINT

- Only sunscreens that have SPF 15 or higher and broad spectrum protection are known to reduce the risk of both skin cancer and signs of photoaging.

Bibliography

FDA announces changes to better inform consumers about sunscreen [press release]. Silver Spring MD: Food and Drug Administration (FDA). http://www.fda.gov/NewsEvents/Newsroom/PressAnnouncements/ucm258940. Published June 14, 2011. Accessed June 23, 2014.

Item 21   Answer: D

Educational Objective: Diagnose intertrigo.

This patient has intertrigo, a chronic, recurrent skin condition often seen in obese patients. It is caused by moist conditions in skin fold (intertriginous) areas and is exacerbated by heat and exercise. The rash is confined to the intertriginous area and does not extend beyond these boundaries. Secondary infection with *Candida* may occur, as in this patient; a clinical clue to this situation is the appearance of multiple small red papules on the periphery of the rash, referred to as "satellitosis." Treatment consists of keeping the areas dry and well ventilated, with avoidance of occlusive clothing and possibly the use of drying agents (such as powders). Low-potency topical glucocorticoids and antifungal creams may be used to relieve acute flares by reducing the inflammation and treating secondary yeast infection, respectively.

Allergic contact dermatitis in these areas is a diagnostic possibility; however, the multifocal recurrent nature of the rash and its limitation to areas under the breasts and groin make this less likely.

Atopic dermatitis is a red scaly eruption that arises in childhood and presents with periodic flares throughout life. It may occur on flexor surfaces of the arms and legs but does not typically appear under the breasts or in the groin. Atopic dermatitis is extremely pruritic and is frequently associated with allergic rhinitis and asthma.

Cellulitis may often cause an erythematous rash in various parts of the body; however, the findings would be unilateral rather than bilateral or multifocal. It tends to be painful; lack scale, maceration, or other surface changes; and not be accompanied by satellitosis/candidal infection. Also, the recurrent nature of the patient's rash is not typical of cellulitis.

KEY POINT

- Intertrigo is an inflammatory process found in intertriginous areas; the rash consists of confluent, well-demarcated erythema, generally symmetrically distributed.

Bibliography

Yosipovitch G, DeVore A, Dawn A. Obesity and the skin: skin physiology and skin manifestations of obesity. J Am Acad Dermatol 2007 Jun;56(6):901-16. [PMID: 17504714]

Item 22   Answer: A

Educational Objective: Manage generalized pruritus without a primary skin rash.

The next step in managing this patient's pruritus is to obtain a chest radiograph for possible Hodgkin lymphoma, which is the malignant disease most strongly associated with pruritus. When primary skin lesions are absent, especially when pruritus is generalized, systemic causes of pruritus are suspected. A systemic disease or medication reaction is found in 14% to 24% of patients with generalized pruritus without a primary skin rash. The investigation begins with the history, including a medication history, since medications can cause pruritus. A review of systems should be performed to investigate for thyroid disorders, lymphoma, kidney and liver diseases, and diabetes mellitus. Initial laboratory evaluation for occult systemic disease includes a complete blood count with differential, thyroid function studies, and measurement of serum alkaline phosphatase, bilirubin, creatinine, and blood urea nitrogen levels. A CT scan of the chest, abdomen, and pelvis is not recommended without earlier studies that indicate the need for widespread imaging.

A skin biopsy of normal appearing skin is unlikely to contribute useful information; however, a biopsy would be indicated if the patient had pruritus and primary skin changes.

No further testing is not an appropriate choice since the patient has an impaired quality of life from the pruritus, and up to a 25% of patients with diffuse pruritus without a rash can have an indolent metabolic or malignant process.

KEY POINT

- When pruritus is generalized and primary skin lesions are absent, systemic causes of pruritus should be sought.

Bibliography

Fett N, Haynes K, Propert KJ, Margolis DJ. Five-year malignancy incidence in patients with chronic pruritus: a population-based cohort study aimed at limiting unnecessary screening practices. J Am Acad Dermatol. 2014 Apr;70(4):651-8. [PMID: 24485529]

Item 23   Answer: C

Educational Objective: Diagnose scabies.

The most common cause of skin problems in the homeless is infections and infestations, and this patient has a scabies infection. Scabies usually involves the hands (including the palms and interdigital spaces) and feet as well as "folds" of the body (neck, axillary folds, waist, and upper thighs). Scabies also has a predilection for the areola/breast in women and the male genitals (glans, penile shaft, and scrotum). Head involvement is rare except in young children. The rash associated with scabies consists of pink papules and macules, some with scale or serous crust, as well as some linear macules that are the burrows of the mites. The patient likely became infested when he stayed with the friend with a rash. After infestation, the rash may take up to a month to become clinically obvious.

Allergic contact dermatitis may involve the dorsal hands, finger web spaces, and skin on the volar wrists, particularly when the palms are spared, but more commonly presents with erythema, edema, and papulovesicles, which are not present in this patient. Lesions are frequently geometric and have sharp cut-offs and a linear component to the morphology. There is typically a delayed onset of 1 to 3 days after exposure.

Bedbugs (genus *Cimex*) are another parasite of humans, but while the scabies mite lives on the human host, the bedbug lives off the human body. The bedbug is active during the night and typically bites areas of skin that are not covered by nightclothes. The face (including the eyelid), neck, hands, arms, and waist may have evidence of bites in the morning or may be delayed by 7 to 10 days. The bites are itchy and may be small pink-red papules or urticarial plaques 1 to 2 cm in diameter. Bedbugs live in crevices of mattresses, furniture cushions, suitcases, and walls.

Tinea manuum is a dermatophyte infection involving the hands and feet. Tinea manuum characteristically involves only one hand (and two feet). The findings are characterized by a dry scale, and if chronic, nails can be involved. The diagnosis of tinea manuum is unlikely if the feet are not involved.

KEY POINT

- The rash associated with scabies consists of pink papules and macules, some with scale or serous crust as well as some linear macules that are the burrows of the mites.

Bibliography
Heukelbach J, Feldmeier H. Scabies. Lancet. 2006 May 27;367(9524):1767-74. [PMID: 16731272]

Item 24   Answer: A

Educational Objective: **Diagnose allergic contact dermatitis.**

A pruritic geometric patch typical of allergic contact dermatitis, and in this patient, the clonidine patch is the likely cause. Contact dermatitis is an example of an "outside job" when a rash is in linear or geometric patterns because the rash corresponds exactly to where the allergen touches the skin from the outside. Allergic contact dermatitis is a hypersensitivity reaction to a specific chemical. With repeated exposure to the chemical, a pruritic eczematous dermatitis develops on the area that was exposed. In exuberant cases, pinpoint flesh-colored to red papules develop in the vicinity of exposure or diffusely over the body. The clonidine patch has been associated with allergic contact dermatitis. Although many

transdermal drug delivery systems may cause allergic contact dermatitis, the clonidine patch tends to have a higher incidence, possibly owing to its formulation that allows the patch to be left in place for up to 7 days. The patient's adjacent areas of hyperpigmentation likely represent resolving inflammation from prior applications of the patch.

A fixed drug eruption is typically a purple patch that is painful and is not localized to the area underneath a patch. Fixed drug eruptions occur in the same location (fixed) each time a patient is exposed to the same medication. Lips, genitals, and hands are commonly involved. Common drug culprits include over-the-counter medications such as pseudoephedrine, NSAIDs, sulfonamide medications, and other antibiotics.

Irritant contact dermatitis is a direct toxic effect on the epidermis from exposure to a chemical such as a cleaning agent, other caustic substance, or repeated wetting and drying and is not mediated by the immune system. Irritant contact dermatitis would present with a generalized dermatitis in all of the exposed areas but not in a geometric pattern.

Tinea corporis is a dermatophyte infection that may occur in healthy people, although patients with compromised immune systems (such as with diabetes mellitus) may be more susceptible. The classic findings are a pruritic, circular or oval, erythematous, scaling patch or plaque that spreads centrifugally with central clearing. This patient's skin findings are not consistent with this diagnosis.

KEY POINT

- Allergic contact dermatitis is a hypersensitivity reaction to a specific chemical, and with repeated contact with the chemical, a geometric pruritic eczematous dermatitis develops on the area that was exposed.

Bibliography
Corazza M, Mantovani L, Virgili A, Strumia R. Allergic contact dermatitis from a clonidine transdermal delivery system. Contact Dermatitis. 1995 Apr;32(4):246. [PMID: 7600788]

Item 25   Answer: D

Educational Objective: **Treat toxic epidermal necrolysis.**

This patient has toxic epidermal necrolysis (TEN), and he should be admitted to the hospital and any medications that are possible triggers (minocycline) should be stopped immediately. The most commonly implicated medications are antiepileptic agents, especially carbamazepine, lamotrigine, and phenytoin. Sulfonamides, fluoroquinolones, β-lactam antibiotics, minocycline, pantoprazole, sertraline, NSAIDs (oxicam and acetic acid type), tramadol, and allopurinol are also frequent causes. The treatment of TEN begins with drug cessation and aggressive ICU or burn center care.

Stevens-Johnson syndrome (SJS) and TEN are related clinical syndromes that are characterized by acute epidermal necrosis. The classification of SJS and TEN is determined by the percentage of body surface area with epidermal detachment: SJS involves less than 10%, SJS-TEN overlap involves

10% to 30%, and TEN involves greater than 30%. TEN is a rare disease, with a prevalence of 1:1,000,000. TEN is almost exclusively caused by medications, whereas erythema multiforme and SJS can also be triggered by vaccines or infection. SJS and TEN occur within 8 weeks of drug initiation, often between 4 and 28 days. Patients may have flu-like symptoms for 1 to 3 days prior to the skin eruption. Initially, red-purple macules or patches develop on the trunk and extremities, which enlarge and coalesce. Skin pain is prominent, in contrast to the pruritus associated with a common drug exanthema. Vesicles, bullae, and erosions reflect the epidermal necrosis seen on biopsy. Nikolsky sign (the shearing off of the epidermis with lateral pressure on the skin) is present. Two or more mucosal surfaces, such as the eyes, nasopharynx, mouth, and genitals, are involved in more than 80% of patients. Systemic inflammation can result in pneumonia, hepatitis, nephritis, arthralgia, and myocarditis.

Infliximab is a monoclonal antibody that is used for several conditions including psoriasis; however, it has no role in the management of TEN. There is evidence to show that treatment with systemic glucocorticoids, such as intravenous methylprednisolone, can increase mortality rates in patients with TEN. Infection is a risk for patients with SJS or TEN because of the extensive damage to the skin barrier; however, antibiotics, such as vancomycin and ceftriaxone, are not started without signs or symptoms of infection.

KEY POINT

- The treatment of toxic epidermal necrolysis begins with discontinuing the offending drug and providing aggressive supportive care, such as that received in an ICU or burn center.

Bibliography

Bastuji-Garin S, Fouchard N, Bertocchi M, et al. SCORTEN: a severity-of-illness score for toxic epidermal necrolysis. J Invest Dermatol. 2000; 115:149–53. [PMID: 16679892]

Item 26 Answer: D

Educational Objective: Diagnose subacute cutaneous lupus erythematosus.

This patient has a typical eruption of subacute cutaneous lupus erythematosus (SCLE). Although associated with systemic lupus erythematosus (SLE), it is a distinct disorder that may present with different cutaneous findings than those usually associated with SLE. There are two presentations of SCLE: annular scaly patches on the upper back and sun-exposed areas or a more psoriasiform eruption that can have less distinctive morphology but also occurs in sun-exposed areas. SCLE is associated with a number of medications believed to trigger the disorder, including hydrochlorothiazide, calcium channel blockers, ACE inhibitors, terbinafine, and the tumor necrosis factor α (TNF-α) inhibitors. This patient is taking hydrochlorothiazide, which was the first drug reported in association with SCLE and remains a common cause of drug-induced SCLE. Patients with SCLE tend to be very

photosensitive, may have antinuclear antibody positivity, and are often positive for anti–Ro/SSA antibodies (and may be positive for anti–La/SSB antibodies). Patients with drug-induced SCLE may be antihistone antibody positive (about one third to one half of patients), but antihistone antibody positivity is not necessary to make the diagnosis. Compared patients with SLE, those with SCLE tend to have fewer systemic findings, although a subset of patients may have kidney involvement. Notably, all women with anti-ro/SSA and anti-La/SSB antibodies are at risk for having newborns with neonatal lupus, and pregnant patients or mothers of newborns with this pattern of skin eruption or serologic antibody profiles should be counseled and their babies screened accordingly. For drug-induced SCLE, discontinuing the inciting medication is essential to treatment.

Dermatomyositis may present without muscle inflammation, but this patient's skin eruption is characteristic of SCLE. The rash of dermatomyositis is accentuated around the eyes (heliotrope rash), around the lateral shoulders ("shawl sign"), and involves the knuckles of the metacarpal and interphalangeal joints (Gottron sign).

Pemphigus foliaceus is an autoimmune blistering disease in which the autoantigen is in the upper regions of the epidermis, leading to superficial blisters that rapidly rupture and cause dried crusts over inflamed skin, which have been described as looking like "cornflakes." The morphology and distribution of the eruption described in this patient would be atypical, and patients with pemphigus foliaceus are not often positive for anti–Ro/SSA antibodies or high-titer antinuclear antibodies.

Psoriasis generally occurs over joints or at areas of trauma or friction, is not generally annular, and should not be photodistributed. Classic plaque psoriasis is characterized by pink plaques with silvery scale over the knees, elbows, and often around the umbilicus and gluteal cleft.

KEY POINT

- Patients with subacute cutaneous lupus erythematosus have annular scaly patches that are typically drug or sunlight induced.

Bibliography

Lowe G, Henderson CL, Grau RH, Hansen CB, Sontheimer RD. A systematic review of drug-induced subacute cutaneous lupus erythematosus. Br J Dermatol. 2011 Mar;164(3):465–72. [PMID: 21039412]

Item 27 Answer: D

Educational Objective: Treat a hospital-acquired skin infection.

This patient should be treated with vancomycin. Hospital-acquired skin and soft-tissue infections should be treated as a methicillin-resistant *Staphylococcus aureus* (MRSA) infection until culture results are received and therapy can be tailored appropriately. Hospital-acquired skin infections are increasingly caused by MRSA, and coverage against this organism in the hospital setting is important to prevent

CONT.

further morbidity and mortality, particularly in high-risk patients. Once culture and sensitivity results are known, antibiotic therapy can be focused toward a specific organism. In the patient described here, a local abscess and surrounding cellulitis with corresponding fever and leukocytosis suggests the potential for systemic involvement.

Amoxicillin-clavulanate should not be used because these antibiotics do not provide coverage against MRSA organisms.

Similarly, cephalexin is often effective against multiple skin and soft-tissue infections and may be considered first-line therapy for an abscess and cellulitis in the ambulatory setting; however, it too is ineffective against MRSA.

Although meropenem is a potent antibiotic with broader antimicrobial coverage, it is not effective against MRSA infection and thus would not be an appropriate choice for this patient.

Several strategies may be used to attempt to reduce rates of MRSA infection in hospitalized patients. Routine screening and active surveillance cultures for MRSA colonization are obtained in some institutions to identify carriers and to guide use of contact precautions and possibly attempted decontamination with intranasal mupirocin. However, the efficacy of this practice is not clear except in the setting of an acute outbreak. Daily chlorhexidine bathing has been shown to decrease the risk of colonization and infection with drug-resistant and other organisms in ICU settings.

KEY POINT

- Vancomycin, an empiric antibiotic therapy against methicillin-resistant *Staphylococcus aureus*, is the treatment of choice for most hospitalized patients with skin and soft-tissue infections until culture results are available.

Bibliography

Daum RS. Clinical practice. Skin and soft-tissue infections caused by methicillin-resistant Staphylococcus aureus. N Engl J Med. 2007 Jul 26;357(4): 380-90. [PMID: 17652653]

Item 28   Answer: A

Educational Objective: Diagnose localized alopecia areata.

This patient has alopecia areata, a chronic autoimmune disease that results in smooth, hairless patches of skin. Tapered "exclamation point" hairs may be seen at the periphery; these hairs have shafts that are thicker at the distal portion and narrower near the scalp. Older patients may demonstrate sparing of white/gray hairs, and in some patients the hair regrowth in existing patches begins with fine, white/fair hairs. The scalp is the most common site. Individual patches can spontaneously resolve within 12 months; however, new patches may develop. An autoimmune mechanism is supported by the increased rate of other autoimmune diseases, such as type 1 diabetes mellitus and autoimmune thyroid disease, in patients with alopecia areata as well in their family members.

Androgenetic alopecia is a type of diffuse nonscarring alopecia that can affect both men and women. In men, the bilateral temples and vertex are often affected. Androgenetic alopecia results in hair follicles that are thinner in caliber or "miniaturized" and loss of the hair follicle; however, androgenetic alopecia causes a decreased density of hair but not areas of complete loss of hair as seen in alopecia areata.

Discoid lupus erythematosus is the most common type of chronic cutaneous lupus. On the scalp, discoid lupus erythematosus manifests as scaling, erythematous, and hyper- and hypopigmented patches with alopecia. Multiple lesions are more likely than a single lesion.

Telogen effluvium is a diffuse nonscarring form of hair loss that is usually triggered by a systemically stressful event such as a serious illness, surgery, or childbirth. Approximately 3 to 5 months after the inciting event, numerous hairs are shed, leading to noticeably thinned hair. A small hair bulb may be visible at the scalp end of the shed hair. The hair loss tends to be patchy and diffuse; foci of total alopecia are not seen as in alopecia areata.

Tinea capitis causes scaling, inflammation, pustules, and pruritus, none of which are present in alopecia areata.

KEY POINT

- Alopecia areata is a chronic autoimmune disease that results in smooth, hairless patches of skin, most commonly appearing on the scalp.

Bibliography

Mounsey AL, Reed SW. Diagnosing and treating hair loss. Am Fam Physician. 2009 Aug 15;80(4):356-62. [PMID: 19678603]

Item 29   Answer: A

Educational Objective: Diagnose calciphylaxis.

This painful black eschar with slight surrounding angulated purpura in a patient on dialysis is consistent with calciphylaxis. Calciphylaxis is an uncommon syndrome that typically occurs in patients with advanced kidney dysfunction and an elevated calcium-phosphorus product (>60-70 mg^2/dL^2), which may be present in this patient who has difficulty with medication adherence. Calciphylaxis results from abnormal deposition of calcium within the lumen of the arterial vasculature, compromising blood flow with distal ischemia resulting in painful tissue necrosis. It has a poor prognosis with a 60% to 80% 1-year mortality rate, with patients often succumbing to infectious complications. Management requires pain control, meticulous skin care, and surveillance for associated infection due to increased risk of tissue ischemia. Directed therapy is preferably multi-interventional and typically includes aggressive lowering of the calcium-phosphorus product (by dialysis and non-calcium phosphate binders) to less than 55 mg^2/dL^2, administration of sodium thiosulfate (mechanism unclear), and lowering of the parathyroid hormone level (by surgery or cinacalcet). Hyperbaric oxygen, careful debridement, and bisphosphonates may also be helpful.

Vasculitis is inflammation of the blood vessels and can affect any size vessels. The most common cutaneous vasculitis is a small vessel vasculitis, which manifests as palpable purpura (nonblanching red papules). Medium vessel vasculitis (such as polyarteritis or granulomatosis with polyangiitis) can lead to ulcers in the skin, but the lesions are often strikingly inflamed with an active erythematous-to-red border and often surrounding livedo-like changes. A single, thick black eschar, as seen in this patient, would be uncommon.

Spider bites are exceedingly rare and overdiagnosed in clinical practice. Bites that do occur usually follow an exposure to secluded, dark, neglected areas such as a woodshed. Many patients living in environments rich in brown recluse spiders never receive a bite, and most patients diagnosed with bites have alternative diagnoses. Additionally, only a small percentage of brown recluse spider bites become necrotic. In those that do, the bite is usually exquisitely painful, rapidly progressing with deep tissue necrosis and accompanying systemic symptoms. Most necrotic bites are smaller than the lesion seen in this patient and usually stop expanding and start healing within about 10 days.

Pyoderma gangrenosum is a neutrophilic dermatosis in which the host's neutrophils cause autoinflammation in the skin, leading to painful, exudative, rapidly progressive ulcers. The ulcers typically start as a pustule or shallow erosion in response to minor trauma and rapidly expand. Classic PG ulcers will have a rim of violaceous erythema and edema; an overhanging lip; thin, anastomosing strands of intact epidermis hanging over the ulcer base; and excessive serous exudates that can lead to fibrinous "slough" over the ulcer base. This patient's skin findings are not consistent with pyoderma gangrenosum.

KEY POINT

- A painful black eschar with slight surrounding angulated purpura in a patient on dialysis who has calcium and phosphorus abnormalities is consistent with calciphylaxis.

Bibliography

Ross EA. Evolution of treatment strategies for calciphylaxis. Am J Nephrol. 2011;34(5):460-7. [PMID: 21986387]

Item 30   Answer: C

Educational Objective: Treat impetiginized insect bite.

The most appropriate treatment for this patient is mupirocin ointment for localized impetigo. Impetigo is a superficial bacterial infection most commonly caused by *Staphylococcus aureus* and, to a lesser extent, β-hemolytic streptococci. The patient initially had an insect bite that became secondarily infected, likely due to the skin trauma associated with scratching the bite. Because there are no signs of systemic illness and the patient has a localized infection, treatment with topical antibacterial agents, such as mupirocin, is considered first-line therapy. Bleach baths may be a treatment option (put 1/4 to 1/2 cup of common liquid bleach into the bath water to create a chlorinated bath), which decreases colonization of *S. aureus*). Topical retapamulin cream also has been demonstrated to have effective antimicrobial properties against *Staphylococcus* and *Streptococcus* spp. and can be effective in patients with mupirocin-resistant organisms.

Although cephalexin can be effective for impetigo, localized infections should be treated with topical antibiotics whenever possible to avoid systemic side effects and potential resistance with overuse of oral antibiotics. If the infection was systemic or more severe, cephalexin would be appropriate. In addition, if topical mupirocin failed to resolve the infection, oral therapy can be considered.

Doxycycline is effective against methicillin-resistant *Staphylococcus aureus* but provides poor coverage against *Streptococcus*, which is another organism that can lead to impetigo. In addition, topical therapy is considered first-line therapy for localized impetigo.

Triamcinolone ointment is not effective against impetigo. Triamcinolone ointment can be used for symptomatic treatment of insect bites; however, when pain and honey-colored crust is present, impetigo needs to be considered and treated.

KEY POINT

- A topical antibacterial agent, such as mupirocin, is the first-line therapy for localized impetigo.

Bibliography

Drucker CR. Update on topical antibiotics in dermatology. Dermatol Ther. 2012 Jan-Feb;25(1):6-11. [PMID: 22591495]

Item 31   Answer: C

Educational Objective: Manage pityriasis rosea in a patient at risk for syphilis.

This patient should have a rapid plasma reagin test. He has scaling plaques on the trunk and proximal extremities after a recent upper respiratory tract infection, which is most typical of pityriasis rosea. The clinical appearance of scaling papules and plaques is similar to that of secondary syphilis, although pityriasis rosea typically spares the face, palms, and soles, whereas syphilis often affects the palms and soles. In a sexually active patient who is not consistently using protection and has palm involvement, secondary syphilis must be ruled out. The primary chancre is typically painless in syphilis and therefore may go unnoticed.

Hepatitis C virus testing is indicated for patients with lichen planus (LP), especially if oral. LP is an acute eruption of purple, pruritic, polygonal papules that most commonly presents on the flexural surfaces, especially the wrists and ankles. LP can also present in the mucous membranes (mouth, vaginal vault, and penis) with white plaques that, if uncontrolled, may ulcerate. This patient's physical findings are not consistent with LP.

Herpes simplex virus infection presents with grouped vesicles and erosions and no scaling plaques, and so polymerase chain reaction test is not necessary.

Because testing should be performed if there is any clinical concern for syphilis, not doing a work-up is not an acceptable treatment option.

KEY POINT

- The clinical appearance of pityriasis rosea is similar to that of secondary syphilis, and rapid plasma reagin testing should be performed if there is any clinical concern for syphilis.

Bibliography

Wollenberg A1, Eames T. Skin diseases following a Christmas tree pattern. Clin Dermatol. 2011 Mar-Apr;29(2):189-94. [PMID: 21396559]

Item 32   Answer: A

Educational Objective: Manage dysplastic nevus syndrome.

The patient has dysplastic nevi, and he should be taught how to perform monthly self-examinations and should be referred to a dermatologist for close clinical monitoring. Dysplastic nevi are benign melanocytic lesions most commonly found on the trunk and extremities. In contrast to common nevi, they have one or more atypical clinical features that may make them difficult to distinguish from malignant melanoma. Histologically, they possess varying degrees of cytologic atypia and architectural disorder. Although benign, they often serve as a marker for persons who have a higher than average risk of developing melanoma. Any lesions suspicious for melanoma should be removed and sent for histologic evaluation.

Partial biopsy of multiple pigmented lesions is not recommended since it leaves room for sampling error and the possibility of nevus recurrence. If a given pigmented lesion is worrisome for melanoma, it should be removed in its entirety whenever possible and sent for pathologic analysis.

Patients with dysplastic nevus syndrome often have large numbers of nevi. Removal of either the largest lesions or nevi en masse has not been shown to reduce the risk of developing melanoma, is often not practical, and is not cost effective; therefore, neither procedure is recommended. In patients with numerous dysplastic nevi who develop melanoma, approximately two thirds of the time the melanoma will arise on normal appearing skin rather than within a preexisting nevus. Thus, even if all of a patient's nevi were removed, the overall risk would only be partially reduced.

KEY POINT

- Dysplastic nevi are benign melanocytic lesions most commonly found on the trunk and extremities that have atypical clinical and histologic features that may make them difficult to distinguish from malignant melanoma.

Bibliography

Duffy K, Grossman D. The dysplastic nevus: From historical perspective to management in the modern era. Part I: Historical, histologic, and clinical aspects. J Am Acad Dermatol. 2012; 67: 1e1-1e16. [PMID: 22703916]

Item 33   Answer: D

Educational Objective: Treat pyoderma gangrenosum.

This patient has peristomal pyoderma gangrenosum (PG), and a topical potent glucocorticoid, such as clobetasol, is the preferred treatment. PG is an autoimmune ulcerative process that may occur idiopathically or in conjunction with an underlying disease; the most common disease association is inflammatory bowel disease (IBD). This patient has IBD and had recent surgery; 20% to 30% of patients with PG may exhibit "pathergy" or induction of lesions in response to trauma, such as surgery. Peristomal PG is a common manifestation, and early recognition is essential to avoid expansion, thereby limiting ostomy appliance adherence and devastating patients' quality of life. PG ulcers are typically painful, may rapidly expand, and are often exudative. When appropriate therapy is instituted, the lesions often dry out and become less painful over 1 to 2 weeks. Even when the PG inflammation is controlled, patients are left with a large ulcer that must then heal, and local care is critical. PG is treated with glucocorticoids (oral, topical, or intralesional), cyclosporine, or infliximab (a tumor necrosis factor α inhibitor) as first-line therapy for most patients. Active IBD should be treated as well.

Replacing the ostomy to the opposite side would entail major surgery, which, in the setting of active PG, could worsen the problem and may lead to PG at the new site. Removing the ostomy would not address the PG ulcer.

Rituximab is not indicated for PG, as rituximab targets CD20+ cells (B cells), which have little role in the pathogenesis of PG.

Because of the nature of the disease, PG lesions should not be debrided. PG lesions will worsen after debridement. It is not uncommon for PG to be diagnosed after repeated, unsuccessful debridements for a presumed infection result in dramatic worsening of the initial ulcer. Regardless, there is no necrotic tissue here to debride.

KEY POINT

- Glucocorticoids (oral, topical, intralesional) are first-line therapy for peristomal pyoderma gangrenosum.

Bibliography

Miller J, Yentzer BA, Clark A, Jorizzo JL, Feldman SR. Pyoderma gangrenosum: a review and update on new therapies. J Am Acad Dermatol. 2010 Apr;62(4):646-54. [PMID 20227580]

Item 34   Answer: C

Educational Objective: Diagnose pretibial myxedema.

This patient has clinical features of pretibial myxedema, generally seen in patients with Graves hyperthyroidism. Also termed thyroid dermopathy, pretibial myxedema results from the accumulation of glycosaminoglycans in the dermis that leads to the characteristic thickening and development of firm but compressible plaques described in this patient. The pretibial thickening generally occurs 1 to 2 years after the onset of Graves hyperthyroidism. The mechanisms of development of both pretibial myxedema and Graves ophthalmopathy are similar, and the findings often develop within a year of one another. The mechanisms of pretibial myxedema are not well understood but may be related to the interaction of thyrotropin-receptor antibodies with antigen-specific T cells and dermal fibroblasts causing inflammation and increased glycosaminoglycan production. Similar to increasing the risk for ocular disease, tobacco use may also increase the risk for pretibial myxedema in patients with Graves disease; almost all patients with pretibial myxedema have evidence of ophthalmopathy. The skin lesions typically occur on the shins, but rarely may occur elsewhere. Some patients may develop elephantiasis and severe leg deformity from the extent of myxedema. Once the lesions occur, they tend to persist regardless of the status of the thyroid disease. Skin-directed therapy may be required for improvement, although the lesions are generally of cosmetic concern and do not pose health risks.

Lipodermatosclerosis is a severe form of stasis in which the skin becomes thickened and may develop an "inverted champagne bottle" appearance with the skin on the distal legs being very tight and "woody."

Necrobiosis lipoidica (NL) is another skin manifestation of an endocrine condition that can occur on the anterior shins. NL presents as atrophic, orange-colored patches often associated with visible vasculature from skin thinning; the lesions may ulcerate. NL may develop in patients with diabetes mellitus, and when present may be a sign of end-organ damage, as patients with NL are more likely to have retinopathy or nephropathy.

Stasis dermatitis occurs in the setting of lower extremity edema. It is characterized by a ruddy-brown complexion in the setting of chronic venous backup and fluid filling the legs in response to proximal compression. This is typically seen in patients with heart failure.

KEY POINT

- Pretibial myxedema is generally seen in patients with Graves hyperthyroidism; dermal-based mucinous deposits in the skin of the anterior shins leads to the characteristic thickening and other skin changes.

Bibliography
Fatourechi V. Pretibial myxedema: pathophysiology and treatment options. Am J Clin Dermatol. 2005;6(5):295-309. [PMID: 16252929]

Item 35   Answer: A
Educational Objective: Diagnose bedbug infestation.

This patient has bedbug bites, and the most appropriate treatment is topical glucocorticoids. Bedbugs (*Cimex lectularius*) are parasites that feed on human blood, often producing pruritic papules in a characteristic grouped pattern ("breakfast, lunch, and dinner"). Bites occur in exposed skin areas and are more pronounced in the morning because bedbugs are nocturnal and feed at night, usually without being noticed. Bedbugs are about the size of a dog tick and are brownish in color with flat bodies. They frequently inhabit spaces in furniture such as mattresses and cushions. Bedbug bites can be extremely pruritic, and topical glucocorticoids provide anti-inflammatory and symptomatic relief. However, the lesions will self-resolve, so treatment is not mandatory. Professional exterminators are required for evaluation and removal of the bedbugs with pesticides, and eradication can be difficult, making their infestation a significant public health concern. Travel is a risk factor for bedbug infestation, and often multiple family members, if they share the same sleeping quarters, can be affected.

Body lice (pediculosis) also can lead to pruritic papules, but do not occur in a characteristic grouped pattern. Pruritic lesions can occur diffusely, as body lice usually live within the seams of clothing and not on the skin.

Flea bites also result in pruritic papules, but these lesions are not typically grouped. Additionally, because fleas are external parasites and do not live on humans, bites are more commonly present on the lower extremities because fleas typically jump from another location (such as a dog or cat) and bite the legs.

Scabies is an infestation of a mite that lives on the human skin and results in intensely pruritic papules and eruptions involving the waistline, genitals, finger web spaces, wrists, and axillae. A hypersensitivity reaction also can occur. The distribution of lesions in the patient described here is uncommon for scabies infestation.

Spider bites can result in pruritic lesions, but they typically occur as an isolated finding without evidence of multiple or recurrent bites. The number of bites and frequency in which the patient is developing lesions would be atypical for spider bites.

KEY POINT

- Bedbug bites can be recognized by their characteristic grouping in a linear series pattern ("breakfast, lunch, and dinner"); the lesions are painless, pruritic, urticaria-like papules.

Bibliography
Haddad V Jr, Cardoso JL, Lupi O, Tyring SK. Tropical dermatology: Venomous arthropods and human skin: Part I. Insecta. J Am Acad Dermatol. 2012 Sep;67(3):331.e1-14. [PMID: 22890734]

Item 36   Answer: C
Educational Objective: Diagnose erythroderma.

This patient has erythroderma, which is a term used to describe erythematous inflammation of at least 80% to 90% of the skin surface and is a dermatologic urgency. Erythroderma is most often due to an uncontrolled existing dermatosis such as cutaneous T-cell lymphoma, graft-versus-host disease, psoriasis, or pityriasis rubra pilaris. Medications are the second most common cause; thus, taking a history of current and recently discontinued medications is also important. Men are affected more often than women, and the average age of onset is 55 years. Although the diagnosis of erythroderma is usually straightforward, in some patients it may be difficult to determine the cause, particularly in patients without a known preexisting condition that may be responsible. In these patients, a combination of clinical evaluation and careful clinicopathologic correlation is needed. Owing to compromise of the skin barrier, affected patients are at risk for dehydration, electrolyte abnormalities, protein loss, heat loss, and infection. Peripheral edema, erosions from severe pruritus, scaling, and lymphadenopathy are common findings.

Angioedema is soft-tissue swelling that may be mast cell or bradykinin mediated. It may occur independently, with urticaria, or may be associated with anaphylaxis. Angioedema tends to affect less dense connective tissue, including the face, lips, throat, and extremities, but is not associated with erythroderma. This patient's presentation is therefore not consistent with angioedema.

Drug-induced subacute cutaneous lupus erythematosus (SCLE) can be triggered by hydrochlorothiazide. Other medications that can cause this eruption are calcium channel blockers, ACE inhibitors, statins, proton-pump inhibitors, and tumor necrosis factor α inhibitors. Although this patient is taking hydrochlorothiazide, the appearance of his rash is not consistent with SCLE. Drug-induced SCLE typically presents as annular pink-red patches with fine scale, predominantly affecting the photodistributed areas of the upper chest, back, and shoulders.

Pityriasis refers to flaking of the skin, and a number of cutaneous conditions incorporate this descriptive term into their name. Pityriasis rosea (PR) is a relatively common inflammatory reaction of the skin and may be caused by a viral infection; however, a specific virus causing this condition has not been identified. It generally occurs in patients younger than 30 years old and does not cause an erythrodermic eruption. Typically, PR begins as a single annular patch or plaque with fine scaling (the so-called herald patch). About 1 week later many smaller pink macules, patches, and papules erupt over the trunk and proximal extremities.

KEY POINT

- Erythroderma is characterized by erythema of at least 80% to 90% of the skin surface and is a dermatologic urgency.

Bibliography

Khaled A, Sellami A, Fazaa B, et al. Acquired erythroderma in adults: a clinical and prognostic study. J Eur Acad Dermatol Venereol. 2010 Jul;24(7):781-8. [PMID: 20028449]

Item 37   Answer: C

Educational Objective: Manage potential complications of herpes zoster infection.

This patient has herpes zoster infection involving the forehead and has a vesicular lesion on the tip of the nose (Hutchinson sign) suggesting the possibility of ocular involvement, and she should be referred for urgent ophthalmologic evaluation. This clinical scenario is consistent with herpes zoster infection involving the V1 distribution of the trigeminal nerve, which

can result in eye involvement (herpes zoster ophthalmicus) and ophthalmologic complications including keratitis, scleritis, uveitis, and acute retinal necrosis. When grouped vesicles on an erythematous base involve the V1 distribution or extend to the tip of the nose, concurrent management with an ophthalmologist is indicated to help treat and prevent any of these complications. Management of these patients usually involves antiviral therapy and topical glucocorticoid eye drops to reduce inflammation.

The herpes zoster vaccine is recommended for persons 60 years or older to prevent herpes zoster and its complications. The administration of the vaccine after an episode of zoster is debated. The Centers for Disease Control recommends providing the vaccine even after an initial herpes zoster infection. However, a recent article states that the cellular immune response to varicella zoster virus (VZV) during the first 3 years after vaccination is similar to that after an episode of herpes zoster. As a result, deferring vaccination for up to 3 years in patients who are immunocompetent, such as this patient, is recommended, as vaccination during the episode will not be as effective.

Mupirocin is an antibiotic used for the treatment of bacterial skin infections such as impetigo, furuncles, or methicillin-resistant *Staphylococcus aureus*. Herpes zoster is a viral infection, and mupirocin would not be appropriate.

Otolaryngology consultation is not necessary. The distribution of the vesicles in the central face is not concerning for underlying hearing or other otolaryngologic involvement. Herpes virus infection may involve the ear canal and hearing may be affected and a facial nerve palsy or vertigo also can result. This complex of findings is known as Ramsay Hunt syndrome, and systemic glucocorticoids and antiviral agents may be necessary to treat this complication, usually with co-management with an otolaryngologist.

KEY POINT

- Herpes zoster infection involving the V1 distribution of the trigeminal nerve can result in ophthalmologic complications including keratitis, scleritis, uveitis, and acute retinal necrosis.

Bibliography

Cohen JI. Clinical practice: herpes zoster. N Engl J Med. 2013 Jul 18;369(3):255-63. [PMID: 23863052]

Item 38   Answer: A

Educational Objective: Diagnose drug reaction with eosinophilia and systemic symptoms.

This patient should discontinue the trimethoprim-sulfamethoxazole, and a complete blood count and liver chemistry tests should be ordered. She has a widespread morbilliform eruption with fever, facial edema, and lymphadenopathy that started 6 days after taking trimethoprim-sulfamethoxazole. This is typical of a systemic drug hypersensitivity syndrome, otherwise known as drug reaction with eosinophilia and systemic symptoms (DRESS) syndrome. It is a rare, potentially

CONT.

life-threatening drug-induced hypersensitivity reaction. The presentation of DRESS typically includes a skin eruption, hematologic abnormalities, lymphadenopathy, and internal organ involvement (including the liver, kidneys, and lungs). The presence of DRESS should be suspected in patients with a morbilliform rash, fever, facial swelling, and lymphadenopathy that occur 5 to 10 days after starting a potentially offending medication. The initial diagnostic approach in suspected DRESS is to assess for evidence of systemic organ involvement, and this is accomplished by obtaining a complete blood count, which may show atypical lymphocytosis and eosinophilia, and liver chemistry studies, which may show aminotransferase elevations. Patients with extensive cutaneous reactions or evidence of organ involvement may require hospitalization and possibly treatment with systemic glucocorticoids. Even if the rash fades, the patient can still progress to liver failure.

Lymph node biopsy may show a range of findings that may be suspicious for lymphoma. Lymph node biopsy is rarely required for the diagnosis or management of DRESS.

Skin biopsy may show lymphocytic infiltration and edema in DRESS and may confirm the diagnosis, although it is not helpful in assessing the severity of systemic organ involvement.

No further testing following discontinuation of the likely causative medication is appropriate in patients without evidence of significant organ involvement. However, exclusion of significant systemic involvement is necessary before a supportive approach is taken.

KEY POINT

- Patients with suspected drug hypersensitivity syndrome, also known as drug reaction with eosinophilia and systemic symptoms, should have a complete blood count with differential to evaluate for eosinophilia or atypical lymphocytosis and liver chemistry tests to assess for evidence of systemic organ involvement.

Bibliography

Cacoub P, Musette P, Descamps V, Meyer O, Speirs C, Finzi L, Roujeau JC. The DRESS syndrome: a literature review. Am J Med. 2011 Jul;124(7):588-97. [PMID: 21592453]

Item 39   Answer: A

Educational Objective: Manage lichen sclerosus in a postmenopausal woman.

The patient should be treated with a topical high-potency glucocorticoid (class I or II), such as clobetasol, mometasone, or betamethasone. Her clinical presentation of white atrophic patches circumferentially involving the anus and vagina with associated pruritus and dyspareunia is consistent with lichen sclerosus. Lichen sclerosus is a benign, chronic, and progressive dermatologic condition of unclear etiology that tends to affect peri- and postmenopausal women. It manifests with marked inflammation and epithelial thinning that is pruritic; because of its usual location, lichen sclerosus is

usually associated with pain during intercourse. Skin findings are characteristic, and the diagnosis is confirmed on biopsy showing epidermal thinning, scarring, and evidence of inflammation. The appropriate first-line therapy for this disease is a potent topical glucocorticoid, such as clobetasol, daily for 2 to 3 months (or until resolved) and then intermittently to prevent recurrence. Not treating lichen sclerosus will result in permanent scarring (including all anatomic structures such as the clitoris and vaginal opening), and there is evidence of early scarring with resorption of the labia minora in this patient. Close monitoring also is essential to evaluate for cutaneous squamous cell carcinomas that can occur with chronic inflammation.

A low-potency glucocorticoid, such as hydrocortisone 1% ointment, is not adequate to treat lichen sclerosus. Continued inflammation with this treatment will result in permanent scarring.

Vulvar lichen sclerosus is not caused by a bacterial infection; therefore systemic (cephalexin) or topical (mupirocin) antibiotics are not indicated.

Occasional co-infection with vaginal candidiasis can occur, which would present with foul-smelling and thick white discharge. Vulvar candidiasis can also occur, which would present with bright red patches and satellite pustules. These infections should be treated with intravaginal or oral antifungal agents. Topical nystatin is an antifungal agent used to treat candidiasis but would not be effective for treatment of vulvar lichen sclerosus.

KEY POINT

- The use of potent topical glucocorticoids is considered first-line treatment for lichen sclerosus.

Bibliography

Virgili A, Borghi A, Minghetti S, Corazza M. Mometasone fuoroate 0.1% ointment in the treatment of vulvar lichen sclerosus: a study of efficacy and safety on a large cohort of patients. J Eur Acad Dermatol Venereol. 2014 Jul;28(7):943-8. [PMID: 23879234]

Item 40   Answer: B

Educational Objective: Diagnose fixed drug eruption.

This patient likely has a fixed drug eruption (FDE). A painful purple patch that occurs in the same location repeatedly is a classic sign of a FDE. Patients with an extensive eruption may have central bullae that occur in the same location (fixed) each time the patient is exposed to the same medication. Lips, genitals, and hands are commonly involved. There may be only one spot with the first exposure; but if reexposed, the lesion may recur along with new areas. Common drug culprits are over-the-counter medications such as NSAIDs, pseudoephedrine, sulfonamide medications, and other antibiotics. The patient's periodic recurrent lesion is likely associated with his periodic use of ibuprofen. Drug discontinuation is the appropriate treatment, with resolution of the rash expected to occur over days to weeks.

Contact dermatitis is a delayed hypersensitivity reaction to a specific chemical. With repeated exposure to the chemical, a diffuse, pruritic eczematous dermatitis develops on the area that was exposed. The characteristic rash is typically reddish, scaly, and crusting, and when occurring on the penis may be associated with condom use. However, this patient's rash is not typical for eczematous dermatitis.

Herpes simplex virus infection usually presents with a vesicular rash if acute or erosion if chronic, as may be seen in patients with HIV infection. Recurrent genital herpes is similar to oral herpes with a prodrome, followed by grouped vesicles on an erythematous base, erosions, and crusting. This patient's presentation is not consistent with recurrent herpes simplex virus infection.

Primary syphilis presents as a chancre, classically a shallow nonexudative ulcer with an indurated border that is not painful. This patient's lesion is not consistent with a chancre.

KEY POINT

- The classic sign of a fixed drug eruption is a painful purple patch that occurs in the same location repeatedly; the lips, genitals, and hands are commonly involved.

Bibliography

Mizukawa Y, Shiohara T. Fixed drug eruption: a prototypic disorder mediated by effector memory T cells. Curr Allergy Asthma Rep. 2009 Jan;9(1):71-7. [PMID: 19063828]

Item 41   Answer: D

Educational Objective: Diagnose Sweet syndrome.

This patient has the typical skin findings characteristic of Sweet syndrome, also known as acute febrile neutrophilic dermatosis. The lesions are well demarcated with a sharp cut-off separating normal and inflamed skin. Because of the intense neutrophilic inflammatory infiltrate and accompanying papillary dermal edema, the lesions are often referred to as appearing "juicy." Patients often have a leukocytosis with a predominance of neutrophils and bands; there may be an accompanying, albeit nonspecific, elevation in inflammatory markers such as erythrocyte sedimentation rate. Patients with Sweet syndrome may have idiopathic disease (common in older white women) or paraneoplastic Sweet syndrome, most commonly seen in patients with hematologic malignancies, particularly acute myeloid leukemia or myelodysplastic syndrome. The sharply demarcated, indurated red papules, plaques, or nodules almost always develop in the setting of fever and are often mistaken for infection. Patients may develop these lesions at any time during their treatment course. Sweet syndrome may also occur as a reaction to certain medications, particularly granulocyte colony-stimulating factors. The condition is extraordinarily responsive to treatment with glucocorticoids, with the fever stopping immediately and the lesions fading within 1 to 2 days.

Candidiasis would not be expected to occur this early in this patient's neutropenic course, and the skin lesions of disseminated candidiasis are generally small red papules,

sometimes with a prominent white or translucent center; plaques are not common in disseminated candidiasis.

Keratoacanthoma is a subtype of squamous cell carcinoma that often presents with an isolated, rapidly growing, red nodule with a central keratin-filled core, resembling a "volcano" with the center composed of crusted dried keratin. The "juicy" red nodule shown would be atypical for a keratoacanthoma.

Pyogenic granulomas are small, benign vascular papules that can occur almost anywhere but tend to be seen on the extremities around the nails and on the face. They tend to occur more commonly in patients treated with certain types of medications (such as certain acne medications and antiretroviral agents) and in pregnant women.

KEY POINT

- The lesions in Sweet syndrome are "juicy" red papules, plaques, or nodules with sharp borders, appearing on the upper trunk and proximal extremities in the setting of fevers.

Bibliography

Dabade TS, Davis MD. Diagnosis and treatment of the neutrophilic dermatoses (pyoderma gangrenosum, Sweet's syndrome). Dermatol Ther. 2011 Mar-Apr;24(2):273-84. [PMID: 21410617]

Item 42   Answer: C

Educational Objective: Diagnose eosinophilic pustular folliculitis.

This patient has eosinophilic pustular folliculitis, a rash most commonly seen in patients with HIV infection, and usually in those with a CD4 cell count less than 300/µL. The lesions are typically intensely pruritic papules (and rarely pustules) clustered on the chest and face, generally in areas with a high concentration of sebaceous glands. Biopsy will reveal an eosinophilic infiltrate in the hair follicle, and peripheral eosinophilia may develop in up to 50% of patients. The exact etiology is unknown, but the condition is relatively common. Diagnosis is usually based on the presence of the typical skin rash in an appropriate clinical context. The rash usually responds to antiretroviral therapy, although high-potency glucocorticoids and systemic antihistamines may be used for symptomatic treatment.

Acne is characterized by comedonal lesions (plugged pores, blackheads) and, when drug induced, often involves the shoulders and back; this patient is not taking any drugs typically associated with drug-induced acne (glucocorticoids, bromides, lithium, certain oncologic agents [particularly epidermal growth factor-receptor antagonists], and more).

Drug reaction with eosinophilia and systemic symptoms (DRESS), also referred to as drug-induced hypersensitivity syndrome, would appear within 2 to 8 weeks of starting a new drug and would include fevers, a widespread morbilliform eruption often involving the face accompanied by facial edema, complete blood count abnormalities (eosinophilia or atypical lymphocytosis), and systemic inflammation (generally lymphadenopathy and hepatitis, although nephritis, pneumonitis, and myocarditis can occur). This patient lacks the fever and systemic symptoms of DRESS, and the rash would be atypical for this diagnosis.

Scabies can also cause intense pruritus and eosinophilia. However, patients rarely have lesions above the neck and generally have involvement of the finger web spaces, umbilicus, and, in men, the genitals.

KEY POINT

- Eosinophilic pustular folliculitis causes intensely pruritic papules on the face and chest and is most commonly seen in patients with HIV infection, generally with a CD4 cell count less than 300/µL.

Bibliography

Nervi SJ, Schwartz RA, Dmochowski M. Eosinophilic pustular folliculitis: a 40 year retrospect. J Am Acad Dermatol. 2006 Aug;55(2):285-9. [PMID: 16844513]

Item 43   Answer: A

Educational Objective: Manage a superficial skin infection.

The most appropriate first step in management is to culture a pustule to identify the causative organism prior to institution of antibiotic therapy. Bacterial skin infections are most commonly caused by *Staphylococcus* and *Streptococcus* spp. and may present in a variety of ways. This patient has recurrent folliculitis and furunculosis but is otherwise healthy. The history of recurrent infections and being part of a wrestling team would suggest that infection may be secondary to community-acquired methicillin-resistant *Staphylococcus aureus* (MRSA). Community-acquired MRSA, defined as MRSA infections that occurs in the absence of health care exposure, tends to have enhanced virulence compared with other strains and is currently the most common organism causing skin infection requiring medical therapy. However, because of the recurrent nature of the patient's skin infections and his exposure to previous courses of antibiotics, a culture to identify the causative organism and its susceptibility pattern would be the most appropriate next step to guide further management.

In addition to systemic therapy, topical antibiotic therapies, including benzoyl peroxide wash, chlorhexidine, or topical mupirocin, can be used. Bleach baths may be a treatment option (put 1/4 to 1/2 cup of common liquid bleach into the bath water to create a chlorinated bath), which decreases colonization of *S. aureus*).

A Tzanck smear can be performed if a herpes simplex virus or varicella infection is suspected. Both infections can occur in wrestlers but would typically present as painful vesicles or punched-out erosions as opposed to furuncles or folliculitis.

Linezolid is effective against many strains of MRSA and streptococci. However, its use should be limited to patients with a documented infection who have not benefitted from sensitive antibiotics because of potential toxicities or cost.

Oral cephalexin (or other cephalosporins or penicillins) should not be used because these antibiotics would not be effective against MRSA if used empirically. In addition, antimicrobial therapy in this patient would more appropriately be guided by culture and sensitivity results.

Parenteral therapy for skin and soft-tissue infections should be considered in patients with extensive involvement, in patients with evidence of systemic involvement, or patients who are immunocompromised. Although vancomycin is effective against possible MRSA, parenteral therapy would not be appropriate in a stable, otherwise healthy man without any signs of systemic infection, particularly without a confirmed MRSA infection.

KEY POINT

- In managing a superficial skin infection, a culture of the pustule is important to determine both the causative organism and the antibiotic susceptibility pattern.

Bibliography

Daum RS. Clinical practice. Skin and soft-tissue infections caused by methicillin-resistant Staphylococcus aureus. N Engl J Med. 2007 Jul 26;357(4): 380-90. [PMID: 17652653]

Item 44   Answer: B

Educational Objective: Recognize livedo reticularis.

The patient has livedo reticularis, and her clinical presentation is consistent with the antiphospholipid antibody syndrome. Livedo reticularis is a subtle, lacy network of faintly blue or purple vessels, usually seen on the lower legs, caused by the prominence of the vasculature under the skin. It is a very nonspecific finding and is most often seen in patients without an underlying condition. Livedo reticularis can sometimes be elicited by keeping a leg in the dependent position; if livedo resolves when the leg is straightened horizontally, it is likely not a pathologic process. However, it can also be a component of a variety of systemic diseases, typically those that cause a slow-flow or hypercoagulable state. Associated conditions include autoimmune diseases (systemic lupus erythematosus, rheumatoid arthritis, dermatomyositis), vasculitis (polyarteritis nodosa, giant cell arteritis), paraproteinemias (multiple myeloma, cryoglobulinemia), hematologic diseases (polycythemia vera, thrombocytosis), and infections. Livedo reticularis also has a strong association with the antiphospholipid antibody syndrome, and there is evidence that its presence suggests increased risk of cerebral or ocular ischemia. This patient's livedo reticularis and history of prior miscarriages are suggestive of antiphospholipid antibody syndrome. According to the revised Sapporo criterion, a diagnosis of antiphospholipid antibody syndrome requires at least one clinical criteria (vascular thrombosis excluding superficial venous thrombosis or pregnancy morbidity) and at least one laboratory criterion (the presence of antiphospholipid antibodies on two or more occasions at least 12 weeks apart).

Amyloidosis is an infiltrative disease that causes skin thickening and is more often associated with development of petechiae and ecchymoses than with changes consistent with livedo reticularis.

Autoimmune thyroid disease, particularly Graves disease, may uncommonly be associated with pretibial myxedema, an accumulation of glycosaminoglycans in the dermis, usually over the lower legs. This patient's clinical findings are not consistent with this diagnosis.

Systemic sclerosis involves excessive production of extracellular matrix with increased collagen production resulting in skin thickening. Livedo reticularis is not a common manifestation of this disorder.

KEY POINT

- Antiphospholipid antibody testing should be performed in persons with fixed livedo reticularis that persists despite position and temperature changes, or those with signs, symptoms, or history suggestive of thromboses.

Bibliography
Thornsberry LA, LoSicco KI, English JC 3rd. The skin and hypercoagulable states. J Am Acad Dermatol. 2013 Sep;69(3):450-62. [PMID: 23582572]

Item 45   Answer: D

Educational Objective: Diagnose seborrheic keratosis.

This patient's lesion is a seborrheic keratosis. Seborrheic keratoses are benign skin lesions that commonly occur in older persons. They typically have a waxy or scaly texture and often have a "stuck-on" appearance. They are usually oval and brown and may occasionally itch or bleed.

Dermatofibromas are benign firm brown or reddish papules that most commonly occur on the lower extremities. They generally lack the scale seen with seborrheic keratoses. They extend deeper into the skin than seborrheic keratoses and exhibit the "dimple sign" when squeezed.

Malignant melanomas may occasionally resemble seborrheic keratoses, and thus lesions that are questionable should be removed and sent for histologic evaluation. Although some features of seborrheic keratoses may be suggestive of malignant melanoma, such as elevations above the skin and inconsistent coloration, melanomas tend to progress more rapidly, are darker in color, have more blurred borders, and lack the scaly "stuck-on" appearance characteristic of seborrheic keratoses.

Pigmented basal cell carcinomas may mimic seborrheic keratoses, but they tend to be more translucent and less scaly.

Solar lentigines ("liver spots") are flat brown macules that occur on sun-exposed skin of older persons, particularly the face and dorsal hands rather than the trunk. They resemble large freckles.

KEY POINT

- Seborrheic keratoses are benign skin lesions commonly occurring in older persons; they typically have a waxy or scaly texture with a "stuck-on" appearance.

Bibliography
Noiles K, Vender R. Are all seborrheic keratoses benign? Review of the typical lesion and its variants. J Cutan Med Surg. 2008 Sep-Oct;12(5):203-10. [PMID: 18845088]

Item 46   Answer: B

Educational Objective: Manage a patient with acute urticaria.

The most appropriate therapy for this patient is a second-generation H_1 antihistamine, such as cetirizine. He has acute urticaria, characterized by evanescent red, pruritic plaques and wheals that last less than 24 hours after a probable viral upper respiratory tract infection. Newer-generation H_1 antihistamines are preferred to first-generation agents (diphenhydramine, hydroxyzine) primarily because they are long-acting and are more likely to suppress the urticaria consistently. They also do not readily cross the blood-brain barrier and therefore have less sedating and anticholinergic side effects that may be dose-limiting in some patients.

Amoxicillin can be used if there is concern for a bacterial infection, but the clinical history of nonpurulent cough, rhinitis, and self-resolution is not consistent with a bacterial infection.

Glucocorticoids, such as prednisone, are effective therapy for urticaria, but have considerable systemic side effects. Although their use may be appropriate in patients with angioedema, antihistamines are the preferred initial treatment option owing to their effectiveness and safer side-effect profile.

Ranitidine is an H_2 antihistamine used primarily for gastric acid suppression and would not be appropriate antihistamine monotherapy for this patient. The combination of an H_1 and H_2 antihistamine is often used, particularly in patients with severe urticaria, although there is limited evidence of effectiveness of this practice.

KEY POINT

- Treatment of urticaria is most effective with long-acting antihistamines since they help treat active disease and prevent new flares.

Bibliography
Zuberbier T1, Asero R, Bindslev-Jensen C, Canonica G et al. EAACI/GA(2) LEN/EDF/WAO guideline: definition, classification and diagnosis of urticaria. Allergy. 2009 Oct;64(10):1417-26. [PMID: 19772512]

Item 47   Answer: B

Educational Objective: Treat seborrheic dermatitis.

This patient should be treated with ketoconazole cream. Scaling and redness, specifically on the eyebrows, nasolabial folds, and sides of the chin, are characteristic of seborrheic dermatitis. The redness and scaling are a response to commensal yeasts in the skin, and topical ketoconazole targets these yeasts. Patients may believe that their skin findings are due to dry skin on the face. However, the redness of the eyebrows and nasolabial folds extending onto the cheeks and chin with scaling is typical of seborrhea and often does not respond to moisturization only.

Benzoyl peroxide is approved for treatment of acne vulgaris, which is characterized by open and closed comedones and inflammatory lesions, but not the redness and scaling associated with seborrheic dermatitis.

Metronidazole is used to treat rosacea, which usually presents with flushing and central facial erythema, telangiectasias, papules, and pustules but not typically with scaling.

Mupirocin is a topical antibiotic that targets gram-positive organisms, but there are no pustules, crusting, bullae, or erosions that would be diagnostic of impetigo in this patient.

Triamcinolone would decrease the inflammatory response and redness of seborrheic dermatitis but is too potent to be used consistently on the face.

KEY POINT

- The redness and scaling of seborrheic dermatitis are a response to commensal yeasts in the skin, and topical ketoconazole targets these yeasts.

Bibliography

Dessinioti C, Katsambas A. Seborrheic dermatitis: etiology, risk factors, and treatments: facts and controversies. Clin Dermatol. 2013 Jul-Aug;31(4): 343-51. [PMID: 23806151]

Item 48   Answer: B

Educational Objective: Diagnose basal cell carcinoma.

This patient has basal cell carcinoma (BCC), the most common type of skin cancer. BCC typically presents as translucent ("pearly") telangiectatic papules on sun-exposed areas in fair-skinned persons with a history of extensive sun exposure. It is usually asymptomatic and enlarges slowly over time. Although it rarely metastasizes, BCC can cause significant local tissue destruction if not removed in a timely fashion. BCC has a wide variety of morphologies, some of which can be challenging diagnostically.

Angiofibromas (fibrous papules of the nose) are common solitary lesions that are often seen in patients with rosacea. They tend to be flesh colored, lack pearliness or telangiectasias, and are stable in size and appearance over time.

Sebaceous hyperplasia present as small papules found on the face in patients with rosacea. They often have a central umbilication, which is a characteristic feature. They lack the pearliness seen in BCC, have less prominent telangiectasias, and often have a yellowish color.

Squamous cell carcinoma (SCC) may resemble BCC in many aspects; however, SCC tends to be much scalier, lack the pearliness seen in BCC, and have less prominent telangiectasias. It also tends to grow more rapidly than BCC.

KEY POINT

- Basal cell carcinoma presents as asymptomatic translucent telangiectatic papules on sun-exposed areas in fair-skinned patients; extensive tissue damage may occur if not removed.

Bibliography

Rubin AI, Chen EH, Ratner D. Basal cell carcinoma. N Engl J Med 2005 Nov 24;353(21):2262-9. [PMID: 16306523]

Item 49   Answer: A

Educational Objective: Treat mild acne in a pregnant woman.

This woman should be treated with azelaic acid cream. Women of childbearing age need special consideration, as treatment of some of the most common diseases, including acne, involves the use of teratogenic medications. The FDA pregnancy safety category of all medications should be considered when prescribing to women who are pregnant, breastfeeding, or trying to conceive. Several commonly used systemic and some topical dermatologic drugs are contraindicated for use in pregnancy. Azelaic acid cream is rated pregnancy category B and is the safest of the listed acne therapies. Acne is a chronic inflammatory skin condition characterized by open and closed comedones (blackheads and whiteheads, respectively) and inflammatory lesions, including papules, pustules, or nodules. Androgens stimulate increased sebum production, so pregnancy-associated hyperactivity of the hypothalamic–pituitary–gonadal axis can trigger acne exacerbations. This patient has mild comedonal and inflammatory acne, and topical treatment is preferred; however, it is important to consider the safety of topical acne treatments during pregnancy. Topical erythromycin can also be used to manage acne, since it is a pregnancy category B medication.

Doxycycline is rated pregnancy category D and can cause defects in the formation of teeth and bone in the fetus. Both tazarotene and tretinoin are topical retinoids and have been rated as pregnancy category X and D, respectively. They should not be used during pregnancy.

KEY POINT

- Azelaic acid cream is rated FDA pregnancy category B and is safe to use for mild comedonal and inflammatory acne during pregnancy.

Bibliography

Strauss JS, Krowchuk DP, Leyden JJ, et al; American Academy of Dermatology/American Academy of Dermatology Association. Guidelines of care for acne vulgaris management. J Am Acad Dermatol. 2007 Apr;56(4):651-63. [PMID: 17276540]

Item 50   Answer: B

Educational Objective: Diagnose herpes simplex virus infection.

This patient has a herpes simplex virus (HSV) infection, and direct-fluorescent antibody testing (DFA) should be performed. The patient is immunocompromised due to HIV infection, and establishing the diagnosis is important in these patients. Although the diagnosis of HSV infection can often be made clinically, ancillary tests are available to confirm the diagnosis. Of these, DFA and polymerase chain reaction (PCR) are tests that can be rapidly completed (in less than 24 hours). They are also able differentiate between the various types of herpesvirus infections: HSV1, HSV2, and varicella infection. DFA and PCR are done by unroofing a vesicle and swabbing the base of the vesicle to provide an adequate sample.

Bacterial culture is incorrect as the lips are often contaminated with bacteria, given the presence of multiple bacteria in oral flora. In addition, the patient's lesions do not have honey-colored crust, suggesting that these are not impetiginized. Performing serologic testing (HSV IgG) is not recommended to diagnose herpes virus infections, as the seroprevalence for both HSV1 and HSV2 is high, and a positive result is not indicative of active infection.

Viral culture had been considered the gold standard in the past, but it can take over 48 hours (sometimes up to 1 week) for results to return. Culture is useful if resistance testing is necessary for recalcitrant infections. However, the recommended initial tests are now DFA and PCR to help establish or confirm the diagnosis.

KEY POINT

- Although diagnosis of herpes simplex virus (HSV) infections can be made clinically, direct-fluorescent antibody and polymerase chain reaction testing can provide results in less than 24 hours and can differentiate between HSV1, HSV2, and varicella infections, which is important when treating immunocompromised patients.

Bibliography

Frisch S, Guo AM. Diagnostic methods and management strategies of herpes simplex and herpes zoster infections. Clin Geriatr Med. 2013 May;29(2):501-26. [PMID: 23571042]

Item 51   **Answer:**   **C**

Educational Objective: Diagnose miliaria.

This patient's rash is consistent with a diagnosis of miliaria crystallina. Miliaria, or "heat rash," is characterized by the eruption of fine red papules and pustules specifically located on the back, typically after immobilization in the supine position. Miliaria is caused by superficial clogging of the eccrine sweat glands, which leads to the development of minute pustules that rupture easily and can be wiped off. The clogging may be partially due to overgrowth of *Staphylococcus epidermidis*. Treatment involves implementing measures to decrease sweating and topical measures such cool baths and the use of loose clothing.

Allergic contact dermatitis on the back would appear as an eczematous dermatitis with pruritus on the area exposed to the allergen. This patient does not have pruritus or clinical findings consistent with an allergic contact dermatitis.

Candida albicans infections occur in hot, moist occluded areas, such as the armpits, groin, and beneath the breasts. The rash is not usually diffuse and will typically have some desquamation at the edges. The papules cannot be wiped off as with miliaria crystallina.

Staphylococcal folliculitis will cause more deep-seated follicular pustules, and the area would be red, swollen, and painful. Although *Staphylococcus aureus* is responsible for a wide range of skin infections such as folliculitis, abscesses, furuncles, carbuncles, impetigo, cellulitis, ecthyma, staphylococcal scalded skin syndrome, and erysipelas, this patient's clinical presentation is not consistent with an infection with this organism.

KEY POINT

- Miliaria, or "heat rash," is characterized by the eruption of fine red papules and pustules specifically located on the back, typically after immobilization in the supine position.

Bibliography

Haas N, Martens F, Henz BM. Miliaria crystallina in an intensive care setting. Clin Exp Dermatol. 2004 Jan;29(1):32-4. [PMID: 14723716]

Item 52   **Answer:**   **C**

Educational Objective: Manage arterial ulcers.

This patient has an arterial ulcer, and determination of the ankle-brachial index would be the next appropriate step in management. Arterial ulcers occur in the setting of significant peripheral vascular disease and result from inadequate perfusion of the lower extremities. Ulceration tends to occur at the distal aspects of the arterial supply (such as the distal toes) or in areas of trauma (such as overlying the metatarsal heads or shins and ankles). The ulcers are usually tender, have a well-demarcated border with a "punched out" appearance, and are surrounded by erythematous, tight skin. Dry, shiny skin is often present, and elevation of the legs often results in worsening pain. Changes consistent with venous stasis, such as stasis dermatitis and lipodermatosclerosis, are usually lacking. The presence of peripheral vascular disease may be suggested by a decreased ankle-brachial index, with a value less than or equal to 0.9 suggestive of significant arterial occlusion. If the ankle-brachial index is decreased in this patient, lower extremity Doppler ultrasound arterial studies are indicated to confirm impaired arterial flow as a cause of the ulceration. If significant arterial compromise is found, referral to a vascular surgeon is indicated for consideration of a revascularization procedure.

Biopsy is not useful for distinguishing between venous stasis ulcers and arterial ulcers, although it can be useful to rule out other causes of ulceration such as infection or malignancy. Skin biopsy in the setting of arterial insufficiency can lead to an enlargement of the ulcer and thus should be performed with caution.

External compression, a mainstay of treatment for venous stasis ulcers, is contraindicated for arterial ulcers as it may further interfere with perfusion. As venous stasis and arterial insufficiency may sometimes coexist, vascular studies should be considered prior to starting compression

Answers and Critiques

therapy for venous stasis if there is significant concern for the presence of arterial disease.

Oral antibiotics are useful when overt signs of infection are present; however, they are not indicated otherwise. Common signs of infection include purulent discharge, swelling, and increasing tenderness. Overuse of antibiotics has been shown to lead to the development of resistant bacteria, a situation that is particularly problematic in the setting of chronic wounds.

KEY POINT

- Determination of the ankle-brachial index (ABI) is helpful in diagnosing suspected arterial insufficiency.

Bibliography

Greer N, Foman NA, MacDonald R, Dorrian J, Fitzgerald P, Rutks I, Wilt TJ. Advanced wound care therapies for nonhealing diabetic, venous, and arterial ulcers: a systematic review. Ann Intern Med. 2013 Oct 15;159(8):532-42. [PMID: 24126647]

Item 53   Answer: B

Educational Objective: Treat cutaneous larva migrans.

This patient has cutaneous larva migrans, and the most appropriate treatment is oral ivermectin. Cutaneous larva migrans (creeping eruption) is a parasitic skin disease caused by migration of the hookworm larvae within the superficial layers of the skin. It presents as a pruritic serpiginous, linear, or arciform red plaque that migrates at a rate of a few millimeters to centimeters per day and represents a hypersensitivity reaction to the hookworm, most commonly *Ancylostoma braziliense.* The clinical appearance of a migratory pruritic plaque after exposure to a beach is characteristic of cutaneous larva migrans. Although cutaneous larva migrans can be self-limited, treatment with oral ivermectin (or albendazole) is the medication of choice.

Oral cephalexin is an antibiotic that is used for bacterial skin infections, which may occur secondarily in patients with cutaneous larva migrans at times, but the lack of honey- or yellow-colored crust and surrounding erythema in this patient make a bacterial infection unlikely.

Oral prednisone may be helpful for the symptoms associated with cutaneous larva migrans, but it is not necessary or first-line treatment (topical glucocorticoids can be used for severe pruritus); oral prednisone would be the treatment of choice for allergic contact dermatitis, which can be geometric (rectangular, circular, even serpiginous) in shape, but should not migrate.

Terbinafine is the treatment of choice for dermatophyte infections, such as tinea pedis, which presents on the feet and ankles. Dermatophyte infections can be annular in appearance but differ from the clinical picture here in that it usually has superficial scale in a "moccasin" distribution or annular configuration, maceration between the web spaces and does not migrate. It would not be effective against this parasitic infection.

KEY POINT

- Although cutaneous larva migrans can be self-limited, oral antiparasitic agents (ivermectin as the preferred agent or albendazole as an alternative) can help resolve the eruption.

Bibliography

Feldmeier H, Schuster A. Mini review: Hookworm-related cutaneous larva migrans. Eur J Clin Microbiol Infect Dis. 2012 Jun;31(6):915-8. [PMID: 21922198]

Item 54   Answer: A

Educational Objective: Recognize the prognostic features of malignant melanoma.

The depth of invasion (Breslow depth) of a melanoma is the most important prognostic feature and correlates most strongly with the risk of recurrence and metastasis. The 2009 American Joint Committee on Cancer (AJCC) staging system defines the primary tumor stage based on the Breslow depth, with 10-year survival rate decreasing progressively with increasing depth.

Other features have also been identified as secondary negative prognostic indicators, including an elevated mitotic rate (defined as more that 1 mitotic figure per mm^2) and the presence of ulceration. The presence or absence of these two factors are used to subdivide the tumor stages based on depth into further prognostic categories

The radial diameter of the lesion has not been found to correlate with prognosis; many melanomas are quite wide, and yet if they have not developed an invasion component, the risk of metastasis is very small.

KEY POINT

- The Breslow depth (or depth of invasion) of a melanoma is the most important prognostic feature and correlates most strongly with the risk of recurrence and metastasis.

Bibliography

Balch CM, Gershenwald JE, Soong SJ, et al. Final version of 2009 AJCC melanoma staging and classification. J Clin Oncol. 2009 Dec 20;27(36): 6199-206. [PMID: 19917835]

Item 55   Answer: E

Educational Objective: Manage a patient with acute urticaria.

No further diagnostic evaluation is indicated for this patient. This patient has urticaria, which affects up to 20% of the adult population at some point in time. She presents with red wheals and urticarial plaques on the trunk that appear and disappear. In addition to the rings, urticarial lesions are often in arcuate forms with "C" and "S" shapes. The lesions also last less than 24 hours, which is typical for urticaria. Common causes include infections, allergic reactions to medications, foods, or insect exposure (stings and bites), and nonallergic responses to medications (such as opioids or NSAIDs). Skin lesions in urticaria are characterized by erythematous papules and plaques that are pruritic and transient with no associated systemic symptoms. Acute urticaria is defined as being of less than 6 weeks' duration. The history should focus on the severity of the reaction (such as the presence of angioedema or anaphylaxis), identification of a potential trigger, and whether there is evidence of an underlying systemic disorder associated with urticaria. The physical examination should confirm the presence of urticaria and evaluate for evidence of angioedema or other systemic involvement. In patients with uncomplicated acute urticaria, laboratory studies are almost always normal, and no further diagnostic evaluation is required in most patients before initiating therapy, if needed.

Although infections, liver or kidney disease, thyroid dysfunction, and lymphoma have been associated with urticaria, in a healthy patient with a negative review of systems and normal physical examination, further diagnostic evaluation for an underlying cause is not generally indicated.

Food allergies can present with urticaria, but unless there is consistent ingestion of the food on a daily basis, the urticaria should not be consistent for 1 week. Testing for other allergic causes may be appropriate for confirmation if there is a clearly identifiable trigger or for refractory urticaria believed to be allergic in nature; however, allergy testing is not indicated for acute, uncomplicated urticaria.

KEY POINT

- In patients with uncomplicated acute urticaria, laboratory studies are almost always normal, and no further diagnostic evaluation is required in most patients before initiating therapy, if needed.

Bibliography

Zuberbier T, Bindslev-Jensen C, Canonica W, et al. EAACI/GA2LEN/EDF. EAACI/GA2LEN/EDF guideline: definition, classification and diagnosis of urticaria. Allergy. 2006 Mar;61(3):316-20. [PMID: 16436140]

Item 56   Answer: C

Educational Objective: Diagnose subungual melanoma.

This patient has melanonychia, and she requires a nail matrix biopsy. Melanonychia refers to a brown or black discoloration of the nail plate. It is a common normal variant in persons with darker skin types, but it may also occur as a result of systemic disease, medication, infection, or an underlying melanocytic lesion. Typically, multiple nails are affected. A single nail with longitudinal melanonychia is suggestive of an underlying melanocytic lesion. In this setting, it is important to rule out subungual melanoma. Clinical signs of subungual melanoma include Hutchinson sign (pigmentation expanding onto the proximal nail fold) and a wider diameter of the longitudinal pigment stripe proximally as compared with distally (indicative of an expanding underlying pigmented lesion in the nail matrix). Subungual melanoma may also present as diffuse nail discoloration and is often initially misdiagnosed as onychomy-

cosis or subungual hematoma. Although rare in patients with fair skin, subungual acral lentiginous melanoma is the most common type of melanoma in Asian and black patients.

Onychomycosis is the result of dermatophytes invading the nail plate and causing thickening and discoloration. The diagnosis of onychomycosis can be confirmed by potassium hydroxide (KOH) examination of the nail, a fungal culture, or by histologic examination of the nail clippings. The finding of a pigmented linear streak is not consistent with the diagnosis of onychomycosis, and these studies are not indicated.

A culture of the nail clipping is not appropriate because the nail plate changes are not consistent with an infection such as onychomycosis.

Histopathologic examination of the nail clipping is not sufficient to determine the presence or absence of a melanoma since other disorders can cause pigment deposition in the nail plate. Observation is not appropriate in this situation, since a delay in diagnosis can have potentially serious consequences.

KEY POINT

- A single nail with longitudinal melanonychia is suggestive of an underlying melanocytic lesion that should be evaluated with a nail matrix biopsy.

Bibliography

Levit EK, Kagen MH, Scher RK, Grossman M, Altman E. The ABC rule for clinical detection of subungual melanoma. J Am Acad Dermatol. 2000 Feb;42(2 Pt 1):269-74. [PMID: 10642684]

Item 57   Answer: A   H

Educational Objective: Diagnose bullous pemphigoid.

This patient has bullous pemphigoid. Bullous pemphigoid is a chronic autoimmune blistering disease that predominantly affects older patients and presents with urticarial plaques with tense bullae often on the trunk and upper legs. Mucosal involvement can occur in 10% to 40% of patients. Associated peripheral eosinophilia also is common. Microscopic examination of a blistering lesion usually reveals the presence of eosinophils with the separation of tissue layers subepidermally causing tense bullae (as opposed to an intraepidermal blister that causes more flaccid bullae seen in pemphigus). Bullous pemphigoid is caused by autoantibodies directed against collagen XVII, which is bullous pemphigoid antigen 180 (BP180); direct immunofluorescence shows linear IgG deposition at the basement membrane zone.

Pemphigus foliaceus is a chronic autoimmune blistering disorder with autoantibodies against desmoglein 1. It results in very superficial intraepidermal, flaccid bullae, which are often easily ruptured, as opposed to the tense bullae in bullous pemphigoid. The lesions in pemphigus foliaceus often present as superficial erosions with a "corn flake"–like crust, as opposed to bullae. Mucosal involvement is also uncommon.

Pemphigus vulgaris is a chronic autoimmune blistering disorder that has autoantibodies predominantly against desmoglein 3, also resulting in flaccid bullae with mucous membrane involvement.

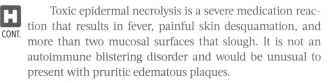

Toxic epidermal necrolysis is a severe medication reaction that results in fever, painful skin desquamation, and more than two mucosal surfaces that slough. It is not an autoimmune blistering disorder and would be unusual to present with pruritic edematous plaques.

KEY POINT

- Bullous pemphigoid is a chronic autoimmune blistering disease that predominantly affects elderly patients and presents with urticarial plaques with tense bullae often on the trunk and upper legs.

Bibliography

Ruocco E, Wolf R, Caccavale S, Brancaccio G, Ruocco V, Lo Schiavo A. Bullous pemphigoid: associations and management guidelines: facts and controversies. Clin Dermatol. 2013 Jul-Aug;31(4):400-12. [PMID: 23806157]

Item 58   Answer: C

Educational Objective: Recognize striae and atrophy from potent topical glucocorticoids.

This patient has striae distensae or stretch marks. The groin is a common area for developing stretch marks, and one of the main risks of topical glucocorticoids is the development of striae. Potential cutaneous complications associated with the use of topical glucocorticoids include thinning of the skin, development of striae, development of purpura, pigmentary changes (hypo- or hyperpigmentation), acneiform eruptions, and increased risk of infections. The risk increases when glucocorticoids are used for prolonged periods, are applied under occlusion or in skin folds where there is natural occlusion, or when high-potency glucocorticoids are applied to areas of thin skin, as in this patient. This patient was appropriately prescribed potent topical glucocorticoids for the control of his plaque psoriasis on his elbows and knees, but potent glucocorticoids are too strong for the groin and can rapidly lead to striae and atrophy.

Contact dermatitis typically has a geometric pattern in response to the area of contact with an allergen, and not along lines of stress as in this patient. Additionally, the skin is more edematous and often weeps serous fluid, and the area is intensely pruritic.

Inverse psoriasis refers to psoriatic changes occurring in intertriginous areas (as opposed to its more usual presence on extensor surfaces) where it can appear somewhat atypical, often lacking the characteristic surface scale because of the moistness of the skin creases. Inverse psoriasis results in broad areas of erythema confluent through the skin folds.

Tinea cruris presents as broad patches of erythema with fine scale (most often at the edges) and usually has a macerated appearance deep in the skin creases.

KEY POINT

- Prolonged use of topical glucocorticoids in areas of thin, moist, occluded skin can lead to striae and atrophy.

Bibliography

Beer K, Downie J. Sequelae from inadvertent long-term use of potent topical steroids. J Drugs Dermatol. 2007 May;6(5):550-1. [PMID: 17679193]

Item 59   Answer: D

Educational Objective: Manage severe, recalcitrant acne vulgaris.

This patient has recalcitrant nodulocystic acne, and the most appropriate next step in therapy is to discontinue his current medications and start oral isotretinoin. Acne is a chronic inflammatory skin condition characterized by open and closed comedones (blackheads and whiteheads, respectively) and inflammatory lesions, including papules, pustules, or nodules. Patients with severe acne can develop large, painful cysts; nodules; and interconnecting sinus tracts on the face, neck, and trunk. It is important to treat this disease aggressively as it can cause permanent scarring that can be disfiguring. Isotretinoin is an oral retinoid that is extremely effective in treating severe nodular acne. However, it is associated with significant side effects, including teratogenicity, mucocutaneous effects (cheilitis, pruritus, photosensitivity, or desquamation), skin thinning, myalgia, liver toxicity, and hyperlipidemia. Because of this, its use is limited to patients with recalcitrant disease. When used in women of childbearing age, prescribers and patients must participate in an FDA-mandated risk management program to minimize the risk of possible fetal exposure to isotretinoin. This patient has severe nodular acne that has been recalcitrant to oral antibiotic treatment; therefore, isotretinoin is an appropriate next step in treatment. In some patients, isotretinoin may be used as first-line treatment for severe, nodulocystic acne, and may also be appropriate for treatment of less severe inflammatory acne that is recalcitrant to multimodality therapy with topical retinoids and oral antibiotics.

Topical metronidazole is first-line therapy for rosacea; however severe nodular acne is usually treated initially with systemic antibiotics. It is important to educate patients that antibiotic treatments often take 6 to 8 weeks to demonstrate an effect. This patient has been on an oral antibiotic for 6 months and continues to have severe acne on his face and neck.

A change to an alternative topical retinoid (such as tazarotene) or another oral antibiotic (such as minocycline) is not expected to dramatically improve his acne. In addition, guidelines recommend that the duration of oral antibiotic therapy be limited; specifically, oral antibiotics should be used for 3 months and the patient reassessed for response. For patients who respond, antibiotics are discontinued.

KEY POINT

- Isotretinoin is first-line treatment for severe, nodulocystic acne and for inflammatory acne that is recalcitrant to multimodality therapy with topical retinoids and oral antibiotics.

Bibliography

Strauss JS, Krowchuk DP, Leyden JJ, et al; American Academy of Dermatology/American Academy of Dermatology Association. Guidelines of care for acne vulgaris management. J Am Acad Dermatol. 2007 Apr;56(4):651-63. [PMID: 17276540]

Item 60   Answer: D

Educational Objective: Diagnose porphyria cutanea tarda.

This patient has porphyria cutanea tarda (PCT). PCT is a rare skin disease that typically occurs in the setting of underlying liver disease, which in this patient is likely due to heavy alcohol use. It may also develop in patients with chronic hepatitis C infection and hemochromatosis. PCT is caused by decreased activity of hepatic uroporphyrinogen decarboxylase, an enzyme in the heme biosynthesis pathway that leads to accumulation of porphyrins in the tissues. Only 20% of cases of PCT are due to inherited enzyme mutations, the remainder is acquired. The acquired forms appear to be related to increased oxidative stress in hepatocytes, possibly associated with iron deposition, although the exact mechanisms of decreased enzyme activity have not been elucidated. Patients with PCT often have darkening of the skin, hypertrichosis, and fragility of the skin, particularly in sun-exposed and frequently traumatized areas, such as the dorsal hands. Numerous scars and small milia (tiny proteinaceous cysts) are often seen on the dorsal hands; intact blisters are rare, but often exist transiently before being spontaneously ruptured following mild trauma.

Allergic contact dermatitis may lead to blisters, but not scarring or milia, and there is no history to suggest an environmental trigger in this patient. The lesions of contact dermatitis typically will be sharply demarcated and geometric in appearance, corresponding to the area affected by the causative agent.

Bullous lupus erythematosus is a rare form of cutaneus lupus in which patients develop small blisters within and in addition to their other cutaneous lupus lesions; the blisters are generally small and often rupture with some residual dyspigmentation and scarring. Signs of systemic lupus erythematosus should be present when making a diagnosis of bullous lupus erythematosus.

Bullous pemphigoid is an autoimmune blistering disease common in the elderly that presents with urticarial plaques and tense, intact bullae; there is no association with liver disease.

KEY POINT

- Porphyria cutanea tarda, which may develop from extensive alcohol use, hemochromatosis, or hepatitis C virus infection, presents with skin fragility and small, transient, easily ruptured vesicles in sun-exposed areas such as on the hands.

Bibliography

Balwani M, Desnick RJ. The porphyrias: advances in diagnosis and treatment. Blood. 2012 Nov 29;120(23):4496-504. [PMID: 22791288]

Item 61   Answer: C

Educational Objective: Manage urticarial vasculitis.

This patient's presentation is suggestive of urticarial vasculitis, and a skin biopsy is indicated. He has an urticarial eruption with joint pain and low-grade fevers suggesting systemic inflammation. Typical urticarial wheals last for less than 24 hours (with individual lesions lasting only a few hours), resolve without cutaneous sequelae, and are pruritic and not painful. In contrast, this patient has painful wheals that last for more than 24 hours and leave bruise-like changes when they resolve, which is atypical for usual urticaria, and is characteristic of urticarial vasculitis. Patients with urticarial vasculitis may have an underlying autoimmune disease, most often lupus erythematosus, but even in the absence of an associated autoimmune disease, patients with urticarial vasculitis (particularly hypocomplementemic urticarial vasculitis) are at risk of multisystem disease, including nephritis. A skin biopsy is important in making the diagnosis, and guiding further work-up and treatment.

A gluten-free diet is unlikely to have any impact on urticarial vasculitis, and only rarely will gluten intake impact urticarial skin conditions. Gluten avoidance is important in patients with dermatitis herpetiformis, which is often associated with insensitivity to gluten.

Radioallergosorbent testing (RAST) may be appropriate in patients with a typical urticarial eruption from a likely food or environmental trigger; however, this patient is presenting with atypical urticarial lesions with signs and symptoms concerning for urticarial vasculitis. RAST plays no role in the diagnosis of urticarial vasculitis.

Thyroid function testing is indicated in the evaluation of chronic urticaria in which patients have regular episodes of typical urticaria over a period of more than 6 weeks. Because of the atypical presentation of this patient's wheals and the lack of clinical findings suggestive of thyroid disease, testing would not be the most appropriate next step.

KEY POINT

- In contrast to typical urticaria, urticarial vasculitis presents with painful wheals that last for more than 24 hours and leave bruise-like changes behind.

Bibliography

Micheletti R, Rosenbach M. An approach to the hospitalized patient with urticaria and fever. Dermatol Ther. 2011 Mar-Apr;24(2):187-95. [PMID: 21410608]

Item 62   Answer: D

Educational Objective: Diagnose stasis dermatitis.

This patient has stasis dermatitis. Stasis dermatitis, especially in the acute setting, can present with brightly erythematous, edematous plaques, as shown in the figure, that are tender to palpation and can be slightly warm to touch. Overlying scale and serum crust also can develop as a consequence of fluctuating edema (as seen in the figure). Differentiating

Answers and Critiques

CONT.

stasis dermatitis from cellulitis can be difficult; however, the presence of similar-appearing erythematous plaques bilaterally in an afebrile patient with no lymphadenopathy or other symptoms or signs of infection would be unusual for cellulitis. Because stasis dermatitis usually results from decreased venous drainage or excess fluid in dependent areas causing increased vascular permeability and stretching of the skin, the clinical scenario of a patient with heart failure who has recently stopped taking a diuretic also is supportive of a diagnosis of stasis dermatitis. Chronic stasis dermatitis will cause more brown discoloration, suggesting a longer term process, but acute stasis dermatitis can present as bright red patches/plaques. Treatment typically includes optimization of volume status or external compression stockings to decrease fluid volume and skin stretching in dependent areas.

Cellulitis presents as a painful, erythematous, well-demarcated patch that is warm to touch. The presence of fever, lymphadenopathy, or other evidence of infection, such as an elevated leukocyte count, also would suggest this diagnosis. It is important to consider alternative diagnoses when there are erythematous patches on both legs.

Contact dermatitis may present with localized inflammation at the site of exposure to an irritant and may cause erythema and edema. However, it is often pruritic and may be accompanied by bullae and oozing. Contact dermatitis may also be preceded by a history of application of a sensitizing agent in the area.

Deep venous thrombosis can present as a swollen, erythematous leg. Although bilateral deep venous thromboses can occur, this is a less likely cause in this patient.

KEY POINT

- Stasis dermatitis is sometimes confused with cellulitis; however, patients with stasis dermatitis will have no leukocytosis or lymphadenopathy and will be afebrile.

Bibliography
Bailey E, Kroshinsky D. Cellulitis: diagnosis and management. Dermatol Ther. 2011 Mar-Apr;24(2):229-39. [PMID: 21410612]

Item 63   Answer: C

Educational Objective: Diagnose *Staphylococcus aureus* infection of atopic dermatitis.

This patient has atopic dermatitis with new pustules typical for a *Staphylococcus aureus* infection. Staphylococcal colonization is very common, being present at the site of skin involvement in almost all patients with atopic dermatitis. Scratching of the skin and breakdown of the skin barrier are conducive to infection, and this is a common occurrence in patients with atopic dermatitis. However, efforts to identify or eradicate the organisms causing the colonization have not been shown to decrease the risk of infection. Therefore, routine skin or nasal swab testing or decolonization procedures for *S. aureus* are not recommended in these patients, although these procedures may be helpful in selected patients

in whom there is recurrent infection or failure of an infection to respond to antimicrobial therapy. Most *S. aureus* infections may be treated with a topical antibiotic such as mupirocin, with more extensive infections requiring systemic antibiotic therapy.

Herpes simplex virus can superinfect atopic dermatitis (eczema herpeticum), but typically presents with painful groups of vesicles on an erythematous base, "punched-out" erosions, and hemorrhagic crusting. Intact herpetic vesicles may transition to pustules and may be difficult to distinguish from a staphylococcal infection. A viral cause should be suspected in a patient with superinfected atopic dermatitis who does not respond to appropriate antibiotic therapy.

Soap allergy can lead to widespread eczematous dermatitis with pruritus and edema. It would appear on the exposed area and would not be localized just to the areas of atopic dermatitis. Soap allergy also presents with vesicles or bullae, not pustules.

Although topical glucocorticoids are associated with multiple potential side effects, including skin thinning, purpura, and changes in pigmentation, their use is not directly associated with the occurrence of staphylococcal infection. Glucocorticoids may help reestablish the skin barrier by decreasing the inflammatory response of atopic dermatitis but would not directly cause staphylococcal infection.

KEY POINT

- Atopic dermatitis with new pustules in addition to breakdown of the skin barrier is indicative of *Staphylococcus aureus* infection.

Bibliography
Eichenfield LF, Ellis CN, Mancini AJ, Paller AS, Simpson EL. Atopic dermatitis: epidemiology and pathogenesis update. Semin Cutan Med Surg. 2012 Sep;31(3 Suppl):S3-5. [PMID: 23021783]

Item 64   Answer: D

Educational Objective: Treat postinflammatory hyperpigmentation due to acne in a patient with darker skin.

This patient has postinflammatory hyperpigmentation (PIH) resulting from her inflammatory acne papules, and she should be treated with a topical retinoid. The first step in management is to treat her acne, which is the source of the discoloration, rather than initially treating the discoloration with a bleaching cream such as hydroquinone. After any injury to the skin such as inflammation or trauma, dark skin may become hypo- or hyperpigmented. For this reason it is important to advise patients not to pick at their acne, as this can contribute to postinflammatory discoloration. Patients often report "scarring," when in fact there are only postinflammatory changes. The duration of postinflammatory pigmentary changes varies, depending on the location and degree of inflammation. Hyperpigmentation on the lower legs can take several years to fade. Some postinflammatory pigment changes are permanent. Treatment of postinflammatory pigment changes includes treatment of any underlying skin inflammation, sun avoidance or sun protection, and consideration of a bleaching cream, such as hydroquinone. Topical retinoids are the standard of care for acne therapy, as they can prevent acne. They should be applied to the entire area affected by acne, not used as a "spot treatment."

This patient has moderate acne with more than a dozen inflammatory papules distributed over her face. A topical antimicrobial agent would not be the first choice in acne management since it has no preventive properties and there are no clinical signs of infection, such as impetiginization of the acne lesions. Topical glucocorticoids would not be a treatment for this patient because they can exacerbate acne.

KEY POINT

- Topical retinoids are the standard therapy for acne and postinflammatory hyperpigmentation, especially when paired with depigmenting agents.

Bibliography

Thiboutot D, Gollnick H, Bettoli V, et al. New insights into the management of acne: an update from the Global Alliance to Improve Outcomes in Acne group. J Am Acad Dermatol. 2009 May;60(5 suppl):S1-50. [PMID: 19376456]

Item 65   Answer: B

Educational Objective: **Treat superficial dermatophyte infections (tinea).**

This patient has tinea pedis, which is characterized by superficial scaling in a "moccasin" distribution on the feet, maceration in the toe webs spaces, and often dystrophic toenails corresponding to onychomycosis. The recommended treatment is a topical antifungal agent such as clotrimazole. Other azole-based agents or topical terbinafine (squalene epoxidase inhibitors) may also be used. Over-the-counter and prescription preparations are equally effective in treating tinea pedis. A 2- to 4-week course in conjunction with washing footwear to help remove any fomites also is necessary. Other associated management may include use of foot powder as a drying agent to prevent maceration, avoidance of occlusive footwear, and treating shoes with antifungal powders before being worn.

Topical betamethasone is a topical glucocorticoid that is beneficial in treated eczematous dermatitis. Although it may initially help with the inflammation of tinea pedis, it may result in a florid infection and potentially a pustular eruption known as Majocchi granuloma.

Although FDA approved, clotrimazole-betamethasone combination cream also is not the preferred treatment for dermatophyte infections as it can lead to increased side effects because of the potent topical glucocorticoid. Although this combination of a glucocorticoid and an antifungal agent is commonly prescribed, the combined agents can partially suppress a superficial dermatophyte infection but may ultimately make the infection more severe and deeper, requiring systemic antifungal agents to treat the disease. The use of this combination cream should be avoided because it can lead to

treatment failures and skin atrophy related to prolonged topical glucocorticoid use, and has an increased cost compared with topical antifungal agents alone. It can be effective in treating chronic paronychia.

Although topical nystatin is an antifungal medication, it is effective only against *Candida* spp. and is ineffective against other dermatophytes. Tinea pedis is secondary to dermatophytes, not *Candida*, so nystatin should not be used in this patient.

KEY POINT

- Treatment of most superficial dermatophyte infections includes topical antifungal agents such as azole-based preparations or squalene epoxidase inhibitors (terbinafine); over-the-counter preparations are cost-effective options and have good efficacy.

Bibliography

Moriarty B, Hay R, Morris-Jones R. The diagnosis and management of tinea. BMJ. 2012 Jul 10;345:e4380. [PMID: 22782730]

Item 66   Answer: D

Educational Objective: **Diagnose cutaneous vasculitis.**

This patient's skin findings are most likely caused by vasculitis of the cutaneous blood vessels. Inflammation of the blood vessels may lead to vascular injury with hemorrhage into the skin. The resulting clinical lesions are described by their size. Petechiae are pinpoint macules (<3 mm in diameter), which are seen most commonly in platelet disorders, while purpura causes more widespread areas of involvement (up to 1 cm in diameter). Ecchymoses are confluent purpuric areas larger than 1 cm in diameter. Vasculitic lesions are nonblanchable, and when vasculitis involves the small cutaneous vessels, they may be palpable, resulting in the characteristic diagnostic finding in cutaneous vasculitis of palpable purpura. Small vessel vasculitis may be idiopathic but may also occur in association with systemic diseases, including infection, sepsis, a more diffuse vasculitic process or autoimmune disorder, medication reactions, or rarely malignancy. Because vasculitic skin findings may reflect a significant underlying disease process, a thorough evaluation is required, particularly in this patient with fever, joint and muscle pain, and possible focal weakness.

Erythema multiforme (EM) is believed to be a cell-mediated immune process that occurs in response to a specific trigger, which is most commonly infectious (and particularly associated with herpes simplex virus infection). EM often manifests as a three-ring target on the palms, and the center of the target can have a dark red or purple appearance; the dusky center may become necrotic and can form a discrete blister or eschar. Lesions range in size from several millimeters to several centimeters. Few to hundreds of lesions develop within several days and are most commonly located on the extensor surfaces of the extremities, particularly the hands and feet. EM, however, does not cause widespread purpura.

CONT.

Lichen planus (LP) is an inflammatory skin disorder of unclear etiology that can affect the skin, mucous membranes, scalp, and/or nails. The hallmark lesion of LP is the pruritic, purple, polygonal papule; these papules are usually distributed symmetrically on the wrists, flexural aspects of the arms and legs, lower back, and genitals. A reticulated network of gray-white lines (Wickham striae) may be visible on the surface of the papules. LP does not cause purpura.

Traumatic ecchymosis can cause extensive purpura, especially in older patients who have age-related thinning of the skin and vascular structures and are more likely to take antiplatelet or anticoagulant medications; however, traumatic bruising is more often localized and may have a pattern that suggests the external cause of injury.

KEY POINT

- Purpura and ecchymosis are signs of vascular injury and may be associated with systemic disease including more widespread vasculitis.

Bibliography

Wysong A, Venkatesan P. An approach to the patient with retiform purpura. Dermatol Ther. 2011 Mar-Apr;24(2):151-72.

Item 67   Answer: A

Educational Objective: **Treat hand dermatitis.**

Less frequent washing and application of a thick emollient such as petrolatum are the treatments of choice for this patient. Irritant hand dermatitis often occurs through friction, removal of the protective skin barrier, and irritation from the surfactant properties of the soap in persons who overwash their hands. Overwashing is common in patients with obsessive-compulsive disorder. Irritant dermatitis will be especially marked on the dorsal hands where the stratum corneum is thinner than that of the palms. Topical petrolatum moisturizer is an inexpensive and effective way of repairing the damaged skin barrier by softening the stratum corneum, reducing skin water loss, and helping maintain a barrier to decrease further irritation. The petrolatum moisturizer should be applied several times daily, particularly after hand washing when it is most necessary.

Topical diphenhydramine is an antihistamine but irritant dermatitis is not driven by histamine. Therefore, an antihistamine will not be effective.

Although topical lidocaine may relieve the pain, it will not heal the skin barrier and it should not be applied repeatedly to fissured skin because of possible absorption.

Neomycin is not indicated since this patient does not have an infection. There is no purulence or crusting, and there are no pustules or erosions to indicate bacterial infection.

KEY POINT

- Less frequent handwashing and application of a thick emollient such as petrolatum are the treatments of choice for irritant hand dermatitis caused by overwashing.

Bibliography

Stein DJ, Hollander E. Dermatology and conditions related to obsessive-compulsive disorder. J Am Acad Dermatol. 1992 Feb;26(2 Pt 1):237-42. [PMID: 1552059]

Item 68   Answer: A

Educational Objective: **Diagnose drug hypersensitivity syndrome.**

This patient most likely has systemic drug hypersensitivity syndrome, otherwise known as drug reaction with eosinophilia and systemic symptoms (DRESS). DRESS is a severe and potentially life-threatening type IV hypersensitivity reaction. Similar to most type IV reactions, onset of the syndrome is delayed, usually occurring 10 days to several weeks after the start of the causative medication. The most common medications that trigger this reaction are sulfonamide antibiotics, allopurinol, and anticonvulsants, but many others have been implicated. In DRESS, patients develop an exanthem rash on the face, trunk, and extremities, and they often have facial edema. Due to systemic inflammation, patients may have fever, lymphadenopathy, and, in severe reactions, hypotension. When these findings occur in a patient being treated with antibiotics, the systemic inflammatory nature of the reaction may make it difficult to differentiate between a response to an antimicrobial agent or inadequate control of the underlying infection, as in this patient. The treatment of DRESS is to stop the suspected medication immediately, switch to another medication that is unlikely to cross-react, and start systemic glucocorticoids, which can reduce systemic inflammation and lower the risk of end-organ damage.

Morbilliform (meaning measles-like) drug exanthems are the most common pattern of a cutaneous drug reaction. This reaction occurs in up to 8% of hospitalized patients and appears 5 to 15 days after exposure to the causative drug. The characteristic findings include erythematous papules coalescing into plaques, often with some pruritus, and no accompanying systemic symptoms. Facial edema, fever, and laboratory abnormalities are not expected.

Stevens-Johnson syndrome (SJS) is an inflammatory reaction with prominent skin findings that is more commonly triggered by medications than infections. Patients may also have flu-like symptoms, and these may precede the onset of the rash. SJS can be differentiated by the presence of mucosal erosions. Patients with SJS have two or more mucosal sites involved, associated with erythema, pain, and often bloody discharge, none of which this patient has. SJS also has different cutaneous findings including annular erythematous plaques that may have purpuric and eroded centers. These are found on the face, trunk, and extremities including the palms and soles, and involve no more than 10% of the body surface area.

Medications can cause a cutaneous or systemic vasculitis; however, the appearance of this patient's skin findings is not consistent with vasculitis. Purpuric or nonblanching

CONT.

erythematous macules, papules, or plaques are indicative of vasculitis.

KEY POINT

- Drug reaction with eosinophilia and systemic symptoms is a systemic drug hypersensitivity reaction that presents with new rash and flu-like symptoms.

Bibliography

Husain Z, Reddy BY, Schwartz RA. DRESS syndrome: Part I. Clinical perspectives. J Am Acad Dermatol. 2013 May;68(5):693.e1-14. [PMID: 23602182]

Item 69   Answer: D

Educational Objective: Diagnose psychogenic itch.

This patient has psychogenic itch, which is localized pruritus associated with a concomitant diagnosis (or symptoms of) depression, anxiety, or somatoform disorders. Self-reported depression is present in about 40% of persons with psychogenic pruritus. Most patients are able to identify a precipitating psychological trigger. Patients with psychogenic pruritus excessively pick and scratch normal skin and report constant pruritus. Physical examination findings include linear crusted lesions and hypopigmented scars. It is important to examine patients carefully and completely to avoid missing a dermatologic or systemic cause of itch in those with concomitant psychiatric disorders.

Morbilliform drug eruptions can be pruritic; however, this patient has only secondary skin changes (linear erosions) and does not have a primary finding that would be expected with a drug eruption.

Localized itching with less prominent skin lesions suggests neuropathic pruritus, which results from inflammation or damage to sensory nerves. The most common forms are notalgia paresthetica and brachioradial pruritus. With notalgia paresthetica, there is recurrent and persistent itching on the medial back, usually around the scapula. Brachioradial pruritus causes itching on the extensor forearms, arms, or upper back. The itch in these conditions is often described as burning or stinging, and some patients experience a crawling sensation. The skin is initially normal but may become excoriated, lichenified, and hyperpigmented from recurrent rubbing and scratching. Patients often obtain relief with application of ice, and this may be a distinguishing characteristic.

Patients with generalized pruritus who lack primary skin lesions may have an associated medical condition or internal malignancy. However, hematologic or hepatobiliary malignancies are more likely diagnoses than colorectal adenocarcinomas.

KEY POINT

- Psychogenic itch is localized pruritus associated with a concomitant diagnosis (or symptoms) of depression, anxiety, or somatoform disorders and is typically associated with linear cutaneous lesions and scars.

Bibliography

Yosipovitch G, Bernhard JD. Clinical practice. Chronic pruritus. N Engl J Med. 2013 Apr 25;368(17):1625-34. [PMID: 23614588]

Item 70   Answer: A

Educational Objective: Recognize the association of dermatitis herpetiformis with celiac disease.

This patient has dermatitis herpetiformis, which is associated with celiac disease. Dermatitis herpetiformis is a chronic, extremely pruritic autoimmune disorder associated with gluten-sensitive enteropathy, or celiac disease. Although not all patients have gastrointestinal symptoms, nearly 100% of patients will have some underlying abnormality associated with celiac disease. Dermatitis herpetiformis classically presents as extremely pruritic vesicles and papules in a symmetric distribution involving the elbows, knees, buttocks, and scalp. At times, excoriations predominate, and intact vesicles may not be visualized. Although dermatitis herpetiformis is an uncommon skin finding, the association with celiac disease is very high, and the diagnosis should be suspected if the characteristic skin findings are present. Patients with dermatitis herpetiformis are also at risk for other autoimmune conditions, including autoimmune thyroid disease, type 1 diabetes mellitus, and pernicious anemia. There is also a potential association of dermatitis herpetiformis with lymphoma. Treatment is gluten avoidance, although improvement of the rash may occur very slowly over months to years. Dapsone can be used to treat dermatitis herpetiformis and is very effective; however, it can allow persistence of celiac disease, which can result in small bowel lymphoma with chronic inflammation. As a result, dapsone should be used in conjunction with gluten-free diets as first line treatment.

Hepatitis C can occur in association with porphyria cutanea tarda, which presents as vesicles in sun-exposed areas such as the dorsal hands, and resultant milia (small white cysts). Associated hypertrichosis also can be seen.

Non-Hodgkin lymphoma is associated with paraneoplastic pemphigus, which presents as painful oral, conjunctival, or esophageal erosions with associated erythema and blistering on the skin. Paraneoplastic pemphigus always has mucosal involvement, which was absent in this patient's presentation.

Inflammatory bowel disease, including ulcerative colitis, can occur in association with epidermolysis bullosa acquisita, which presents as painful bullae and erosions in areas of trauma, often on extensor surfaces; these lesions heal with scarring and milia. This patient's extreme pruritus makes epidermolysis bullosa acquisita unlikely.

KEY POINT

- Dermatitis herpetiformis is a chronic, extremely pruritic autoimmune disorder associated with gluten-sensitive enteropathy, or celiac disease.

Bibliography

Kárpáti S. Dermatitis herpetiformis. Clin Dermatol. 2012 Jan-Feb;30(1):56-9. [PMID: 22137227]

Item 71   Answer: D

Educational Objective: Diagnose sarcoidosis.

This patient has sarcoidosis. Sarcoidosis is a granulomatous, infiltrating disease that is more common in black persons and may be incidentally discovered by detection of lymphadenopathy, often in the chest. A chronic, nonproductive cough is the most common pulmonary symptom of sarcoidosis, as occurs in this patient. The cutaneous manifestations of sarcoidosis result from granulomatous infiltration in the skin with papule formation at the site of disease. Lesions tend to be grouped around the nose and are sometimes seen around the eyes or mouth. Sarcoidal involvement of tattoos and scars is not uncommon. Smoking may alter the pulmonary immune milieu, and smokers tend to have a lower incidence of sarcoidosis, with some patients occasionally developing sarcoidosis after smoking cessation. However, smoking is not recommended as a preventive or therapeutic measure. Medium-potency topical glucocorticoids are the usual first-line therapy for cutaneous sarcoidosis on the face, with high-potency agents used in other lower risk sites. Intralesional glucocorticoids are also a treatment option.

Dermatomyositis presents with cutaneous findings of erythema over skin folds or flexures, such as the metacarpal and proximal and distal interphalangeal joints, the elbows, the shoulders and back ("shawl sign"), posterior neck, the upper chest ("V sign"), lateral hips, and around the eyes. Patients may have an interstitial lung disease; however, the skin lesions described in this patient are not characteristic of dermatomyositis.

Hodgkin lymphoma can cause hilar lymphadenopathy and may cause severe pruritus. The resulting pruritus can lead to extensive skin excoriations; these lesions are usually elongated, jagged, angled erosions and scars due to self-induced scratching. The pruritus from Hodgkin lymphoma may be striking and severe, and lymphoma is one of the potential culprits to consider as an internal source of pruritus in select patients.

Limited systemic sclerosis, or CREST syndrome, is characterized by cutaneous calcinosis, Raynaud phenomenon, esophageal dysmotility, sclerodactyly or tapering of the digits, and telangiectasias. None of these features are present in this patient.

Systemic lupus erythematosus often presents with skin findings. The classic acute rash of systemic lupus is a bright red symmetric patch over the cheeks and central face, the "butterfly" malar rash. Subacute cutaneous lupus presents with annular red scaly patches in photodistributed areas, especially prominent on the upper back, chest, and arms. Chronic cutaneous lupus lesions are generally the characteristic "discoid lupus" lesions with pink-to-violaceous erythema, scaling, and dyspigmentation and atrophic scarring. While pleuritis can occur with lupus, the combination of papular skin lesions and dry cough is characteristic of sarcoidosis.

KEY POINT

- Classic cutaneous sarcoidosis appears as violaceous papules around the nose including the ala, or periorbitally and periorificially; lesions may also develop in sites of trauma, such as scars or tattoos.

Bibliography

Haimovic A, Sanchez M, Judson MA, Prystowsky S. Sarcoidosis: a comprehensive review and update for the dermatologist: part I. Cutaneous disease. J Am Acad Dermatol. 2012 May;66(5):699.e1-18. [PMID: 22507585]

Item 72   Answer: B

Educational Objective: Treat chronic cutaneous lupus erythematosus.

Hydroxychloroquine is first-line systemic treatment for patients with chronic cutaneous lupus erythematosus, such as discoid lupus. The cutaneous manifestations of lupus may present focally, as with the classic "butterfly" malar rash, or with more diffuse findings. A unique form of lupus-associated skin disease is discoid lupus. Discoid lupus may occur in patients with clearly defined lupus but may also present in other patients with few other clinical manifestations of lupus. This patient has had chronic lesions for 3 years limited to a relatively small area on the head and neck. She lacks other symptoms of systemic lupus erythematosus (SLE). Low titer antinuclear antibody positivity may occur in patients with skin-limited chronic cutaneous lupus. Topical therapy with glucocorticoids and calcineurin inhibitors is the usual initial treatment approach. For patients who fail to improve, systemic antimalarial therapy such as hydroxychloroquine, which is the systemic treatment of choice for most manifestations of cutaneous lupus, is indicated. There is some evidence that treatment with hydroxychloroquine can diminish the risk of progression to overt SLE in some patients.

Dapsone is a sulfonamide that has efficacy in treating specific types of lupus-associated skin disease. However, along with methotrexate, mycophenolate mofetil, and systemic retinoids, dapsone is considered second-line therapy for cutaneous lupus.

Although systemic glucocorticoids such as prednisone are sometimes used in systemic lupus, this patient does not have SLE (negative titers for anti-Smith and antidouble-stranded DNA, normal complete blood count and urinalysis, and no extracutaneous signs or symptoms). Because of this and the potential associated adverse effects of systemic glucocorticoids, they are not routinely used in the management of lupus skin disease.

Vitamin D supplementation, even in high dosages, has not shown efficacy in preventing or treating the cutaneous manifestations of lupus.

KEY POINT

- Hydroxychloroquine is the first-line systemic treatment for patients with chronic cutaneous lupus erythematosus, such as discoid lupus.

Bibliography

Okon LG, Werth VP. Cutaneous lupus erythematosus: diagnosis and treatment. Best Pract Res Clin Rheumatol. 2013 Jun;27(3):391-404. [PMID: 24238695]

Index

A NAME AND ADDRESS (Please complete.)

Last Name   First Name   Middle Initial

Address

Address cont.

City   State   ZIP Code

Country

Email address

ACP®
American College of Physicians
Leading Internal Medicine, Improving Lives

Medical Knowledge Self-Assessment Program® 17

TO EARN *AMA PRA CATEGORY 1 CREDITS*™ YOU MUST:

1. Answer all questions.
2. Score a minimum of 50% correct.

==

TO EARN *FREE* INSTANTANEOUS *AMA PRA CATEGORY 1 CREDITS*™ ONLINE:

1. Answer all of your questions.
2. Go to **mksap.acponline.org** and enter your ACP Online username and password to access an online answer sheet.
3. Enter your answers.
4. You can also enter your answers directly at **mksap.acponline.org** without first using this answer sheet.

To Submit Your Answer Sheet by Mail or FAX for a $15 Administrative Fee per Answer Sheet:

1. Answer all of your questions and calculate your score.
2. Complete boxes A–F.
3. Complete payment information.
4. Send the answer sheet and payment information to ACP, using the FAX number/address listed below.

B **Order Number**
(Use the Order Number on your MKSAP materials packing slip.)

C **ACP ID Number**
(Refer to packing slip in your MKSAP materials for your ACP ID Number.)

COMPLETE FORM BELOW ONLY IF YOU SUBMIT BY MAIL OR FAX

Last Name   First Name   MI

Payment Information. Must remit in US funds, drawn on a US bank.

The processing fee for each paper answer sheet is $15.

☐ Check, made payable to ACP, enclosed

Charge to   ☐ **VISA**   ☐ **MasterCard**   ☐ **AMERICAN EXPRESS**   ☐ **DISCOVER**

Card Number _____

Expiration Date _____ / _____
     MM   YY

Security code (3 or 4 digit #s) _____

Signature _____

Fax to: 215-351-2799

Mail to:
Member and Customer Service
American College of Physicians
190 N. Independence Mall West
Philadelphia, PA 19106–1572

1 Ⓐ Ⓑ Ⓒ Ⓓ Ⓔ
2 Ⓐ Ⓑ Ⓒ Ⓓ Ⓔ
3 Ⓐ Ⓑ Ⓒ Ⓓ Ⓔ
4 Ⓐ Ⓑ Ⓒ Ⓓ Ⓔ
5 Ⓐ Ⓑ Ⓒ Ⓓ Ⓔ

6 Ⓐ Ⓑ Ⓒ Ⓓ Ⓔ
7 Ⓐ Ⓑ Ⓒ Ⓓ Ⓔ
8 Ⓐ Ⓑ Ⓒ Ⓓ Ⓔ
9 Ⓐ Ⓑ Ⓒ Ⓓ Ⓔ
10 Ⓐ Ⓑ Ⓒ Ⓓ Ⓔ

11 Ⓐ Ⓑ Ⓒ Ⓓ Ⓔ
12 Ⓐ Ⓑ Ⓒ Ⓓ Ⓔ
13 Ⓐ Ⓑ Ⓒ Ⓓ Ⓔ
14 Ⓐ Ⓑ Ⓒ Ⓓ Ⓔ
15 Ⓐ Ⓑ Ⓒ Ⓓ Ⓔ

16 Ⓐ Ⓑ Ⓒ Ⓓ Ⓔ
17 Ⓐ Ⓑ Ⓒ Ⓓ Ⓔ
18 Ⓐ Ⓑ Ⓒ Ⓓ Ⓔ
19 Ⓐ Ⓑ Ⓒ Ⓓ Ⓔ
20 Ⓐ Ⓑ Ⓒ Ⓓ Ⓔ

21 Ⓐ Ⓑ Ⓒ Ⓓ Ⓔ
22 Ⓐ Ⓑ Ⓒ Ⓓ Ⓔ
23 Ⓐ Ⓑ Ⓒ Ⓓ Ⓔ
24 Ⓐ Ⓑ Ⓒ Ⓓ Ⓔ
25 Ⓐ Ⓑ Ⓒ Ⓓ Ⓔ

26 Ⓐ Ⓑ Ⓒ Ⓓ Ⓔ
27 Ⓐ Ⓑ Ⓒ Ⓓ Ⓔ
28 Ⓐ Ⓑ Ⓒ Ⓓ Ⓔ
29 Ⓐ Ⓑ Ⓒ Ⓓ Ⓔ
30 Ⓐ Ⓑ Ⓒ Ⓓ Ⓔ

31 Ⓐ Ⓑ Ⓒ Ⓓ Ⓔ
32 Ⓐ Ⓑ Ⓒ Ⓓ Ⓔ
33 Ⓐ Ⓑ Ⓒ Ⓓ Ⓔ
34 Ⓐ Ⓑ Ⓒ Ⓓ Ⓔ
35 Ⓐ Ⓑ Ⓒ Ⓓ Ⓔ

36 Ⓐ Ⓑ Ⓒ Ⓓ Ⓔ
37 Ⓐ Ⓑ Ⓒ Ⓓ Ⓔ
38 Ⓐ Ⓑ Ⓒ Ⓓ Ⓔ
39 Ⓐ Ⓑ Ⓒ Ⓓ Ⓔ
40 Ⓐ Ⓑ Ⓒ Ⓓ Ⓔ

41 Ⓐ Ⓑ Ⓒ Ⓓ Ⓔ
42 Ⓐ Ⓑ Ⓒ Ⓓ Ⓔ
43 Ⓐ Ⓑ Ⓒ Ⓓ Ⓔ
44 Ⓐ Ⓑ Ⓒ Ⓓ Ⓔ
45 Ⓐ Ⓑ Ⓒ Ⓓ Ⓔ

46 Ⓐ Ⓑ Ⓒ Ⓓ Ⓔ
47 Ⓐ Ⓑ Ⓒ Ⓓ Ⓔ
48 Ⓐ Ⓑ Ⓒ Ⓓ Ⓔ
49 Ⓐ Ⓑ Ⓒ Ⓓ Ⓔ
50 Ⓐ Ⓑ Ⓒ Ⓓ Ⓔ

51 Ⓐ Ⓑ Ⓒ Ⓓ Ⓔ
52 Ⓐ Ⓑ Ⓒ Ⓓ Ⓔ
53 Ⓐ Ⓑ Ⓒ Ⓓ Ⓔ
54 Ⓐ Ⓑ Ⓒ Ⓓ Ⓔ
55 Ⓐ Ⓑ Ⓒ Ⓓ Ⓔ

56 Ⓐ Ⓑ Ⓒ Ⓓ Ⓔ
57 Ⓐ Ⓑ Ⓒ Ⓓ Ⓔ
58 Ⓐ Ⓑ Ⓒ Ⓓ Ⓔ
59 Ⓐ Ⓑ Ⓒ Ⓓ Ⓔ
60 Ⓐ Ⓑ Ⓒ Ⓓ Ⓔ

61 Ⓐ Ⓑ Ⓒ Ⓓ Ⓔ
62 Ⓐ Ⓑ Ⓒ Ⓓ Ⓔ
63 Ⓐ Ⓑ Ⓒ Ⓓ Ⓔ
64 Ⓐ Ⓑ Ⓒ Ⓓ Ⓔ
65 Ⓐ Ⓑ Ⓒ Ⓓ Ⓔ

66 Ⓐ Ⓑ Ⓒ Ⓓ Ⓔ
67 Ⓐ Ⓑ Ⓒ Ⓓ Ⓔ
68 Ⓐ Ⓑ Ⓒ Ⓓ Ⓔ
69 Ⓐ Ⓑ Ⓒ Ⓓ Ⓔ
70 Ⓐ Ⓑ Ⓒ Ⓓ Ⓔ

71 Ⓐ Ⓑ Ⓒ Ⓓ Ⓔ
72 Ⓐ Ⓑ Ⓒ Ⓓ Ⓔ
73 Ⓐ Ⓑ Ⓒ Ⓓ Ⓔ
74 Ⓐ Ⓑ Ⓒ Ⓓ Ⓔ
75 Ⓐ Ⓑ Ⓒ Ⓓ Ⓔ

76 Ⓐ Ⓑ Ⓒ Ⓓ Ⓔ
77 Ⓐ Ⓑ Ⓒ Ⓓ Ⓔ
78 Ⓐ Ⓑ Ⓒ Ⓓ Ⓔ
79 Ⓐ Ⓑ Ⓒ Ⓓ Ⓔ
80 Ⓐ Ⓑ Ⓒ Ⓓ Ⓔ

81 Ⓐ Ⓑ Ⓒ Ⓓ Ⓔ
82 Ⓐ Ⓑ Ⓒ Ⓓ Ⓔ
83 Ⓐ Ⓑ Ⓒ Ⓓ Ⓔ
84 Ⓐ Ⓑ Ⓒ Ⓓ Ⓔ
85 Ⓐ Ⓑ Ⓒ Ⓓ Ⓔ

86 Ⓐ Ⓑ Ⓒ Ⓓ Ⓔ
87 Ⓐ Ⓑ Ⓒ Ⓓ Ⓔ
88 Ⓐ Ⓑ Ⓒ Ⓓ Ⓔ
89 Ⓐ Ⓑ Ⓒ Ⓓ Ⓔ
90 Ⓐ Ⓑ Ⓒ Ⓓ Ⓔ

91 Ⓐ Ⓑ Ⓒ Ⓓ Ⓔ
92 Ⓐ Ⓑ Ⓒ Ⓓ Ⓔ
93 Ⓐ Ⓑ Ⓒ Ⓓ Ⓔ
94 Ⓐ Ⓑ Ⓒ Ⓓ Ⓔ
95 Ⓐ Ⓑ Ⓒ Ⓓ Ⓔ

96 Ⓐ Ⓑ Ⓒ Ⓓ Ⓔ
97 Ⓐ Ⓑ Ⓒ Ⓓ Ⓔ
98 Ⓐ Ⓑ Ⓒ Ⓓ Ⓔ
99 Ⓐ Ⓑ Ⓒ Ⓓ Ⓔ
100 Ⓐ Ⓑ Ⓒ Ⓓ Ⓔ

101 Ⓐ Ⓑ Ⓒ Ⓓ Ⓔ
102 Ⓐ Ⓑ Ⓒ Ⓓ Ⓔ
103 Ⓐ Ⓑ Ⓒ Ⓓ Ⓔ
104 Ⓐ Ⓑ Ⓒ Ⓓ Ⓔ
105 Ⓐ Ⓑ Ⓒ Ⓓ Ⓔ

106 Ⓐ Ⓑ Ⓒ Ⓓ Ⓔ
107 Ⓐ Ⓑ Ⓒ Ⓓ Ⓔ
108 Ⓐ Ⓑ Ⓒ Ⓓ Ⓔ
109 Ⓐ Ⓑ Ⓒ Ⓓ Ⓔ
110 Ⓐ Ⓑ Ⓒ Ⓓ Ⓔ

111 Ⓐ Ⓑ Ⓒ Ⓓ Ⓔ
112 Ⓐ Ⓑ Ⓒ Ⓓ Ⓔ
113 Ⓐ Ⓑ Ⓒ Ⓓ Ⓔ
114 Ⓐ Ⓑ Ⓒ Ⓓ Ⓔ
115 Ⓐ Ⓑ Ⓒ Ⓓ Ⓔ

116 Ⓐ Ⓑ Ⓒ Ⓓ Ⓔ
117 Ⓐ Ⓑ Ⓒ Ⓓ Ⓔ
118 Ⓐ Ⓑ Ⓒ Ⓓ Ⓔ
119 Ⓐ Ⓑ Ⓒ Ⓓ Ⓔ
120 Ⓐ Ⓑ Ⓒ Ⓓ Ⓔ

121 Ⓐ Ⓑ Ⓒ Ⓓ Ⓔ
122 Ⓐ Ⓑ Ⓒ Ⓓ Ⓔ
123 Ⓐ Ⓑ Ⓒ Ⓓ Ⓔ
124 Ⓐ Ⓑ Ⓒ Ⓓ Ⓔ
125 Ⓐ Ⓑ Ⓒ Ⓓ Ⓔ

126 Ⓐ Ⓑ Ⓒ Ⓓ Ⓔ
127 Ⓐ Ⓑ Ⓒ Ⓓ Ⓔ
128 Ⓐ Ⓑ Ⓒ Ⓓ Ⓔ
129 Ⓐ Ⓑ Ⓒ Ⓓ Ⓔ
130 Ⓐ Ⓑ Ⓒ Ⓓ Ⓔ

131 Ⓐ Ⓑ Ⓒ Ⓓ Ⓔ
132 Ⓐ Ⓑ Ⓒ Ⓓ Ⓔ
133 Ⓐ Ⓑ Ⓒ Ⓓ Ⓔ
134 Ⓐ Ⓑ Ⓒ Ⓓ Ⓔ
135 Ⓐ Ⓑ Ⓒ Ⓓ Ⓔ

136 Ⓐ Ⓑ Ⓒ Ⓓ Ⓔ
137 Ⓐ Ⓑ Ⓒ Ⓓ Ⓔ
138 Ⓐ Ⓑ Ⓒ Ⓓ Ⓔ
139 Ⓐ Ⓑ Ⓒ Ⓓ Ⓔ
140 Ⓐ Ⓑ Ⓒ Ⓓ Ⓔ

141 Ⓐ Ⓑ Ⓒ Ⓓ Ⓔ
142 Ⓐ Ⓑ Ⓒ Ⓓ Ⓔ
143 Ⓐ Ⓑ Ⓒ Ⓓ Ⓔ
144 Ⓐ Ⓑ Ⓒ Ⓓ Ⓔ
145 Ⓐ Ⓑ Ⓒ Ⓓ Ⓔ

146 Ⓐ Ⓑ Ⓒ Ⓓ Ⓔ
147 Ⓐ Ⓑ Ⓒ Ⓓ Ⓔ
148 Ⓐ Ⓑ Ⓒ Ⓓ Ⓔ
149 Ⓐ Ⓑ Ⓒ Ⓓ Ⓔ
150 Ⓐ Ⓑ Ⓒ Ⓓ Ⓔ

151 Ⓐ Ⓑ Ⓒ Ⓓ Ⓔ
152 Ⓐ Ⓑ Ⓒ Ⓓ Ⓔ
153 Ⓐ Ⓑ Ⓒ Ⓓ Ⓔ
154 Ⓐ Ⓑ Ⓒ Ⓓ Ⓔ
155 Ⓐ Ⓑ Ⓒ Ⓓ Ⓔ

156 Ⓐ Ⓑ Ⓒ Ⓓ Ⓔ
157 Ⓐ Ⓑ Ⓒ Ⓓ Ⓔ
158 Ⓐ Ⓑ Ⓒ Ⓓ Ⓔ
159 Ⓐ Ⓑ Ⓒ Ⓓ Ⓔ
160 Ⓐ Ⓑ Ⓒ Ⓓ Ⓔ

161 Ⓐ Ⓑ Ⓒ Ⓓ Ⓔ
162 Ⓐ Ⓑ Ⓒ Ⓓ Ⓔ
163 Ⓐ Ⓑ Ⓒ Ⓓ Ⓔ
164 Ⓐ Ⓑ Ⓒ Ⓓ Ⓔ
165 Ⓐ Ⓑ Ⓒ Ⓓ Ⓔ

166 Ⓐ Ⓑ Ⓒ Ⓓ Ⓔ
167 Ⓐ Ⓑ Ⓒ Ⓓ Ⓔ
168 Ⓐ Ⓑ Ⓒ Ⓓ Ⓔ
169 Ⓐ Ⓑ Ⓒ Ⓓ Ⓔ
170 Ⓐ Ⓑ Ⓒ Ⓓ Ⓔ

171 Ⓐ Ⓑ Ⓒ Ⓓ Ⓔ
172 Ⓐ Ⓑ Ⓒ Ⓓ Ⓔ
173 Ⓐ Ⓑ Ⓒ Ⓓ Ⓔ
174 Ⓐ Ⓑ Ⓒ Ⓓ Ⓔ
175 Ⓐ Ⓑ Ⓒ Ⓓ Ⓔ

176 Ⓐ Ⓑ Ⓒ Ⓓ Ⓔ
177 Ⓐ Ⓑ Ⓒ Ⓓ Ⓔ
178 Ⓐ Ⓑ Ⓒ Ⓓ Ⓔ
179 Ⓐ Ⓑ Ⓒ Ⓓ Ⓔ
180 Ⓐ Ⓑ Ⓒ Ⓓ Ⓔ

MK4001